COMMUNICATING PREGNANCY LOSS

"Deeply moving and evocative, *Communicating Pregnancy Loss* strikes a perfect chord that will resonate throughout the field of health communication. This courageous collection is unique in its pairing of compelling narratives of loss with critical analyses that contextualize authors' experiences within cutting-edge theory and concepts. Silverman and Baglia's volume is the perfect text for enriching health communication courses, a must-have for researchers in women's health and narrative medicine, and a deep comfort for women and their partners living with pregnancy loss. Bravo to the authors and editors for breaking the silences that surround miscarriage and infertility."

—Laura L. Ellingson, Santa Clara University,
former Senior Editor for Qualitative, Interpretive, and Rhetorical Methods
at *Health Communication* and author of *Communicating in the Clinic:
Negotiating Frontstage and Backstage Teamwork*

"The most exciting development in scholarship on pregnancy loss in years. Moving personal accounts paired with savvy theoretical insights. A must-read for health care providers who may encounter those undergoing pregnancy loss."

—Linda Layne, University of Rochester, National Science Foundation,
and author of *Motherhood Lost: A Feminist Account of Pregnancy Loss in America*

"Bearing witness. Imagining otherwise. Moving audiences and mobilizing resources. The potential of storytelling to transform selves and society is revealed in this poignant collection of stories artfully compiled by Silverman and Baglia. The storytellers who populate this volume write with clarity and raw honesty, inviting readers to consider the social and political dimensions of pregnancy loss. Healthcare practitioners and the general public alike will find *Communicating Pregnancy Loss* an invaluable resource for enacting social support and shifting public dialogue surrounding pregnancy loss specifically and vulnerability writ large."

—Lynn Harter, Ohio University; author
Imagining New Normals: A Narrative Framework for Health Communica

COMMUNICATING
PREGNANCY LOSS

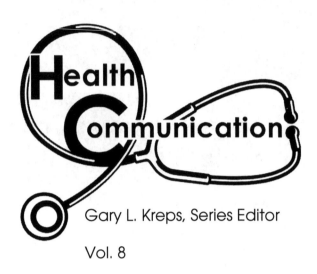

Gary L. Kreps, Series Editor

Vol. 8

The Health Communication series is part of
the Peter Lang Media and Communication list.
Every volume is peer reviewed and meets
the highest quality standards for content and production.

PETER LANG
New York • Bern • Frankfurt • Berlin
Brussels • Vienna • Oxford • Warsaw

COMMUNICATING
PREGNANCY LOSS

Narrative as a Method for Change

EDITORS
RACHEL E. SILVERMAN & JAY BAGLIA

PETER LANG
New York • Bern • Frankfurt • Berlin
Brussels • Vienna • Oxford • Warsaw

Library of Congress Cataloging-in-Publication Data

Communicating pregnancy loss: narrative as a method for change /
edited by Rachel E. Silverman, Jay Baglia.
pages cm — (Health communication; v. 8)
Includes bibliographical references and index.
1. Miscarriage—Psychological aspects.
2. Pregnancy—Complications—Psychological aspects.
3. Patients' narratives—History and criticism. 4. Grief—Psychological aspects.
5. Physician and patient. 6. Loss (Psychology)
I. Silverman, Rachel E., editor. II. Baglia, Jay, editor.
RG648.C58 618.3'92—dc23 2014016408
ISBN 978-1-4331-2397-9 (hardcover)
ISBN 978-1-4331-2396-2 (paperback)
ISBN 978-1-4539-1384-0 (e-book)
ISSN 2153-1277

Bibliographic information published by **Die Deutsche Nationalbibliothek**.
Die Deutsche Nationalbibliothek lists this publication in the "Deutsche
Nationalbibliografie"; detailed bibliographic data are available
on the Internet at http://dnb.d-nb.de/.

The paper in this book meets the guidelines for permanence and durability
of the Committee on Production Guidelines for Book Longevity
of the Council of Library Resources.

© 2015 Peter Lang Publishing, Inc., New York
29 Broadway, 18th floor, New York, NY 10006
www.peterlang.com

Printed in the United States of America

Contents

Contents

Foreword: The Sacred Number Four

PATRICIA GEIST-MARTIN

I was married for seven years the first time and there were no children. My resistance to having children was most certainly one of the many reasons we divorced. The second time around, in a marriage that has lasted twenty-six years, my husband J.C. and I told each other from the beginning "no children." After much debate, we reconsidered. But it wasn't easy. There were months we couldn't broach the topic, others when J.C. spoke to my expressionless face about a potential cousin for his sister's child, and still others when I coaxed J.C. into tales of adventures we would take with a child. Somehow, we found ourselves in agreement, bracing for the ride, wherever it took us.

Nature stepped in, and left us powerless to carry any of our pregnancies to term. J.C. and I are true believers in things happening for a reason—and for us that reason is nature taking its course. Maybe our spirits were not ready; maybe our bodies were moving in another direction, maybe we were connected to some other responsibility on this earth. But for us, nature spoke. The first pregnancy ended after eight weeks, the second, ten weeks, and the third time seemed like a charm when we made it to thirteen weeks, one week into what people told us was the "safe zone" of the second trimester. Each loss felt like both devastation and relief, sort of like getting the wind knocked out of you and dodging a bullet in the same moment. The devastation was like waves of pain that kept recurring—this loss, the accumulated losses, and the prospect that we would always be childless. Relief sat right up front with devastation—relief that nature had spoken, and we trusted her, relief because we had doubts that we could be "good" parents, whatever that means, relief that I should just go ahead and believe what the doctors said about miscarriages being caused by the "advanced age" of my late thirties, and relief that we could go on living our lives as we chose. None of it made much sense when we added it all up.

The day we came back home from the hospital after my third D&C, I felt lost and angry. D&C is such vacant shorthand for the procedure that dilated my uterus and scraped away the "genetic material" that was my healthy son. All three times, what they called "fetal tissue" was, in truth, a healthy baby, with no indications of genetic abnormalities. With "the third time's a charm" mocking me, I felt stupid lying in bed, feeling sorry for myself, with no one I really wanted to call or talk to. J.C. followed me around the house, offering me pleasantries, trying his best to meet me somewhere; I couldn't face him or my grief. I tugged hard on the cord to bring the attic stairs out of our hallway ceiling to the floor; with one lumbering step at a time, I climbed the eight steps to the top, ducked my head two more steps through the sweltering attic air, and sat down in front of the two beat-up trunks that have traveled with me since high school.

I shuffle through family photos, newspaper clippings, and school grade reports. I land on one black-and-white photo with mom and me side by side, leaning into each other, arms slung around each other's necks, standing in a wide-open field, on parent visitation day at Girl Scout camp. Her newly blond, bouffant hair is such a contrast to her typically dark-brown style. I am drawn to her familiar short-sleeve, flowered top, pedal pushers, and beige moccasins. I remember my mom this way. She looks happy. I feel happy staring at this photo, dreamily remembering whatever I can about that event-filled summer day.

I wonder what words of comfort mom would offer me today. I can imagine her two hands reaching out to rest lightly on my shoulders, face to mine, engaging my eyes to look into hers, and she would say in a soft whisper:

"It will be okay. This will happen. I can picture your little girl."

That's what I want her to say as her lips rendezvous with a tear on my cheek. I would place my hands on top of hers and snuggle into her neck. Her lips would move from my cheek to kiss the top of my head. As I lift my head, the photo stares back, not my mom.

"Patricia, what are you doing?" J.C.'s voice flies up the stairway like a distress flare after an accident. "You need to come down from there. It's time for lunch. What sounds good?"

I hold my breath. I know he knows where I am, but I feel like hiding.

"Patricia?"

"Okay." I shift my weight to stand only halfway, back bent so as not to hit my head on the attic's wooden rafters. I realize my left foot has gone to sleep. "I'm coming. Just a minute. I need a minute." I massage my foot deeply and the tingles return sensation. My whole body feels numb as I crouch the two steps to the ladder, and turn to descend. J.C. stands at the base of the ladder, arms outstretched to support me. His gentle hands touch my calves, hips, waist, and back, as my feet hit solid ground. He turns me around to face him and wraps his arms tightly around me, as I drop my forehead to his chest and his chin rests atop my messy mop of hair, unwashed since before the surgery. The stairs become our anchor as we embrace, leaning into each other. No words pass between us and I feel a shiver of perception tumble from my throat to my toes.

I lift my head, and pull away. "I'm not hungry," I sigh. I'm full with sadness, something I hardly ever feel. The heaviness weighs down the spirited optimism that radiates from me most every day.

"That's okay. Let's just take a break." J.C.'s arms pull me back in as he caresses my shoulders and guides me to our black leather sofa, the dusky early evening light tossing shadows across our hardwood floors. We rest together on the couch, leaning into each other, a tear now and then trickling down his cheek, then mine.

"Maybe we weren't meant to be parents," J.C. thinks aloud in an effort to salve our wounds and check in on how I'm faring. We embrace each other and, hesitantly, this truth.

I knew from experience that no one understands the intense pain of losing a wanted and hoped-for child to miscarriage. I can't say how many times I held my tongue when someone in their most soft and caring voice said things like, "Miscarriage is more common than people realize." Believe me, I know. "I have a friend who had nine miscarriages, but now her baby boy is two!" Oh good, only five more miscarriages to go. And the best one of all, "God wanted your babies."

Really? Who does God want next? In my thoughts, I met their patronizing comments with sarcasm. But in my heart I wondered how so many people whom I call my closest friends could try their best to comfort me and fail so miserably to lift my spirits. One close friend came to my house with an Anne Geddes book, *In the Garden*; this book is filled with photographs of infants (many are newborns) swathed in ways to appear as fruit, vegetables, and insects. A beautiful book under any other circumstance. But disarmingly excruciating at this moment. I stared at each photo, flipping the pages aimlessly, trying to picture what our baby would look like. With each page, each delicately wrapped infant, came the haunting words "no heartbeat," "genetic material," and "D&C." What I saw before me, balanced on my lap, was a heavy, hardcover reminder of what was not to be. My friend had no idea that her whispered, "I know, I know, I know" in response to my tears was salt to my wound. She didn't know the wound was inflicted with her intended comfort.

Only one friend found her way to me in the most loving and comforting way. Jan came to my house, sat on my bed, kissed me, hugged me, said little, and gave me Gloria Steinem's *Revolution From Within*. Jan was one of the first people I told of my pregnancies and miscarriages. She too had struggled through infertility, not miscarriage, but the wanting, the aching, and finally a baby girl. We had talked about how infertility sets loose fears and doubts about anything, not just the loss. I don't know whether she knows how much that moment bonded me to her for the rest of our lives.

In the end, she wasn't the only one. The week before my trip to the Western States annual academic conference I contracted poison oak. It spread throughout my body. I was miserable with itching and sorrow. A part of me believed that getting out and being with others might be the best medicine, but by the time I arrived at the hotel, all I wanted to do was soak in a tub and sleep. I arrived at the door of our room in Albuquerque, gave a slight knock, and my friend Amira appeared with open arms. She knew how difficult it was for me to travel to this conference. We talked for a short while, focusing mostly on my loss, until she headed out to the opening reception. When she returned hours later, I was scratching like crazy and was mad with grief, desperation, and fear.

Comfortably situated in our beds, Amira reminded me of the sacredness and completeness of the number four—the four directions, the four seasons, the four elements, and the four birds that are the sacred gatekeepers of the four directions. A Huichol woman named Guadalupe had guided her use of the four directions in her work with women. This guidance was just what I needed when loss seemed inevitable. That night intensified the bond between Amira and me and drew me into a circle of hopefulness and healing. Yet, I couldn't quiet the whisper that there was a reason we were not having a child.

Only a few months later, J.C. and I discovered that getting pregnant the fourth time was as easy as saying, "Hi." The sacred number four turned out to be a baby girl. Makenna May Martin was born March 30, 1993, a month and a half early from her due date of May 15. Amira became Makenna's spiritual godmother.

The fourth was a charm. Momentous! I would tell people that she was born with the souls of the three miscarried babies that lived before her, vibrant even now, twenty years later! There in the birthing suite, J.C. and I lean our heads side by side, eyes locked on the tiny, four-pound, but healthy baby girl I cradle close to my belly as she nibbles on my breast. We both inhale that fresh, powdery, newborn scent and my lips are drawn into her soft, fuzzy,

strawberry-colored hairline. I look up into J.C.'s face and see the same wonder. His eyes unlock from Makenna and search inside mine. "How are you
feeling? You okay?" J.C. asks, as he locks back into our daughter's eyes, his
forefinger tracing the eyebrows, nose, and lips of OUR tiny, little girl.

Such a neat and beautiful ending to a painful, confusing, and complicated
passage to parenthood. But what is not present in this ending is the depth
of pain and depression that followed as I experienced four more miscarriages
when Makenna was two, three, and four years old. We never got pregnant
again after that seventh miscarriage, and we have relished all the time we have
with our one and only, now twenty-one-year-old "baby girl."

* * *

Writing the foreword to this collection was an unexpectedly difficult ex-
pedition for me as I traveled back through the terrain of my own miscarriages.
There was joy and comfort in seeing in others' words my own feeble voice.
There was pain and defiance in reliving what these stories tell; I remember too
well the ways that I felt stifled and silenced. But importantly for me, and any
reader of this collection, there is inspiration, insight, strength, even liberation
in these stories; the words reverberate, resonate, and revive a spark in fibers
that have been deadened by words and actions lacking empathy, understanding, and caring. The metaphor of a spiral staircase invokes the emotional
and embodied knowledge as readers of this book "come round and round
to explore and re-explore, from a flight or two up or down, from a different
perspective, always with different insights to our experiences" (Ilse & Jones,
p. 67, this volume). We walk alongside the authors as they tell their stories
and reveal the diverse, complicated, and enigmatic threads that become their
readings of the paths they have attempted to navigate, and are still traveling.

The chapters capture the voices of a community of women and men whose
identities have suffered through medical jargon that diminishes lives—"products of conception," "remains," "aborted pregnancy," and "nulligravid" are
shorthand words that provide a medical rationality, not a storied world of
colliding identities. Revealed as well are the patterns of unacknowledged and
unattended emotions that flood the up-and-down terrain of infertility and
miscarriage; fear, doubt, guilt, embarrassment, shame, helplessness, unworthi-
ness all shadow every step taken to move forward, recover, and regain "some
semblance of power in the midst of trauma" (Ferdinand, p. 237, this volume).

A unique feature of this collection is that it includes pieces written by a divorced couple, a medical sonographer and patient, and an MD who works with
women experiencing infertility. These perspectives help us move up and down
the staircase and gain ways of knowing from those voices not often included

in stories of miscarriage. When a holistic MD describes her experience with a patient who could not conceive by saying that "her disappointment indicted me; I couldn't make space for her heartbreak because it meant my failure—now and in the past" (Heinz, p. 93, this volume), we learn another side of the story. These other sides illuminate some of the taken-for-granted assumptions and allow us a fuller picture of people implicated and yet voiceless to defend unintentional absences and neglect.

The storytellers in this volume have offered us examples of positive restitution narratives and quest narratives of communicative bodies (Frank, 2013). The restitution—the storyline from health, to illness, and then to some version of restored health—is offered for their intensive suffering. And the quest—separation, initiation, and return—is provided for all others who can learn from their stories and become that so needed "network of trusted individuals" (Hawkins, p. 223, this volume). I am compelled as a reader to bear witness to "the profound human events that unfold every single day in clinical practice" (Bute, p. 37, this volume) and to walk through the "post-death world through remembering" (Ilse & Jones, p. 267, this volume), and make real for others how "the traces of miscarriage ... stick on to our bodies in complex ways" (Rowe, p. 260, this volume). Authors summon us to the days, months, and years of unacknowledged, unattended, and silenced grief so that we may offer our presence and "our capacity to hold the space for disappointment, blame, and grief as it moves into acceptance and grace" (Heinz, p. 93, this volume).

By the end of this volume of stories, we come to recognize all the ways that through the terrain of pregnancy, miscarriage, fertility, infertility, pronatalism, childlessness, and becoming parents our identities can be lost, manipulated, privatized, interrogated, reformed, reclaimed, and newly created. We can see as well that there are cultural forces in society, medicine, and relationships that create our complicity at the same time that they construct our vulnerability. Understanding, even resisting these forces, is predicated on honoring the stories of loss, constructing a more humane ethic of care through miscarriage and infertility, and becoming a community of supporters who reach out and say, "It's okay ... I got you" (Ferdinand, p. 230, this volume).

Acknowledgments

Together, we would like to thank all of the authors who have contributed to this collection. Without your voices, your time and your commitment, this book would have never been possible. We value your engagement with this project and to creating change in the way our world communicates pregnancy loss. In addition, we would like to specifically thank these authors: Michael Arrington, Maria Brann, Jennifer Bute, Jennifer Fairchild, Renata Ferdinand, Jennifer M. Hawkins, Rebecca Kennerly, Michaela Meyer, Julie Novak, Deleasa Randall-Griffiths, Elizabeth Root, Ben Walker, Julie Walker, and Lisa Weckerle, each of whom participated in a peer-strengthening process for each chapter. We would also like to thank the membership of the Organization for the Study of Communication, Language, and Gender (OSCLG) who were instrumental in the growth of this project. We would especially like to thank Elaine Gale, Deborah Ballard-Reisch, Laura Ellingson, Jessica Elton, Robyn Remke, and Maggie Quinlan for their feedback and support of this project. And finally, we would like to thank the people at Peter Lang who made the book a reality. Thank you to our editor, Mary Savigar, who saw promise in our idea as we wandered through the National Communication Association's book showcase pitching the idea of pregnancy loss to a number of presses. We would not have this book without your vision and belief in our project. Thank you to the production team, including Bernadette Shade and Phyllis Korper. And thank you to Gary Kreps, the series editor, for recognizing the importance of pregnancy loss in the realm of health communication.

Rachel

My sister and my mother inspired this collection, and so I would like to thank you both. Your experiences initiated my quest for understanding the culture of loss, a culture I hope this book will help transform. I also want to thank the friends and family who shared their stories of loss with me as I shared with them my interest in better understanding the experience of pregnancy loss. And finally, I would like to thank my partner, Abby, for her compassion and support through the many hours, days, and months it took for this collection to be complete.

Jay

I'd first like to acknowledge Athena du Pré who has served as an unofficial mentor to me. Thank you for your kind words about my research. At DePaul University, the students who populated my "Narratives in Health Care" graduate seminar informed the Afterword with their thoughtful responses to the interdisciplinary world of narrative. I'd like to acknowledge Nikki Zaleski, Kate Bollier, Andrea Dixon, and Michelle Hill. Each time I investigate the communicative body (and its problems) I am compelled to consider those talented professionals who help me look after my own: Brian Stello, Virginia Vidoni, Britt Tagg, Charise Rogoski, and Samantha Lotti. Finally, my partner, Elissa Foster, has dedicated her health communication expertise, her fine writing and editing skills, and her love.

Introduction: The Politics of Pregnancy Loss

RACHEL E. SILVERMAN AND JAY BAGLIA

"The personal is political." So said Carol Hanisch (1970) in the title of a short essay that examined the uses of consciousness-raising and crystallized the relationship among public issues, episodes of personal impact, biography, history, and feminism. Consciousness-raising (CR) was employed as a way of meeting, a method of gathering women together and sharing voices, and a way of verbalizing experiences around topics—such as sex discrimination, domestic abuse, and access to birth control. The power inherent in CR stems from the notion that giving voice to experience generates awareness. The women who populated those early CR groups would bear witness to each other and this action, this simultaneity of listening and speaking through storytelling, resulting not only in awareness, but also in political energy. As co-editors of this volume we—Rachel and Jay—believe that pregnancy loss is personal and political. And through this volume we give voice to a diversity of pregnancy loss *experiences.*

In this introduction to this volume, we offer some terminology related to pregnancy loss, we provide a rationale for this collection, and we situate the collection within the relevant body of literature of pregnancy loss scholarship. These sections are followed by a discussion of how narrative has been employed in the interdisciplinary field of health communication. We close this introduction with a preview of the chapters contained in this book.

Definition: Pregnancy Loss

As editors, we encouraged each storyteller's choice of language, and we also acknowledge our readers' need for consistency and clarity. Here, we offer a general guideline of terminology as well as some statistical information about the prevalence of pregnancy loss in the United States; the glossary of terms offers more detailed definitions and a complete list of related terminology. We use the term "pregnancy loss" to refer to the loss of a desired pregnancy. Terminology such as "baby" and "fetus" invokes debates over reproductive rights and because the focus of our collection is the experience of loss, we find the term "pregnancy loss" to be most inclusive. The assumption that the pregnancy was desired and the loss not by choice is inherent in our contributors' stories. Pregnancy loss includes any and all types of loss, whether the loss refers to miscarriage or the inability to conceive. While some contributors are able to conceive yet unable to sustain a desired pregnancy, others define their pregnancy losses by the struggle to get pregnant as a result of infertility.

According to the American Pregnancy Association (2013), healthy women miscarry in 15% to 20% of all pregnancies. The causes for pregnancy loss are often unknown and responses to loss differ as greatly as the individuality of each carrier. Generally speaking, there are three causes for miscarriage: fetal, parental, and environmental (see the glossary of terms for more detail). Further complicating the definition of pregnancy loss and miscarriage is the issue of infertility. Infertility is commonly understood as an inability to conceive or carry a pregnancy to term. The causes of infertility vary and many occur in conjunction with the causes of miscarriage, and the lines between the two are often blurred. While the definitions change as to what defines infertility or "miscarriage," or how and why infertility/miscarriage/pregnancy loss occurs, or the exact number of women who suffer from either or both, the space in between the statistics, definitions, and the silences that surround this issue, one that affects so many people, is what we hope to begin filling with this collection.

The Case for Pregnancy Loss Narratives

We came together to work on this book project because we share the belief that reproductive rights constitute a fundamental human right, because stories of pregnancy loss cannot be shrouded in the silence of an anti-abortion backlash, and because narrative is an absent methodology in the vast literature on miscarriage and pregnancy loss, including the loss that stems from infertility.

The loss of a desired pregnancy or the inability to experience pregnancy is an intensely personal phenomenon; these losses are also, in our culture at least, extremely (and some would argue, inexplicably) private. Today, there is no shortage of books and scholarly articles that help prospective parents—along with health care workers, social workers, and clergy—through the process of recovering from an unintended pregnancy loss or "dealing with" or "surviving" infertility, whether that infertility is explained or unexplained. In fact, several academic disciplines—including psychology, social work, nursing, medicine, sociology, and communication studies—have explored various aspects of these different but related experiences.

The availability of this research does not mean, however, that there exists a discourse that has resulted in a better understanding of or an open dialogue about pregnancy loss. Indeed—and it has been said many times in a variety of ways—miscarriage and infertility are silent losses, losses that women and men have frequently suffered and survived in solitude. We believe that one possible reason for this silence is the lack of personal narratives in the vast body of literature. While excerpts from interviews abound and a few individual accounts are interspersed in the pages of important books, nowhere have we found a collection of diverse voices who, in their own words, recount their experiences of these varied kinds of losses. There are analyses of pregnancy loss narratives, to be sure, but we feel that narrative as method has evolved to the point at which individual scholars should be able to tell their own stories, in their own space. Personal narratives, write Harter, Japp, and Beck (2005), "function as powerful tools in an effort to enact both social understanding and political recognition" (p. 24).

Our volume is intended to expand the understanding of what happens when individuals and couples who desire a child do not have that aspiration fulfilled. And because the range of experiences of loss is so expansive, we have endeavored to capture that range through narrative. As a third-wave feminist methodology (Kinser, 2004; Yu, 2011; Zimmerman, 1984), personal narrative is consciousness-raising "with a difference" (Siegel, 1997). In their discussion of the rhetorical strategies of third-wave feminism, Sowards and Renegar (2004) explain that consciousness-raising has evolved in style, substance, and function since its private, face-to-face, second-wave roots so that CR now includes books, classrooms, and popular culture, providing "a wider array of perspectives than any one small group" would be able to provide (p. 547). In this collection, the contributors tell their stories in their own words, encouraging what Sowards and Renegar might call a "critical perspective that focuses on personal and social injustices" (p. 537). Our hope is that through the voices in this diverse collection of pregnancy loss experiences, we are able to reach many more whose own stories might become validated as a result of this volume.

Previous Studies: A Brief Overview of Pregnancy Loss Literature

To situate this volume among others in the vast landscape of pregnancy loss scholarship, while simultaneously attempting to demonstrate how this collection is unique, it is both prudent and informative to explore the kinds of studies that have been published in the past twenty-five years.

One of the earliest collections on pregnancy loss is by Ilse and Burns (1985) with *Miscarriage: A Shattered Dream*. Written in the second person voice—"to you who has lost a baby"—Ilse and Burns focus on the definitions of and causes for loss. Borg and Lasker (1982/1989) begin their second edition of *When Pregnancy Fails* with their observation that both legal precedent and support systems had changed significantly since the publication of their first edition in 1982. Both the legal and policy-making aspects of pregnancy loss have continued to evolve, as has an understanding of the coping needs. In their second edition, Borg and Lasker also revealed the statistical significance of pregnancy loss when they reported that up to 900,000 families in the United States may be affected each year.

Like Borg and Lasker, Gilbert and Smart (1992) also composed their book with the testimony of "survivors." In *Coping With Infant or Fetal Loss*, the authors discuss the considerable improvements for support made in the 1980s; prior to this, they report, sources "were private and idiosyncratic" (p. 2). Nevertheless, their study's primary audience is family care nurses and physicians. Allen and Marks's (1993) collection, *Miscarriage: Women Sharing From the Heart*, offers the voices of women and men who have lost pregnancies; however, the stories are disjointed and commentary is woven throughout. To be sure, much of the book's focus is on "eliciting the in-depth emotional experience of women," acknowledging the mourning process, and giving people permission to feel grief. They are clear in establishing the audience of the book as those who are grieving, rather than those in the medical profession who are in need of techniques and guidance to help those who are grieving. Nevertheless, the stories are fragmented and not presented as uninterrupted narratives.

Psychotherapeutic approaches have addressed the ways in which these kinds of losses not only affect women and men differently but marriages and partnerships as well. Leon's (1990) book, *When a Baby Dies*, attempts to fill a void in the mental health field's collection of literature on loss by framing pregnancy loss within the psychology of pregnancy. Kluger-Bell (1998) contextualizes loss and feelings of shame by recounting interviews with people who have suffered from pregnancy loss within a psychotherapeutic frame in

Unspeakable Losses. The collection focuses on five common emotional reactions (numbing, rage, fear, shame, denial) and offers ways to cope with the loss through grieving strategies.

In *A Silent Sorrow*, Kohn and Moffitt (2000) explore the grieving process and point out that until the 1970s it was held in the medical community that "parents were incapable of caring deeply about their unborn baby because they didn't really know their child" (p. 4). While they do offer the voices of those who have lost a pregnancy and assert that the losses and emotional responses are real, much of the book revolves around their expert opinions of other people's losses rather than personal accounts from people who have experienced loss. Layne's (2003a) *Motherhood Lost* offers a "feminist anthropological approach" and moves from definitions of loss and people's reactions to loss to the history of support groups and pregnancy loss as an incomplete ritual. She situates loss within a number of cultural narratives as a means of reaching a vast audience and addresses the underlying religiosity within many pregnancy loss books that often can provoke feelings of discomfort for readers.

Other studies look to the clinical context of loss and aim at making the process and the patient–caregiver experience a more positive one. Cote-Arsenault, Bidlack, and Humm (2001) stress the need for doctors to be more aware of their patients' anxiety when coping with loss. Robinson, Baker, and Nackerud (1999) employ Attachment Theory to understand the experiences of pregnancy loss and also assert the need for clinicians to understand and promote a healthy grieving process to their patients. McCreight (2001) interviewed nurses and found that the experience of loss extends beyond the immediate family and that the emotional labor of the clinical staff also requires a process of grief when a pregnancy is lost. Armstrong (2001) addresses the specific need for nurses to recognize fathers' experiences of loss and to provide them with support as well.

Many studies examine the post-pregnancy loss feelings of guilt and shame. In a rare study from 1989, Hughes and Page-Leiberman interview fathers' experiences with pregnancy loss and describe their bereavement process as "complex" because men are often expected to help their female partners cope and do not know how to cope with their own sense of loss. A similarly rare study by Kavannaugh and Hershberger (2005) interviewed low-income Black women to find out about their experiences of loss. In this study, the authors show how low-income Black women suffer from pregnancy loss more often than do White women and, for these women, there is often less guilt and more focus on aspects of healing than on identifying an underlying reason for loss.

However, it is important to note that overwhelmingly most of the afore-mentioned collections and studies are entirely heterosexist and assume the loss is occurring within a White, married, heterosexual couple. Few account for single women who suffer from loss, lesbian and gay couples who suffer from loss, people of color who suffer from loss, or even unmarried heterosexual couples who suffer from loss. Furthermore, not one of these collections offers a story of loss in its entirety, told by a person who has lost a pregnancy. While we acknowledge that all of these works have significantly contributed to the understanding of pregnancy loss, we believe it is time for a new approach to understanding loss and the complexities of those who have experienced loss—a narrative approach.

A Narrative Approach to Pregnancy Loss

Narrative is both the process and product of applying a structure to characters, scenes, time, and action and conveyed through a particular point of view (Polkinghorne, 1988). In the humanities and the social sciences, narrative is a mechanism for structuring events, a method for collecting data, and a method for applying criteria to interpret existing narratives. The Personal Narratives Group (1989) write, "Since feminist theory is grounded in women's lives and aims to analyze the role and meaning of gender in those lives and in society, women's personal narratives are essential primary documents for feminist research" (p. 4). As a feminist method, narrative maintains the wholeness of an account and protects those aspects of an event that are particular to the individual, always assuming that the teller is the expert of her or his own experience (Ellingson, 2009; Hall & Stevens, 1991; Hesse-Biber, 2007; Yu, 2011).

The surge of narrative in our contemporary culture can be attributed to several causes: the popularity of post-structuralism in the humanities, the "Me" decade of the 1980s, the rise in the number and success of documentaries in the 1990s, and the explosion of reality television in the earliest years of the twenty-first century. All of these phenomena have at their focus storytelling as a crucial component for navigating postmodern lives and the changing concept of the individual. Bochner (2001) argues that for the humanities and social sciences, "the narrative turn represents a radically different vision" of purposes, a new vision of both research objectives and forms (p. 137). Harter and Bochner (2009) introduce a special issue of the *Journal of Applied Communication Research* on Narrative Medicine with the acknowledgment that invoking narrative practices can contribute to the identification of therapeutic possibilities. More specific to our project, Kleinman (1988) suggests that contemporary narratives borne of loss can explain how "cultural values and social relations shape how we perceive and monitor our bodies" (p. xiii). Frank (1995/2013) suggests that the postmodern narrative turn among those experiencing or surviving a bodily disruption begins because they can "recognize that more is involved in their experiences than the medical story can tell" (p. 6). Charon (2006) describes the need for ordinary people to narrate their illness experiences as a craving. Etymologically, *crave* is thought to stem from the Old Norse *krefja*, "to demand." At the risk of perpetuating a Cartesian mind–body split, perhaps it is the body that demands that a story be told.

This edited collection of pregnancy loss narratives will serve as a valuable resource for individuals and couples, academic audiences, and health care professionals. "Bodies need stories," writes Frank (1995/2013) in *The Wounded Storyteller*. The options currently available lack the depth that can come only from a storyteller. Narratives, asserts Charon (2006), have the "ability to capture the singular, irreplaceable, or incommensurable" (p. 45) as opposed to the universal or scientific. More pointedly, Kleinman (1988) explains that narrative methods such as biography, oral history, and ethnography are the methodologies best suited "to create knowledge about the personal world of suffering" (p. 28). The reason for this, he argues, is that the practitioner of the objective clinical sciences has no training in the aspects of meaning-making that are culturally constructed and rooted in the symbolic. Rather, she or he tends to unapologetically reduce the individual subjective experience to a technical issue and dismisses the patient's version of events until those events "can become quantified and therefore rendered more 'objective'" (p. 17). Clinical reasoning, itself a form of narrative, reflects a symptomatic point of view. Symptoms do tell stories; they do, of course, have meanings. But this meaning-making tends to discount the patient's unique history and renders the narrative that accompanies the symptoms "invalid." And so this meaning-making through symptoms is just one lens through which to read a story. This narrative tension between what has been called the biomedical model and its attendant objective "disease" (represented by the physician's chart), and the biopsychosocial model and what is considered a subjective "illness" experience (represented by the patient's narrative) is emblematic of "dialogized heteroglossia," Bahktin's (1981) term for the ways in which a single utterance is interpreted based on distinct linguistic environments or social circumstances. Discussing the political role of illness narratives, Sakalys (2000) argues convincingly these kinds of narratives "inevitably and abundantly portray the hegemonic power of [medicine's] meta-narratives, as well as patient efforts to demystify them" (p. 1471).

Riessman (2008) draws parallels to feminist research methods when she concludes that narrative is "multivocal, cross-disciplinary, and extremely diverse theoretically and methodologically" (p. 151). We begin by acknowledging that individual experiences of pregnancy loss, whether miscarriage or infertility, do not always fit neatly into medical concepts such as "chronic" or "acute" disease. To be sure, the medical profession may treat women and couples as though their infertility is a chronic condition and the experience of miscarriage may be easily categorized as an acute episode by/through the medical system. We fall short of identifying pregnancy loss in its myriad shapes as an "illness." And yet the literature we draw from in this section is almost universally concerned with illness narratives and their role in contemporary society. We recognize the junction between what Hawkins (1999a) calls *pathographies* (or "stories of sickness") and narratives of pregnancy loss as occurring where the self encounters a profound sense of loss (both physical and psychosocial) with and through the body.

Pregnancy loss is a disorder. That is, for couples and individuals who had hoped for a child, pregnancy loss is a "disordering" of the story they had intended to tell, a disruption in an imagined life story. For some storytellers, the body—whether as a Batesonian system of wholeness or component parts—is the vehicle for that disordering. For the storyteller, the realignment of the body with the self is one eventuality of storytelling; the education of a larger public that includes health care professionals is another.

Narrative acts as the conduit that links the storyteller's invisible world of perception and the external world of behavior capable of being interpreted by the senses. There is the realm of action and the realm of consciousness (Bruner, 1986). "There is reality," writes James Carey (1989) p. 20. "and then, after the fact, our accounts of it" (20). For Harter (2009), "Narratives endow experience with meaning by temporally organizing events, distinguishing characters and their relations with one another, and ascertaining causality by virtue of emplotting otherwise disparate events" (p. 141). In their account of narrative's significance in the study of healing, Mattingly and Garro (2000) suggest that stories make sense of experience, offer causal explanations, implicate an audience, and present an avenue for exploring human temporality, allowing narrators to communicate what is significant in their lives. Here we provide brief extrapolations of these aspects.

As a sense-making mechanism, narrative is employed both by storyteller and audience member. Speaking about the patient–caregiver relationship, Coles (1989) recalls a lesson from a former teacher during his training that cautioned him against listening to a patient's stories as a list of symptoms; rather, listening well to stories is a moral responsibility that validates an experience by honoring how the teller represents the truth of that experience. In *The Illness Narratives*, Kleinman (1988) identifies four levels of meaning-making that could be present in a story. The first is related to symptoms.

Symptoms are objective, standardized "truths" and, as such, they are especially valuable to the medical community. The absence of a heartbeat during an ultrasound is a symptom and it provides important information in the diagnosis of a miscarriage. But it is a meaning devoid of the person and, in fact, perpetuates a Cartesian mind–body split. The role of symptoms in meaning-making, more or less, obfuscates the patient. Diagnoses and prognoses that result from symptoms are not typically made with the individual and her or his context in mind. Researchers with diverse foci, such as Jewson (1976), Hydén (1997), and Sakalys (2000), recognize this tendency—the "disappearance" of stories in favor of symptoms—as a shift resulting from the rise in scientific biomedicine. The framing of an illness narrative is always, according to Kleinman, "marked with cultural salience" (p. 18) whether professional, class-based, geographic, or ethnic.

Kleinman's (1988) second level of meaning is concerned, then, with the cultural significance of illness. For the contemporary woman and couples in our pronatalist U.S. culture, the loss of pregnancy can result in a deviation from one's gender identity, a "biographical disruption" (Bury, 2001). In the ways that pregnancy loss can be a departure from the way a woman or couple imagines a future, which includes parenting, "cultural meanings of illness shape suffering as a distinctive moral or spiritual form of distress" (Kleinman, p. 26). Within the "institutional context" (Agar, 1985) of biomedicine, a miscarriage is something that happens approximately 20% of the time and infertility is something that can be traced to the woman's reproductive system 30% of the time, to the man's, 30% of the time, to the couple 30% of the time, and with 10% unexplained. Such a wide gulf between how two cultures—that must work together—can identify the same phenomena is a testament to the versatility of narrative.

The contextual importance within which a pregnancy loss occurs points to Kleinman's (1988) third level, that of the "Life World." Mishler (1984) characterizes the "Voice of the Life World" as experiencing symptoms in the context of the individual patient's history, personal significance, social and relational situations, and how a particular ailment impacts day-to-day existence including how one imagines goals, obligations, ambitions, and dreams. At the risk of an overgeneralization, the twenty-two-year-old graduate student who miscarries has a different context from that of a forty-two-year-old for whom time is running out. We wish to be clear that it is impossible to qualify or quantify the emotional responses to different contexts.

Finally, Kleinman (1988) identifies emotion as the fourth meaning-making level in his four-part framework. The loss of confidence that stems from multiple miscarriages or continually being unable to get pregnant may be included in this category. Whether we are discussing positive and negative coping strategies, self-blame, denial, or frustration, the emotional level of meaning-making is largely an internal level for individuals and couples. And examples of these are especially salient in pregnancy loss narratives. The purpose of telling a narrative of pregnancy loss is often related to the therapeutic benefits of getting it off one's chest. But frequently, we have found, the pregnancy loss narrative is a form of sense-making related to explanation. Emotion work through personal narrative, it must also be declared, loosens the constraints imposed by traditional disembodied social science in medicine (Ellis, 1999).

The culture of confession is the phrase Stone (1997) attaches to the contemporary explosion of storytelling. In providing causal, cultural explanations, stories mediate culture. Kleinman (1988) has argued that the space between the physiological process of bodily disorder and the "mediated" storytelling experience that makes sense of it is occupied by culture. As a methodology, narrative allows culture to speak through the story of the individual (Lupton, 2003; Riessman, 1993, 2008). Explanatory tales—especially in our culture—also provide an opportunity for narrative reconstruction. For pregnancy loss narratives in particular, storytellers demonstrate a tendency not only to ask "Why me?" but also to identify ways of relating to the situation, to transform it into something that becomes an aspect of one's own existence within that culture. Ultimately, the decision to share an illness narrative transcends personal goals.

Insofar as stories are told—whether orally or through a written medium—they assume an audience. One goal of the storyteller is to move the audience. Frank (1994) writes that storytelling "is informed by a sense of responsibility to the commonsense world and represents one way of living *for* the other" (Frank, p. 17, emphasis in the original). To tell a story—to provide a point of view—is to provoke from an audience a confrontation with their own landscapes, both personal and cultural. Stone (1997) suggests that personal narrative involving trauma involves risk in the telling; similarly, the risk of concealment threatens psychological problems.

In the telling of personal narratives, memory looms large. With regard to identity in today's postmodern world, Gergen (1991) argues that it is through writing that we determine "how we comprehend the past" (p. 161). But at the microcosmic level of the story itself, an event happens, and the plot unfolds within a temporal sequence (Ricoeur, 1984). Narratives contain elements of time in plot development and the stories we tell about ourselves take place in the past, are told in the ephemeral present, and are taken into account when we are presented with a future. Narrative, write Garro and Mattingly (2000), "helps shape future actions as well as explore past actions" (p. 19).

The Chapters

In the chapters to come, stories of loss are told.by the people who have experienced loss. We have not summarized or interpreted their stores, we offer no suggestions for what readers should do with the stories, and we have no preconceived ideas about how the stories will affect the people who read this collection or the writers who have contributed to this collection. We do not employ the multitude of frameworks available in the vast literature of illness narratives to cluster these chapters (for examples of frameworks, see Bury, 2001; Frank, 1995/2013; Hawkins, 1999; Hydén, 1997). Each story is a personal narrative written in the words of the author; each author has made her or his own decisions about what to include and what to remove. We have made the decision to place chapters in sections with similar types of narratives. The similarities are broad and the sections do not suggest anything more than an arrangement through which to discover these narratives.

The first section of the book, "Pregnancy Loss and Social Support," offers a variety of narratives that focus on experiences of loss within the current U.S. health care system. The authors express their disappointments and anxieties with the current system of care. The first chapter, by Maria Brann, "Nine Years Later and Still Waiting: When Health Care Providers' Social Support Never Arrives," opens this collection with a call for change. Her narrative details the unsupportive interactions she endured throughout her pregnancy loss and follow-up care, and she offers a variety of suggestions for how to improve the care given to women. Jennifer Bute's chapter, "Honoring Stories of Miscarriage in the Medical Context: A Plea to Health Care Providers," describes a more positive experience with providers than does Brann; she does, however, reiterate many of the points made by Brann concerning the need for more comprehensive care. Bute describes the gnawing feeling of "discontent" she had toward the health care providers during her miscarriage and the feeling of relief that came from understanding the possibilities that narrative medicine has to offer. The next two chapters in the section move away from medical support and toward lay instrumental and emotional support. Jennifer Fairchild and Michael Arrington's chapter, "Looking for Their Light: Advancing Knowledge and Supporting Women by Listening to Their Pregnancy Loss Narratives," describes their encounters with other people's experiences of loss and how the encounter of loss not only shaped them as individuals but also acted as an impetus to discover ways to help others who have experienced loss. Julie and Ben Walker co-construct their narrative of loss in "Unscripted Loss: A Hesitant Narrative of a Reconstructed Family." They reflect on the lack of "social scripts" available for them to follow during the early stages of their pregnancy and resultant loss. In doing so, they hope to offer a "script" for others to follow, in particular for men who are so often seen as secondary characters in stories of pregnancy loss.

In Section 2, "When the Professional Is Personal," readers will find the voices of academic women along with the voices of medical providers. Because so often the work of women is intimately connected to their personal lives, the importance of this section cannot be understated. Each woman describes her work, her life, and her story/stories of loss. The co-authored piece "A Story We Can Live With: The Role of the Medical Sonographer in the Diagnosis of Fetal Demise," by Elissa Foster and Jodi McGivern, examines the experience of a woman who will never forget the moment when she learned her first pregnancy was "no longer viable" and a medical sonographer who has spent her career learning how to ethically dispense bad news, even against "doctor's orders." The compassion given to Foster by her sonographer during her miscarriage led Foster to find the forgotten voices of the people who are at the forefront of pregnancy loss. And McGivern, a longtime sonographer and educator, shares her experiences of familial loss and patient loss and her never-ending process of creating and maintaining an ethic of care. This chapter is followed by "Searching for Grace," co-written by Kristann Heinz, a primary care physician. This chapter begins with a story about Heinz's aunt who miscarried and traverses the difficulties of dealing with unresolved cases and patients who become "lost to follow-up." Heinz discusses the feelings of guilt that emerge from unfinished stories and Elissa Foster completes the chapter with an empathetic and emotional appeal for Heinz to remember all those she has helped rather than those whose cases were never resolved. In another narrative co-authored with a medical practitioner, Lisa Schilling and Rachel Silverman share Lisa's story of infertility while also working as a pediatric nurse. "When the Professional Is Personal: Case Studies of Pregnancy Loss, My Story of Pregnancy Loss" describes the struggles of infertility, adoption, unwanted pregnancies, and professionalism. While Schilling acknowledges the difficulty working with children has had on her personal life, she also knows that being around babies has saved her during some of her darkest moments and that her own experiences have made her a better caregiver. Bridging the gap between providers and academics, Caryn Medved describes the process of accepting a life without children while studying the communication that occurs at the intersections of work and family lives. Medved's chapter, "Infertility, Professional Identity, and Consciousness-Raising," traces her career and her fertility—from a young age when she hoped for children and was unaware of the heterosexist pronatalism inherent in lives of the people she studied, to life as a happy aunt, dog owner, and scholar continually forced to assert her credibility. Her chapter asks the reader to question their assumptions about work and life, and finding a balance in between. The final chapter in the section, Rebecca Kennerly's "Hidden in Plain Sight: Mystoriography, Melancholic Mourning, and the Poetics of [My Pregnancy] Loss," also explores the intersection between a research agenda and a life lived. Kennerly uses "mystory" as a method for understanding the loss of her child and its impetus as her search for, and research about, roadside shrines. This provocative approach to self-analysis and self-discovery demonstrates the way unspeakable losses are experienced and remembered.

The third section of this collection transitions from Kennerly's "mystory" to demonstrate the uniqueness of narrative as a method. The chapters found in "Space, Time, and Pregnancy Loss" describe stories of liminality, myth, and journey. Beginning the section is Michaela Meyer's chapter, "On the Identity Politics of Pregnancy: An Autoethnographic Journey Through/In Reproductive Time." Meyer moves between her two pregnancies to interrogate the idea of reproductive time through personal narrative and demonstrates how identity politics matter as an aspect of communication and trouble assumptions of identity development as linear. Deleasa Randall-Griffiths also explores the notion of time and movement as she describes the story of her miscarriage and journey to Greece. In "The Healing Journey," Randall-Griffiths contemplates the ways in which time and timing matter; from her surprise pregnancy and surprise loss to her intentional voyage through the Mediterranean, she finds that in the end, sometimes things do happen at just the right time. Lisa Weckerle's chapter, "Once Upon a Time: A Tale of Infertility, In Vitro Fertilization, and (Re)Birth," summons fairy tales and the timeless nature of the women within them as a way to situate her loss. Because fairy tales so often include stories of infertility and loss, Weckerle revisions her story of infertility through fairy tale language as a way to connect to familiar stories and move away from her experiences of alienation. Conversely, Elizabeth Root focuses on a time in her life when she felt alienated. In "The Empty Woman: Dealing With Sadness and Loss After a Hysterectomy," Root explores her life post-hysterectomy, when she felt defined by her emptiness—without a uterus and without a support system—Root was physically and emotionally empty.

In Section 4 of the collection, "Without the Sense of an Ending," the narratives describe the unfinished feelings that arise from pregnancy loss and the difficulties that follow those who have experienced loss. Jay Baglia's chapter, "Melancholy Baby: Time, Emplotment, and Other Notes on Our Miscarriage," opens the section by continuing the theme of time while also expanding into the possibility for change. Baglia's narrative about infertility and miscarriage explicitly draws attention to the temporality of loss and in doing so reiterates the fact that a loss is never complete or finished, but always there, as part of our existence. In "Dying Inside of Me: Unexplained Recurrent Early Pregnancy Loss," Jennifer Morey Hawkins reiterates the sense of incompleteness as she recounts her many miscarriages and unanswered questions about fertility. For Hawkins, theories of narrative and narrative medicine help her to understand her uncertainty while simultaneously providing her with the ability to embrace uncertainty as part of her process and her reality. Renata Ferdinand's "Moving Through Miscarriage: A Personal Narrative" also highlights the possibility of uncertainty. Her uncertainty, in many ways, comes from her racial identity. For her, infertility was "White women's mess" until it wasn't. And when it wasn't, she was forced to negotiate her loss without any preparation or literature, leaving her with nothing but questions. Julie Novak and Eduardo Gargurevich's chapter, "Barren and Abandoned: Our Representations Left Unshared and Uncharted," recounts their loss and her resulting state of "*un*well-being" while also raising questions concerning what could have been. The story moves between Novak's voice, the voice of her ex-husband Eduardo, and an example of Mishler's (1984) "Voice of Medicine" as represented on the endless charts that chronicle their infertility. In this restaging of experience, Novak and Gargurevich demonstrate the way narrative medicine and parallel charting (parallel voices) can answer the unasked questions and offer a more compassionate, holistic approach to loss.

Section 5, "Reframing Loss," concludes this collection and in it each author offers a new way of conceptualizing loss. In her chapter "Cruel Optimism and the Problem With Positivity: Miscarriage as a Model for Living," Desiree Rowe describes miscarriage and loss as a sort of depressive realism in which anyone may play a part. She embraces the messiness and the trauma of the experience of loss as a means to heal from the loss and possibly even prevent others from experiencing the pain of loss. A quite different approach at reframing is taken by Sherokee Ilse and Kara L.C. Jones, who, in "Turning Tragedy Into Triumph: A Hero's Journey From Bereaved Parent to International Advocate," move through Ilse's life journey as an advocate and activist for those who have experienced pregnancy loss using Jones's strategy for creative grief exploration. In this chapter, the two women revisit Ilse's life to rediscover the ways in which loss can create growth. And finally, in "Breaking Through the Shame and Silence: A Media-Centered Approach to Consciousness-Raising," Rachel Silverman offers mediated representations of pregnancy loss as a new sort of consciousness-raising. With an understanding of the work of feminist scholars who, in the 1970s, looked to fiction as a way to shift cultural norms, Silverman suggests today's media can offer an alternative approach to understanding the experience of loss and changing the way our culture treats loss.

Combined, these sections and these chapters create a collection unlike anything offered before. We hope this narrative approach to health communication, reproductive rights, and the subject of pregnancy loss will lend our collection to popular readers, academic audiences, and health care professionals. Conversationally, we know that many women and men who have lost pregnancies feel alone in their loss because of the dearth of this kind of literature. So while narrative is a methodology grounded in academic scholarship, it also offers a unique crossover to mainstream audiences. Each story tells a tale of loss and each story offers spaces of connection and reflection for readers everywhere and sufferers of loss anywhere.

Collectively, these chapters imply demands for social change including requests for more reflexivity in how we communicate about pregnancy loss. Sowards and Renegar (2004) suggest that consciousness-raising through personal narrative operates "as a cathartic mechanism for the writers who can share their private thoughts that may have caused them anguish and agony in the course of determining how to resist oppression, objectification, and exclusion" (p. 542). Pregnancy loss is not, of course, a private issue and these chapters go beyond providing a catharsis for the author. Rather, these chapters exemplify the storyteller's ability to bear witness by providing examples for readers to consider, thereby reiterating the personal as political and offering an opportunity to subvert the dominant paradigm of silence.

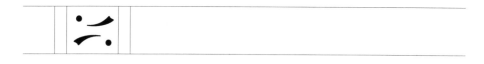

Section 1: Pregnancy Loss and Social Support

1. Nine Years Later and Still Waiting: When Health Care Providers' Social Support Never Arrives

Maria Brann

Nine years ago, I lay in a cold and sterile emergency room nearly nine hundred miles from home bleeding out the once-growing life from inside of me. Throughout the entire experience of losing my baby, I had to be the one to seek out what I needed. I had to care for myself. The providers of care did not give me what I wanted, or what I needed. They did not care for me; they did not support me. Unfortunately, this experience continued after my miscarriage with my follow-up appointment with my own midwife. This lack of support from health care providers is a common experience shared by other women.

Details of the unsupportive interaction with the obstetrics resident and nurses during the loss of my baby are detailed elsewhere (see Brann, 2011, 2013). However, to illustrate how social support is often absent from women's actual experiences, and their recalled narratives, following the physical experience of losing a baby through a miscarriage, I provide the following example highlighting my follow-up appointment with my midwife. In both instances, social support could have provided me, the patient, with comfort to foster healing. Yet, no health care providers, not even my midwife who is trained to provide empathic, woman-focused care (Clift-Matthews, 2007), offered any type of support to me during my mourning. This narrative offers me a way of remembering and provides the reader with a way of knowing, both of which allow us to experience life (Sunwolf & Frey, 2001) and death.

Communicating With My Midwife After Losing My Baby

Two days after the loss of my first child, I sought care from my midwife, Betty (a pseudonym). I went to her to share my experience of losing my precious baby, to make sure my body would heal, to have her hold my hand and tell me that it wasn't my fault and everything would be okay, to find out what to do next ... to have her support me. However, what I sought and what I received were vastly different.

As my husband, Matt, and I sat in the waiting room with all of the other pregnant women and happy couples smiling over ultrasound pictures, I felt my cheeks flush, my eyes fill with tears, and my heart begin to pound. Only a couple of weeks earlier, I sat in the same waiting room, feeling much of the same physiological arousal because of my excitement over being a first-time mom and knowing that a person was growing inside of me. Now, the thoughts that raced through my head faster than a prize-winning greyhound were anxiety-inducing for a very different reason. I was no longer overjoyed; I was saddened. And I was getting annoyed.

Why do I have to sit here with all of these happy women? With all of their healthy babies? Why can't I just go sit in the back? Put me in a room to wait. Please. And why am I waiting so long? Wasn't my appointment more than thirty minutes ago?

As the minutes continued to slowly tick away, I was finally called, by the wrong name, back to see my midwife. There I sat in an exam room looking at my hands clasped in my lap. And I waited. Again. Matt came back to the room with me. I wanted him there, although we didn't say a word to each other. He sat in one chair along the wall, and I sat on the elevated bed, neither of us making eye contact with the other. I knew he was hurting too, but I really just wanted to talk to Betty. I knew she would understand. She was a woman. She helped women with babies, and women without.

Finally, after what seemed like an eternity, the door flew open and there she stood. It was like a scene from a movie; I was just waiting for her hair to blow in the breeze from the swinging door and the lights from behind her to shine forward and make her glow like a superhero about to save the day. I desperately wanted to be rescued from this nightmare I had been living the past two days, and here was my superhero to do just that.

I waited for her to rush to me. To put her arm around me. To comfort me. But instead, she simply stepped into the room as she had every other time we had met, looked down as she flipped through my chart while she was walking past me to the other side of the room, and sat down on the little stool with the rolling wheels. But she didn't wheel herself over to me. She stayed all the way on the other side of the room. This isn't what I wanted, or needed.

"Hi, Maria. So how are you today?"

Is she serious? I just lost my baby two days ago. She just made me wait almost an hour surrounded by happy moms with their round bellies full of life while my baby is gone.

"Um. I don't know."

"Well, you went to the hospital on Saturday, correct?"

"Um hmm. But … I brought this." And I handed her a delicate package. After losing my baby, I went to the emergency room (ER) in my hometown. They told me to keep anything else that was expelled from my body and give it to my health care provider during my next appointment. As heart wrenching as that was, that is what I did. "I don't know exactly what it is, but the doctor at the ER told me to give it to you." And I handed her a bag of tissue fragments that I had released from my womb after visiting the ER.

"Oh yeah. You'll probably keep discarding little things like this until everything is completely out. You don't need to worry about it. It's normal."

What? I don't need to worry about it. I don't need to worry about reminders of my baby being expelled from my body. And that is what I called them—reminders—because I couldn't bear to think about what each piece might really be and what I was supposed to do with them. How is losing my baby from my body normal?

After a quick exam, she said, "Well, I think everything is returning to normal. You should be fine. Do you want to go back on birth control?"

Okay, so I'm still in the movie, right? That surreal feeling is just that … not real, right? It was like Betty was the sweet grandmother who was replaced by the big bad wolf in "Little Red Riding Hood." Where is my superhero? This is not really happening, right?

"No. I want to know why this happened."

"Oh, we'll never know. It just happens. A lot."

"But, I don't know what to do now."

Then Matt, sensing my trepidation, asked Betty whether she had any information she could give us to help us understand what was going on. And he added, "I'm worried about her. Do you have any … can you provide anything to help her?"

"Oh yes. I have a pamphlet of information about miscarriage and the grieving process. Let me go get it."

She quickly left the room, almost as fast as a superhero rushing off to save the day, and my welled-up eyes could no longer hold back the tears. They flowed down my face like water being released from a dam. The tears of sadness were mixed with tears of relief, because finally she was going to provide me with at least some type of support. Although I really wanted her to show emotional support through a gentle touch, reassuring smile, and attentive ear, I would take what I could get. I needed to feel validated, and even if she couldn't match what I wanted, at least she would provide me with information to help me gain some control over my understanding. I had always been a "good patient," doing what the health care provider told me to do without complaining or questioning what was asked, which had previously led to healthy outcomes. So I would be content to get some informational support this time. At least I was going to get some type of support.

When she returned to the room, she handed me my discharge papers and directed me through the maze of hallways so I wouldn't get lost walking to the checkout desk where they would expect me to write them a check for losing my baby.

"What about the pamphlet? The one on grieving."

"Oh yeah. We seem to be out of them. I can't find any. But I will find one and mail it to you."

That was nine years ago, and I am still waiting to receive that piece of mail, or any type of communication or support, from Betty.

Reflections on How Health Care Providers Can Provide Support to Grieving Women

Nine years and two healthy children later, I still grieve for my first child. This is not surprising given that pregnancy loss is recognized as one of the most stressful life events one can experience (Lim & Cheng, 2011). In fact, parental grief over the loss of a child has been identified as one of the most intense and painful experiences a person can face (Davies, 2004; Toller, 2011). One reason that I am still so drastically affected by my loss is because of the lack of support from all of the health care providers during and after my miscarriage experience, most notable being the insufficient support from my midwife. Social support has been defined as "verbal and nonverbal communication between recipients and providers that reduces uncertainty about the situation, the self, the other, or the relationship, and functions to enhance a perception of personal control in one's life experience" (Albrecht & Adelman, 1987, p. 19). Supportive communication may be needed by a woman who has experienced a miscarriage to assist her in understanding the experience and herself. Although she may not be able to control the situation, through support, she may be able to exert some control over her understanding of the situation. Just as I shared my story to open this chapter as a way to relate, explain, create reality, remember, and forecast what is to come (Sunwolf & Frey, 2001), our acts of support hold the same narrative functions. As we communicate social support to each other, we provide opportunities for us to make sense of our lives, shape our realities, control our understanding, and tell our stories.

Social support is part of the story that we need to tell about our losses—a positive response to a negative circumstance. Social support may include the common dimensions of emotional, network, esteem, instrumental, and informational support (Cutrona & Russell, 1990). Action-facilitating support includes instrumental (i.e., direct aid) and informational (i.e., advice or feedback) support, whereas nurturing support includes emotional (i.e., reassurance and comfort), esteem (i.e., confidence bolstering), and network (i.e., social integration) support.

The communication of this support following a miscarriage, particularly from health care providers, leads to improved mental health (Rowlands & Lee, 2010). "Healthcare professionals can powerfully influence how women experience pregnancy loss," and unfortunately, their lack of sensitive and appropriate care often leads to an even more difficult experience (Corbet-Owen & Kruger, 2001, p. 411). This dearth of support often affects women's experience of "disenfranchised grief." Disenfranchised grief is "grief that people experience when they incur a loss that is not or cannot be openly acknowledged, publicly mourned, or socially supported" (Doka, 1989, p. 4). This disenfranchised grief is often prolonged following a miscarriage, and the psychological effect created from the experience (both the miscarriage and the lack of support following the miscarriage) can psychologically distress women (Kong, Lok, Lam, Yip, & Chung, 2010). The psychological morbidity associated with miscarriage is often disregarded by health care providers, and 10% of health care providers have admitted that they were unaware that psychological morbidity was even a potential issue (Kong et al., 2010). The reason may be because caring for women after a miscarriage is one of the most neglected training areas for health care providers (Corbet-Owen & Kruger, 2001; Modiba, 2008). However, health care providers need to be aware that social support is a meaningful narrative response to a tragic situation that does make a difference.

Midwives in particular should be available to support women. I specifically chose midwifery care because of the unique qualities that are often overlooked in traditional obstetric care but are supposedly taught in midwifery care (e.g., "mutual respect, trust, and alliance," guided decision making supplemented with complete information, "ever present support," "reassurance and strength," feelings of value; Thorstensen, 2000, p. 481; see also Clift-Matthews, 2007). And it was being assured of these qualities that led me to choose this particular midwife for my prenatal care. After being highly recommended by multiple women, I met with Betty, and from those initial interactions, I agreed that she would be able to provide me with all the qualities I wanted during my pregnancy. All of the qualities that caring health care providers should possess are underscored by the idea that health care providers support their patients. Although I never anticipated losing my baby, it is also these qualities that would be beneficial to any woman experiencing a loss of this magnitude. Unfortunately, none of these qualities was evident in my interactions with the health care providers, which is similar to so many other women's experiences. Particularly relevant to natural miscarriage (i.e., without medical intervention) are the communication of emotional and informational support to showcase these desired qualities because women who miscarry naturally, like I did, often feel more isolated because of less follow-up treatment (Séjourné, Callahan, & Chabrol, 2010).

Time Does Not Heal All Emotional Wounds

Emotional support is a type of nurturing support that involves communicating caring, comfort, empathy, and sympathy when one is experiencing discomfort. As suggested by Thorstensen (2000), identifying the emotional needs of a woman experiencing a miscarriage is the "basis for sensitive care throughout the management process" (p. 481). For example, when providing emotional support to a grieving mother, it is important to communicate care and willingness to listen so the mother can express any and all emotions she may be experiencing. Recall from my experience how I longed for Betty simply to listen to me, yet she hurried me out of the exam room without providing any comfort.

Emotional support from health care providers is particularly important during and after a miscarriage because this type of support has been linked to effective coping, positive affect, recognition of self-worth, and psychological well-being (Hinson Langford, Bowsher, Maloney, & Lillis, 1997; Jeong et al., 2013). Unfortunately, muted health care providers present the loudest silence of anyone when they fail to provide the support women need, therefore contributing to women's disenfranchised grief. As noted by several women, "the silence [is] deafening" and intensifies the loneliness women feel when they are not supported (Rowlands & Lee, 2010, p. 279; see also Brann, 2011; Gold, 2007; Harvey, Moyle, & Creedy, 2001; Herkes, 2002). Actually, this lack of emotional support is the most frequent criticism of health care providers (Gold, 2007). Not addressing emotional needs through support is the highest-rated reason for dissatisfaction with a health care provider following a miscarriage (Evans, Lloyd, Considine, & Hancock, 2002; Garel, Blondel, Lelong, Bonenfant, & Kaminski, 1994; Geller, Psaros, & Kornfield, 2010). More detrimental than dissatisfaction, however, are the increased feelings of incompetence, depression, anxiety, instability, worthlessness, and unhealthy coping strategies that can occur when needed support is not provided (Corbet-Owen & Kruger, 2001; Hinson Langford et al., 1997).

In fact, women have commented that health care providers ignore their emotional needs even months after the miscarriage (Rowlands & Lee, 2010), much like my experience of being dismissed for years. More than twenty years ago, Neidig and Dalgas-Pelish (1991) recognized that health care providers often overlook, underestimate, or misinterpret the needs of women experiencing miscarriage. Yet, health care providers continue to dismiss these needs either intentionally or unintentionally. This can lead to traumatic outcomes. Women who miscarry are likely to have elevated levels of anxiety and depression for at least a year after the miscarriage, and they do not differ significantly from women who experience late-term pregnancy losses or stillbirths (Nikcevic, Tunkel, & Nicolaides, 1998). They experience similar types of grief, and some even experience post-traumatic stress disorder.

Women who miscarry, however, are likely to have greater psychological morbidity if they did not receive support following a miscarriage, particularly the opportunity to discuss their feelings with their health care provider, than women who did receive support (Nikcevic et al., 1998). This communication about grief with health care providers normalizes the process for grieving women and supports their ability to cope (Thorstensen, 2000). Recall how I went to my appointment with my midwife, who was my primary health care provider, expecting to share my experience and have her listen to me. However, she did not provide any type of active listening cues to suggest she was willing to listen (e.g., eye contact, head nods) nor did she ask any specific questions to illustrate her care or sympathy (e.g., "Would you like to talk about what you are feeling?" "Thank you for bringing in this tissue. Let me explain to you why it is important."). This led to psychological distress for me, and later, my frustration with this lack of care led me to seek care elsewhere with my subsequent pregnancies.

Garel et al. (1994) noted that most women who were dissatisfied with the quality of support they received from their health care providers experienced psychological distress and desired emotional and informational support almost two years after the miscarriage (the last follow-up data collection point for their study). I still experience this nine years later. But Nikcevic et al. (1998) determined that support, even weeks after a loss, is useful following a miscarriage. It is likely if Betty communicated support for me even now that I would benefit from it, and I would likely remember her in the positive light that started our fiduciary relationship when she actually communicated caring and compassion. Even if she confided that she had been saddened or upset over the loss for whatever reasons (e.g., for the loss I was feeling, for the failure she may have felt), her human emotion would illustrate that she could still be a hero to me by sharing that experience. This ongoing support is paramount for well-being and enhanced quality of life (Ried & Alfred, 2013).

Wanting TMI (Too Much Information) but Getting NEI (Not Enough Information)

Not only is the lack of emotional support deafening to women experiencing loss but so, too, is the lack of informational support, which involves the communication of guidance and knowledge (Cutrona & Russell, 1990). Instead of helping patients, many health care providers, through their lack of informational support, make women feel powerless (Lundqvist, Nilstun, & Dykes, 2002). When providing informational support, it may be beneficial to help a grieving mother make sense of her experience by providing information about what to expect, physically and psychologically, during and after the loss. Women report dissatisfaction with the lack of information received from health care providers following a miscarriage. This lack of information leads to poor quality care (Rowlands & Lee, 2010) and increased anxiety (Wong, Crawford, Gask, & Grinyer, 2003), which hinders recovery (Harvey et al., 2001).

Women want information, not just about miscarriage but also about grieving following the miscarriage (Gold, 2007). However, the information, when provided, is often minimal, inadequate, and impersonal (Abboud & Liamputtong, 2005; Thorstensen, 2000). Recall how my midwife provided brief, ambiguous, depersonalizing responses to my questions. For example, she did not follow up with how I was doing when I told her I didn't know. She told me that I would continue to expel pieces of my baby, but she did not tell me why or what I should do with the tissue. She told me that the experience is normal; and yet, although miscarriage is common, I had never had any type of personal experience with miscarriage.

Séjourné et al. (2010) suggested paying particular attention to women's supportive needs, particularly women who miscarry and who do not have physical complications, like me. They recommended providing these women with information, especially about the psychological aspects of miscarriage, even though there are not medical complications, and devoting more attention to their needs because they will likely feel isolated because they may not have a physical need to seek care. Informational support has been shown to be a vital factor in recovery from miscarriage (Stratton & Lloyd, 2008) because it empowers women (Corbet-Owen & Kruger, 2001). Thus, it is imperative that women receive adequate informational support to assist them in controlling their understanding.

Thorstensen (2000) even recommended that *all* women receive information regarding grief and available resources regardless of whether they show initial signs of negative psychological outcomes. Séjourné et al. (2010) determined that an in-depth discussion with a health care provider and an informational brochure about miscarriage were perceived to be the two most useful tools for supporting women following miscarriage. In particular, providing information in both oral and written form regarding grief, loss, bereavement, support, and miscarriage pathology was perceived to be the most helpful (Stratton & Lloyd, 2008). Note that during my interaction with my midwife, I thought that I would ultimately receive both of those types of support. I desired to sit with my provider and have a conversation, but because of her rushed nature, she planned to provide me with written literature. Both types of support could have proved to be very helpful. However, neither was provided. Betty never followed up with me after that meeting, even though she promised she would. This was the last time I ever saw, spoke to, or heard from her.

Providing the "Right" Support at the "Right" Time

Wilson and Leese (2013) argue that nurses and midwives have a professional responsibility to provide support to women at all stages of a fertility journey, from before conception until after the birth, or especially the loss, of a child. In fact, Thorstensen (2000) argued that a midwife's care is invaluable during a miscarriage because midwifery care is characterized by accurate information, encouragement, and sensitivity. However, most health care providers, including midwives, are not providing adequate support. Although Stratton and Lloyd (2008) argue that "good routine care" includes clear emotional and informational support, this type of needed care is often lacking (Rowlands & Lee, 2010; Séjourné et al., 2010). Multiple influences likely affect this lack of care such as inadequate training, uncompensated time, or even unresolved emotion. Regardless of the reason, this lack of support has been shown to contribute to, and even exacerbate, the loss experience (Stratton & Lloyd, 2008).

Social support matching provides "assistance that corresponds directly to the needs of the recipient" (Hullet, 2005, p. 220). This is important because Ried and Alfred (2013) argue that women are disempowered if they do not receive individualized continuous support. In cases involving miscarriage, health care providers are "on the front lines" to provide support to women (Gold, 2007, p. 230), but they must first assess what the woman needs so that they can provide the necessary care she desires. They must be willing to listen to her narrative and respond appropriately. As noted by Stratton and Lloyd (2008), a miscarriage experience is unique to each woman and the psychological outcomes are unique as well (see also Herkes, 2002). Therefore, health care providers "must listen to each woman's perception of her experience and respond to her individual needs" (Stratton & Lloyd, 2008, p. 6).

Still, Corbet-Owen and Kruger (2001) noted that regardless of how women felt about their miscarriage, their short-term needs are always the same, and that is "to have their unique experiences validated by being listened to" (p. 411). Thus, emotional support is vital for women during and after miscarriage. This is not surprising given that Cutrona and Russell (1990) argued that uncontrollable life events require more emotional support than other types of support. However, other types of support may also be needed as well. Toller (2011) determined that bereaved parents benefit from multiple types of social support because loss and grief influence various aspects of life. Thus, health care providers need to adapt the quality, quantity, and timing of support to meet the needs of each woman (Garel et al., 1994; Stratton & Lloyd, 2008). Although health care providers may resist this specificity, each woman's narrative will speak to what will heal her, and a *care*giver must be open to providing this desired care to lessen stressful experiences.

Disconfirming Messages Create Distressful Situations

I experienced the top three distressful situations created by health care providers as described by Stratton and Lloyd (2008), which leads to dissatisfying care: (a) minimizing the loss, (b) not providing adequate medical or supportive information, and (c) receiving no or an unsatisfactory explanation of the reason the miscarriage transpired, all of which may be considered disconfirming messages (Borisoff & Merrill, 1998). When Betty chose not to provide any type of support and made statements such as "You don't need to worry about it. It's normal," she minimized the significance of my loss. This tangential response (Borisoff & Merrill, 1998) provided no comfort. I was worried, and it had never happened to me before so it was not normal to me. Although this may have been routine for her given that 20% of known pregnancies end in miscarriage (National Institutes of Health, 2011), this was the loss of my child for me, and no child should ever be minimized. Even a supportive call, or at least the informational pamphlet she said she would mail to me, would have provided some support and comfort knowing that I was not being dismissed—that I, and my baby, mattered. Instead, it appeared to me that she was denying the significance of my loss, a common complaint from women about their health care providers' communicative actions during a miscarriage

(Rowlands & Lee, 2010). If Betty had acknowledged my loss in a sympathetic way by simply stating that she was sorry for my loss, my experience would have been validated, and I would not have felt like a common medical problem. This humanistic response would not have changed the physical outcome, but it would have acknowledged my disenfranchised grief and empowered me to experience my loss in a supportive atmosphere.

The entire reason for the appointment was so that I would garner support from Betty. I specifically wanted reassurance, comfort, and guidance. She stated she would give me information. However, the supportive attempts were inadequate. By providing the suggested information, she would have communicated that the distress I experienced was real and that she cared enough to help me cope. Instead, she continued to provide disconfirming messages by offering ambiguous responses (Borisoff & Merrill, 1998) that were misleading because she did not follow through with her stated provision of support.

Finally, when I commented that I wanted to know why this happened, Betty simply stated, "It just happens. A lot." This impersonal response (Borisoff & Merrill, 1998) continued to disconfirm my experience. This is not a satisfactory response for any person who loses a loved one. All three of these disconfirming communicative actions accelerated the distress already experienced. Providing emotional and informational support could have squelched those negative feelings of uncertainty, guilt, blame, and discomfort.

Looking Toward a Healthy and Supportive Future

Nine years later, I still feel the need to have my midwife follow up on her promise of support. Although I am confident she no longer recalls who I am and likely does not want to recall any loss of life that she was overseeing because of common feelings of guilt that may ensue (Modiba, 2008), I still vividly remember her and our interaction. Recall how Gold (2007) noted that support has an enormous effect on how women not only cope but also recall their miscarriage experience. The support received, or not received, is a narrative response and will affect how we remember and recount our story of coping.

Women value emotional, informational, and instrumental support when experiencing a miscarriage (Gold, 2007). As noted by Rowlands and Lee (2010), support from health care providers both during and after miscarriage has an intense effect on women (see also Thorstensen, 2000). In fact, Séjourné et al. (2010) noted that women desire *extra* social support from their providers following a miscarriage. Even the most innocuous verbal and nonverbal messages in the public sphere may intensify grief. For example, smaller social triggers may cause distress even when no physical problems continue to exist. As Thorstensen (2000) noted, "Returning to the office to which they came for prenatal care may be difficult for some women, and sensitivity to this is important" (p. 491). I shared during my experience that sitting in the waiting room surrounded by happy and healthy pregnant women was difficult for me, but the recollection of my own feelings of happiness when I was last there was even more overwhelming. Yet, no one even acknowledged that it may be troubling for grieving mothers to be surrounded by healthy life. Something as simple as waiting in another area of the office (whether in a separate waiting area or an exam room) could remove the constant reminder of the life grieving women no longer carry.

Rowlands and Lee (2010) argue that improvements to the medical management of miscarriage are crucial to help women cope with their loss. Instead of assuming that care should cease once the physical management of the miscarriage is complete, health care providers need to be aware that there is more required of them (Harvey et al., 2001). Health care providers need to recognize that a miscarriage is much more than simply a medical procedure, or sometimes not even a medical procedure when women miscarry naturally (Rowlands & Lee, 2010). Because miscarriages are a common medical occurrence, this may affect health care providers' communication of support. In fact, Wong et al. (2003) stated that the commonality of miscarriage likely hinders health care providers' ability to empathize with distraught women. They argued that health care providers normalize miscarriage because of its frequency of occurrence, which negatively affects their ability to communicate, empathize, or even follow up with women.

The answer may be in providing more effective training for health care providers to recognize women's supportive needs and to equip them with the tools to provide that support (see Modiba, 2008, for counseling training recommendations). It has been argued that health care providers are not trained to handle the emotionality related to physical health issues, which contributes to poor care (Rowlands & Lee, 2010). However, as noted by Gold (2007), the support women desire takes only minimal effort by health care providers (e.g., spend time with the woman, allow the woman to emote, provide straightforward information). If my midwife had done any of these minimal acts of support, I would have recognized the care and likely felt validated. This could have led to less psychological distress then and now.

By approaching health from a biopsychosocial perspective (Frankel & Quill, 2005), which privileges the patient narrative, not just the patient chart, and offering holistic care to women (Harvey et al., 2001), health care providers can address not only women's physical needs but also their emotional, psychological, spiritual, and social needs. When providing women with holistic care that involved physical care as well as informational and emotional support, women reported feeling respected and empowered (Ried & Alfred, 2013). "With a thorough understanding of the experience and process of first trimester bleeding and loss [and] an appreciation of its emotional impact and significance, ... midwives [or any health care provider] can provide sensitive and complete care to women at this important time" (Thorstensen, 2000, p. 492). By looking at women and their pregnancy loss experiences more holistically, health care providers can provide the support women need to help them heal in loving, comforting, and informed environments. Then women's narratives can reflect their empowerment instead of their disenfranchisement.

2. Honoring Stories of Miscarriage in the Medical Context: A Plea to Health Care Providers

Jennifer J. Bute

I was eight weeks into my first pregnancy when I started spotting. No gushing blood, no pain or cramping, but I was spotting nonetheless. I knew other people who had spotted during pregnancy and had gone on to delivery beautiful, healthy babies, but I was still panicked. My midwife ordered an ultrasound, and hearing the heartbeat of our first child in the darkened ultrasound room is a moment my husband and I will never forget. We breathed an enormous sigh of relief and braced ourselves for the possibility that I might bleed throughout my entire pregnancy with no other complications.

Two weeks later, I was cleaning the house and planning a romantic evening of dinner and a movie while my husband attended commencement ceremonies for our university. It was a smoldering June day, and I had opted out of participating just to err on the side of caution. Early that afternoon, I felt a sharp pain in my left side and a wave of nausea. I immediately called the nurse's line at my midwife's office. The nurse who answered told me, in a very matter-of-fact-I-hear-this-every-day tone of voice, to drink lots of water and rest lying on my left side. I asked whether I should go to the hospital, and she said, "Only if you see bright red blood." "Which hospital?" I inquired. I was living in a small, rural town at the time, and the local hospital did not allow my midwife to practice there, even though she saw prenatal and gynecology patients at a nearby clinic. She could only deliver babies in a hospital about forty miles away. The nurse instructed me to go to the nearest ER if my condition worsened. It did.

We rushed to the hospital that evening, hearts racing. When I told the admissions clerk that I was ten weeks pregnant and was bleeding profusely, I couldn't hold back the sobs. She patted my arm gently and said, "Don't worry. We'll take care of you." Take care of *you*, take care of *you*, no mention of taking care of the baby. I knew deep down that if I was losing this baby, there was nothing that even the most highly trained medical professional could do, but I wanted some reassurance that someone would try to save my child, my pregnancy. I was quickly escorted to a room, and although I don't recall the precise order of events, I know that the whirlwind involved blood draws to check my HCG levels, a urinalysis, and an IV drip of some sort of saline solution that (I think) was intended to ease the pain in my side.

What I remember most vividly, most agonizingly, is the nurse practitioner who cared for me and his vain attempts to detect the baby's heartbeat. He was perfectly polite, even attentive, throughout my ordeal. He listened to my concerns, ordered the appropriate tests, and provided good care in the sense that he wanted to ensure my physical comfort and minimize my pain. But his efforts to find a heartbeat confound me to this day. We had heard our baby's heartbeat two weeks earlier through a transvaginal ultrasound procedure. When the nurse practitioner entered my room with a Doppler, I had never seen that sort of device before. A Doppler is a handheld ultrasound device used by sonographers and other trained medical personnel to detect a fetal heartbeat. It looked like a small radio with a microphone attached and seemed arcane to me, something I would expect at a small rural hospital. He explained that the device could be used to hear the heartbeat without having to do an ultrasound, but he also warned me that sometimes a Doppler doesn't pick up a heartbeat until around twelve weeks of gestation. He tried for what seemed like an eternity to find a heartbeat, moving the Doppler's wand (the microphone-like piece) slowly over my belly, covering one ear with his hand and closing his eyes. I stared at the ceiling praying that he would hear something, but he didn't. He broke the news but again mentioned that a Doppler sometimes doesn't work at ten weeks. "So, there's no need to panic?" I asked. His response to me was that there was no need to panic because I would be just fine and because "the body is doing what it should."

We left the hospital after midnight. My bleeding was under control, the pain in my side had eased, and there was nothing else to be done. The nurse told me to come back "if anything changes or gets worse." Not quite sure what that meant (how could it get worse?) and feeling too fatigued to ask, we made our way home, calling our families during the ride to share the news. But we were uncertain about what news we should share: I was definitely okay. And the baby? The baby might be okay? We weren't 100% sure and didn't want to make the loss a reality by saying it out loud. Despite everything I knew about pregnancy and miscarriage after studying these issues for almost a decade, I held out a glimmer of promise that the baby might survive. I had interviewed many women who had described such losses to me, and I knew that once a miscarriage had begun, there was absolutely no way to stop it. Yet, I clung to my uncertainty as a source of hope. Just because the nurse practitioner didn't find a heartbeat with the Doppler didn't mean there wasn't one, right? Right? Isn't that what he implied when he told me twice that a Doppler sometimes doesn't detect a heartbeat that early in a pregnancy? To this day, I have no idea why I didn't insist on a transvaginal ultrasound that night. Even though my midwife was prohibited from practicing there, the hospital had a fully functioning maternity ward. Ultrasound equipment sat in a room one floor above the ER. Yet, I was never offered an ultrasound, a procedure that might have given me some sense of certainty about whether my pregnancy was still viable. Nor did I have the presence of mind to demand one.

I woke the next morning to a beautiful day. The bleeding had subsided; the stitch in my side was gone. "Maybe things are all right," I thought. "Maybe I'm still pregnant." I spent the morning on the deck trying to keep my mind occupied by working on a manuscript that was due in a couple of weeks. My mom arrived from Indiana around noon, and she and my husband tried to keep me entertained, to keep my mind occupied. Early that evening, we were sitting on the living room floor, trying to choke down a little food when I felt a gush of blood leave my body. I ran to the bathroom and realized that this was what the nurse meant by things getting worse. Back to the ER we went. I was put in the same room, and cared for by the same nurse practitioner. A blood draw revealed that my hormone levels had dropped significantly since the night before, which meant my pregnancy was "no longer progressing." I consented to a pelvic exam. With a nurse holding one of my hands and my mom the other, the nurse practitioner said, "I believe you have miscarried." At that point, I thought the worst was over. At least I knew. I was no longer pregnant. I could move forward now, whatever that meant. After the exam, I got dressed and was instructed to remain in the room. The worst was yet to come.

The nurse who had assisted with my care returned to the room with a clipboard and a stack of forms. "We need your signature to dispose of the remains," she said, holding out the form. I stared at her in disbelief. I could see my mom crying out of the corner of my eye. The nurse explained that some people choose to have a funeral or some sort of service but that the hospital could take care of everything if I preferred. I was dumbfounded. A service? A funeral? It had never even crossed my mind that there would be "remains" to handle, but now that word is branded in my brain forever—remains that my midwife would later call "the products of conception." The nurse could tell that I was shocked. She put her hand on my arm as I signed the paperwork and said, "I'm sorry." Then she quickly left the room.

The next day I called to make an appointment with my midwife. I felt humiliated as I told the receptionist that I had had a miscarriage over the weekend and needed to be seen as quickly as possible. Despite my best efforts, I couldn't control my emotions, and I was ashamed. Deeply ashamed of my failure. In part, my shame stemmed from my body's inability to hold on to this pregnancy. But mostly, I felt that I should have known better. I'd been interviewing women coping with fertility problems and critiquing discourses of fertility and reproduction for years, and I knew that my age (I was almost thirty-five at the time) put me at "high" risk for a miscarriage. Frankly, I felt stupid that this had happened to me; I felt that somehow all of my knowledge should have prevented it.

My midwife was practicing in another town that day, but I made the drive there so that I could get the appointment over with. Although I'd been seeing her for only a few weeks, it felt odd to visit a different office, to be in an unfamiliar context in the midst of a life-altering trauma. Her nurse, whom I had met on several occasions during my first few prenatal appointments, met me in the waiting room. She was typically a warm and lively young woman who had once confided that vanilla milkshakes were, in her opinion, the best cure for pregnancy-induced nausea. But on that day, she didn't even make eye contact with me. She just called my name and led me to the exam room, curtly saying, "She'll be with you in a moment" and excusing herself from the room. When my midwife entered, I felt a wave of emotion: relief, sadness, fear. "Tell me your story," she said, and I knew I was finally in the right place.

A Nagging Discontent

For months after my miscarriage, I reflected on my interactions with the health care providers I encountered during that period. As someone who has studied communication about reproductive health for most of my scholarly career, I understood the physical process of miscarriage, and I knew that medical technology could never have saved my first child, that the spontaneous abortion was probably a result of a genetic abnormality (though I would never know a precise cause), that my body had, indeed, worked the way it was supposed to. But I had a nagging feeling of discontent with the entire experience. And I'm not referring to the loss itself here, though I in no way want to dismiss the grief that I still feel after the loss of a very much planned, very much wanted child. The term "discontent" comes nowhere close to describing the sense of emptiness, both literal and figurative, triggered by my miscarriage.

The frustration that gnawed at me, still gnaws at me, centers on my conversations with the clinicians. Not because I was treated poorly. Everyone seemed genuinely concerned for my well-being. Not because they were rude or unkind. Even the registration clerk at my first ER visit expressed her sympathy. Yet something was still missing. It wasn't until two years later that I realized what that something was.

On October 26, 2011, I had the distinct privilege of attending a lecture on my campus by Dr. Rita Charon, author of *Narrative Medicine: Honoring the Stories of Illness* (2006). I had admired her work for years, having first encountered it through my friend and colleague Lynn Harter and subsequently incorporating her work into my own courses on health communication. The ideas she presented that day were not entirely new to me, but they sparked an unexpected, even visceral, reaction—an epiphany of sorts. I practically ran to my office after her talk and recorded the story of my miscarriage in a way I never had before (though I have reflected on the intermingling of my personal and professional interests in other outlets; see Bute, 2011, for an example). I took this stroke of inspiration as an opportunity to give myself the time and space to do what Charon (2006) recommends, to make the immaterial material, to bring form and coherence to chaos, by writing, by reflecting for at least a few moments, in an imperfect way, on what happened to me. In this section I reflect on how Charon's call for physicians to bear witness to stories in the clinical context, to open themselves to the suffering of others, and to co-construct meaning alongside their patients has guided my ongoing sense-making about my miscarriage experience.

Charon's words that morning prompted me to think about the care I received in the ER and my interactions with nurses during that fateful weekend in June 2009. And she helped me pinpoint what I found lacking in those interactions. In all of her work on narrative medicine, Charon (cf. 2001, 2006, 2009) calls on physicians (and presumably other health care providers) to come face-to-face with others and to witness the profound human events that unfold every single day in clinical practice. In retrospect, I suffered one of the most profound of all human events: the loss of life. I experienced trouble in its deepest form, the ambiguous and overwhelming loss of what would have been my first child. And though the nurses and nurse practitioner who cared for me during my two ER visits, spoke with me over the phone, and met me in my midwife's office were appropriately courteous and sometimes sympathetic, in my eyes none of them took a moment to connect with me, to share in or even acknowledge my loss, to grieve with me in the way that Charon (2006) would encourage them to.

For instance, when I went to the ER on that first night and the nurse practitioner, with his long curly ponytail and glasses, tried to detect the heartbeat of my unborn child, I thought that his explanation of the Doppler's shortcomings was intended to plant a seed of possibility that my pregnancy might endure. Maybe there was still a heartbeat, but he just couldn't find it. When I said to him, "So, there's no need to panic?" I meant, "So, my baby might be fine?" Instead, he interpreted my question as an inquiry about my own well-being. His response to me was that there was no need to panic because "the body is doing what it should." In that moment, I was stunned into silence. Could I have clarified my question? Could I have been more assertive and insisted on an ultrasound? Yes, of course (also see Brann, 2011, for thoughts on patient empowerment in the midst of miscarriage). But in that moment I was suffering, physically, mentally, and emotionally. I was trying desperately to understand what he was telling me. Was this miscarriage inevitable or was there still hope? Why did he keep telling me that the Doppler might not work in early pregnancy? And in what sense is the loss of a potential child "the body doing what it should"?

When you are terrified that you are losing a baby that you wanted, tried for, planned for, and already love; when you fear disappointing the people you care about the most, then, yes, there is a reason to panic. His response to me absolutely, positively, did not acknowledge that my panic had nothing to do with me and everything to do with my baby. His response was clinical at best—the body doing what it *should*? What it *should*??? My body should be feeding, protecting, and nurturing this baby, not expelling it in a haze of pain and confusion. The implication, of course, was that something had gone wrong in the process—with the fetus, with me, who knows, we rarely have an identified cause in cases of miscarriage, especially in cases of a single miscarriage (Brier, 2004). The benevolent interpretation of his response is that he was trying to assure me and my extremely worried husband that I would be fine, that there was no reason to panic for my own health, and that we would all somehow be better off in the end. But at that moment it was a terrible, terrible thing to hear.

And though this particular conversation with the nurse practitioner is perhaps the most dramatic and traumatic of my encounters that weekend, his perceived lack of concern for the baby and his failure to truly engage with me is indicative of most of my health care interactions throughout the entire ordeal. When I initially felt the stab of pain and phoned the nurse, she was helpful and clear but expressed no genuine concern. She projected an attitude that she gets these sorts of calls every day (and, in fairness, she probably does). The admitting clerk and the nurses in the ER communicated their condolences with "Don't worry," and "I'm sorry." But no one seemed to comprehend that I wasn't concerned with me—I was concerned with the life growing inside me, with the heartbeat I had heard two weeks earlier, with the tiny being in the ultrasound pictures already placed lovingly in a photo album. All of their minimal efforts toward comforting were tantamount to a condescending pat on the head. And while their efforts to comfort me were socially appropriate, they never seemed appropriate to the gravity of the situation. Even worse was the midwife's nurse—with whom I had developed some level of rapport in my first prenatal appointments—refusing to look me in the eye. She was probably uncomfortable, and maybe even felt sorry for me. But I was beyond uncomfortable. I was in mourning. So didn't she have a professional, and perhaps personal, obligation to swallow her discomfort and at least acknowledge me in some way?

A Narrative Medicine Approach

So, from a narrative medicine perspective, what could or should these clinicians have done differently? Scholars of narrative medicine, including Charon (2006) and others in communication studies, offer some insights into the practice of narrative medicine, which Charon calls the ideal in medical practice. "If sickness calls forth stories," writes Charon, "then healing calls forth a benevolent willingness to be subject to them, subjects of them, and subjected to their transformative power" (p. 216). Though I wouldn't call my miscarriage a "sickness" per se, I did suffer a bodily trauma that in some circumstances can become health- or even life-threatening; I endured a "threat to well-being" (Sharf, 2009, p. 133). And I required healing. My miscarriage was what Bruner (1990) would call a moment of rupture, not only from a bodily perspective but also from an emotional, psychological, and relational perspective. The failure of my body to carry my pregnancy to term disrupted our future plans in a way that no health care provider ever took even a mere moment to acknowledge. Only my midwife asked for my story, for our story; no one else expressed a willingness to bear witness to our narrative.

Charon (2001) defined narrative competence as the "ability to acknowledge, absorb, interpret, and act on the stories and plights of the others" (p. 1897). Along with Sharf (2009) and Harter (2009), Charon has called on clinicians to humanize health care by recognizing that information from patients arrives in narrative form. This fact, which Sharf, Harter, Yamasaki, and Haidet (2011) also point out, goes largely unnoticed. In the midst of bloodwork, IV lines, pelvic examinations, paperwork, and a parade of nurses and various assistants traipsing in and out of my ER room, I felt completely dehumanized. If just one person had stopped to acknowledge the enormity of our loss, I am certain that the lingering discontent I've felt for more than four years would not exist. My choice of the word "acknowledge" is intentional here. Across her writings on narrative medicine, Charon goes so far as to call on clinicians to grieve alongside their patients. I'm simply asking for just the smallest of gestures, the slightest bit of recognition that our future hopes and dreams were gone. Instead, my case was very much treated as a routine clinical interaction. I was cared for and sent home. End of (my clinical) story.

Another hallmark of narrative medicine in practice is Charon's (2001) insistence that meaning is "apprehended collaboratively" (p. 1898). As Harter (2009) noted, some scholars have criticized Charon for a failure to attend to the dialogic nature of narrative, particularly in the context of medical encounters that by their very nature involve multiple actors. Yet, Harter points out that Charon does, indeed, acknowledge that shared meanings must arise in interfaces, in conversations between patients and providers. In the best of circumstances, interactants co-construct health encounters and create shared meaning in conjunction with one another. In my experience, my primary care provider that weekend, the nurse practitioner, did not make time to apprehend, let alone comprehend, the life-altering events that were unfolding. As with almost all of the clinicians I encountered, his concern was with my physical well-being and absolutely nothing else. And rightly so, some might say. Yet how much is it to ask that he understand that my panic did not concern me but concerned the baby? He had no idea how much we wanted that baby, how long we had tried to get pregnant, how many of our loved ones were inextricably linked to this potential child. Because he never asked. And even without asking, shouldn't he have sensed that my panic was about so much more than the immediate physical state of my body?

My midwife, on the other hand, did ask. When I saw her the Monday after my trauma, she immediately asked for my story, listened to it attentively and actively, and cried with me as I revealed my very worst fears that a child was just not in my future. In short, she recognized the "physiological and relational ruptures of patients' lives [my life], ever attentive to the plights of those for whom they are summoned to act" (Harter & Bochner, 2009, p. 115).

The Possibilities and Pitfalls of Narrative Medicine

Once I was able to pinpoint an explanation for my nagging discontent with the care I received, I began to wonder what might explain the absence of deep and empathic care. Why might it be challenging for providers to engage in the ways that Charon insists they should? One possible explanation lies with the nature of miscarriage itself, which readers of this volume know is incredibly common. If clinicians regularly encounter a particular condition, then how might that challenge their ability to engage deeply with each individual case? As Harter and Bochner (2009) noted:

> When exercising clinical judgment, providers remain poised between the singularity of lived experience and the generalities of a science-using practice and, thus, must rely on their own interpretive capacities to determine courses of action in inevitably ambiguous moments charged with emotionality, vulnerability, and uncertainty. (p. 113)

Is miscarriage so commonplace and so rarely life-threatening that treating those who suffer is a mundane event? A generality that triggers a routine set of diagnostic and treatment procedures so engrained that it becomes second nature? A miscarriage is typically a shocking and unexpected event for the patient (Brier, 2004; Maker & Ogden, 2003), but perhaps not for health care providers.

Miscarriage is also a medical event shrouded in ambiguity. A definitive cause for a miscarriage is rarely known, the precise moment of loss often remains a mystery, and the loss itself is difficult to articulate (Frost, Bradley, Levitas, Smith, & Garcia, 2007). I often find myself vacillating between describing my own miscarriage as the loss of a "pregnancy," a "baby," or a "child." As "my" loss or "our" loss. Perhaps providers struggle with these same semantics, and thus lack the language necessary to express even a minimal sense of understanding.

The broader context in which these medical encounters are embedded also plays a role in shaping how interactions unfold (Street, 2003). Narrative medicine as Charon envisions it might be better suited to the treatment of chronic conditions or in the context of long-term clinician–patient relationships. Maybe it's too much to expect collaboratively apprehended meaning in the midst of the ER. My midwife, in contrast to the nurse practitioner, had known me for several weeks and talked with me during at least three previous appointments prior to my loss. Did even this limited relational development make her better equipped to hear my story? Even the physical setting itself (an examination room in a clinic versus an ER bed with fabric walls) made narrative engagement feel more possible. And Thompson (2009) has also questioned the ability of all clinicians to perform narrative competencies. Drawing on research suggesting that empathy is a trait rather than a learned skilled, Thompson has suggested that "narrative competence is something at which not everyone excels" (p. 190). My midwife excelled at this skill. Is it possible that some providers simply lack the ability to witness life-altering medical events in thoughtful and meaningful ways? Finally, narrative scholars have noted that although her work is groundbreaking and offers hope for clinical care that feels more humane and less "clinical," Charon still struggles to be understood and influential in her own profession (Sharf et al., 2011). After seeing Charon speak on my campus, I debriefed with several medical school colleagues who were also in attendance. They were far less impressed with Charon's work than I was (indeed, some were wholly unimpressed) and wanted her to provide more concrete evidence linking narrative medicine to specific clinical and psychosocial outcomes.

The Aftermath

Several months after my miscarriage, my husband and I were at a local coffee shop enjoying an evening performance by a colleague's band. Surrounded by good friends and good food, we were in a happy place. I was pregnant again and almost through my first trimester, almost to the safety zone. We had decided to wait until I was well into the second trimester to reveal our current pregnancy, so only a handful of close friends and relatives knew. As the evening wore on, I stood to head to the ladies' room when I saw him: the nurse practitioner whose name I had forgotten, but whose voice, whose touch, I would never forget. I immediately sat down again holding back tears, whispering to my husband and pointing out the man in the corner table who was sipping tea and reading a book. I'd have to walk right past him to get to the lobby. After my miscarriage I had made every effort to avoid anything, web sites, TV shows and movies, even certain professional obligations, any-thing at all that reminded me of my loss. But here in front of me was the man who had searched unsuccessfully for a heartbeat, who had told me I had mis-carried, who had told me that my body was working properly. We decided to leave, and as we walked past his table he glanced up at us and returned to his book, no look of recognition on his face. We slipped out unnoticed. If he had engaged with me that weekend the way Charon might have preferred him to, by grieving alongside me, would he have remembered me? What would he have done if we had run into each other going about our daily lives, as is apt to happen in a small town? Would I have wanted him to stop and talk to me? To ask me how I was doing? That night at the coffee shop, I wanted nothing to do with him. I didn't want to relive that memory. Does the practice of medicine proposed by Charon necessitate a relationship, even a casual one, that extends beyond the therapeutic realm? And is this type of relationship what I want? What other patients want? If my loss had been honored, valued, and explicitly acknowledged, then perhaps I would have stopped to chat and share my joyful news.

Concluding Thoughts

Though in the moment I was relieved to make it home without facing the person who had observed my most profound moment of loss, I still believe in the power and possibility of narrative medicine, of the potential for a more humane ethic of care. If I, as an educated woman, a scholar of health communication, and an expert in discourses of reproductive health, struggled to be clear and directive in communicating my needs and desires during my miscarriage, what does this mean for other women and couples who don't have this background? Although I believe in the promise of the empowered patient, I remain skeptical about the ability to assert one's self in the midst of incredible vulnerability. I know from personal and professional experience how common miscarriage is, but health care providers of all sorts must answer Charon's (2006) call to "enter the room," to imagine the lives of those they care for, to perform deep acts of benevolence as they engage with patients' stories.

I am grateful for what Rita Charon revealed to me that October morning, more than two years after my miscarriage. Her words helped me pinpoint what was missing from those conversations in the ER that weekend. No one was rude, or judgmental, or overtly uncaring. But no one connected with me, no one asked for or listened to my story of trauma; no one truly witnessed my profound suffering. And that made all the difference.

3. Looking for Their Light: Advancing Knowledge and Supporting Women by Listening to Pregnancy Loss Narratives

JENNIFER L. FAIRCHILD AND MICHAEL IRVIN ARRINGTON

This chapter details the process whereby we developed research interests in women's experiences of pregnancy loss. First, Jennifer explains the origins of her interest in the topic. Then Michael, who served as a mentor to Jennifer, recounts interactions that heightened his interest in the topic. Connections between us emerge through reflections on relevant past conversations. Our personal and research experiences were influenced by knowing women who experienced miscarriage firsthand. We sensed their pain but felt powerless to help them. Hence, their experiences served as points of origin for our own stories of inadequate support.

The chapter illustrates encounters that motivate scholars to investigate pregnancy loss and its attendant challenges. Any of our experiences might prompt us to consider our potential to reduce the suffering of others through our scholarship and other actions. The role of the scholar extends beyond the classroom, into our larger social worlds.

Our lived experiences often provide motivations for research. These stories present memorable events that motivated us to try to assist women and their support providers through a traumatic experience. In addition, vis-à-vis pregnancy loss accounts, we highlight the potential utility of the narratives of relative outsiders—a relative, a friend, or even a stranger with a willing ear.

Jennifer's Story—and Ann's Story: 2003

It was a typical afternoon at my small Kentucky college. I was counseling a student—a common occurrence in the Office of Student Life. Lines of students often formed outside my door. Sometimes, it seemed, only some chairs and a stack of outdated magazines differentiated my office from my doctor's.

Ann (a pseudonym) worked next door. We had become friends during our eight years as colleagues. When I was an undergraduate here, she was my sorority's "house mom." Later on, as Interim Dean of Students, Ann helped me find work in the Office of Student Life. I always thought she was smart, kind, and fair. Now, Ann had moved to another position within the college, and she was my colleague, not my boss. Because of our neighboring offices, I saw Ann every day. I enjoyed our chats over coffee and lunch. She struck me as a hard worker who enjoyed her career and regarded it as an important part of her identity. Also, she was one of the most thoughtful people I had ever met. She intuitively knew when someone was suffering, and she was skilled at assessing situations and offering support. She made time to listen to my personal or professional problems without judging me. I often sought her advice and I always appreciated her insight.

Ann peered into my office several times that afternoon. At first, I thought little of her behavior; she knew I was with a student, and she did not want to interrupt my meeting. The third time Ann came into my office, her countenance compelled me to discharge the student and find out what was wrong. At that time, I did not know that she and her husband had been trying to conceive—or that she was pregnant.

"I'm having a miscarriage," she stammered through tears, "and I cannot find my husband. Can you drive me to the doctor, please? I don't want to go alone. I don't think I can drive myself, either."

I tried not to let my expression reveal my shock. She had not told any of her colleagues about her efforts to conceive. Now she was experiencing a miscarriage. I was not her first choice to receive this information or to accompany her to the OB/GYN's office, but we could not find her husband, so I readily stepped in to help.

The urgency of the situation made the silent half-hour drive seem twice as long. Ann's tears flowed through numerous attempts to phone her husband. We reached the doctor's office and sat in the waiting room until her husband arrived. She had finally contacted him by phone and explained the situation. When he arrived, I became a third wheel, an intruder into a private and painful family moment. I left the couple in the waiting room. I knew that Ann was suffering physically and emotionally, but I could not find the words to help. As I left, my thoughts turned from my helplessness to the doctor's staff's ineptitude. How could they treat Ann so nonchalantly? Worse yet, why could she not wait for her doctor in a private room? Why did she have to suffer in the waiting room in front of strangers?

Ann and I did not speak about that day for several months. I did not know how to broach the subject. When Ann felt comfortable enough to re-visit that day with me, her comments comprised a litany of complaints: "The doctor didn't explain what would happen or when it would happen. I didn't know what I needed to do. He just sent me home and said to let it all hap-pen." She described herself as "scared" and "confused." "The only thing I knew, I guess, was that when the physical pain hit me, I figured that I was … well, that must have been when it happened." I failed to mask my sorrow, but again, I knew of nothing that I could offer, other than sympathy.

More than a decade later, thinking of Ann reawakens feelings of helpless-ness. I recall the shock, fear, and sadness on her face—and imagine that my countenance bore the same emotions. We were scared, sad, and confused. I remember trying to make sense of the news that my friend was pregnant but losing her baby. I remember driving to a neighboring city, not knowing what to say while Ann cried incessantly. I remember hurting for a friend who dreamed of being a mother. I was dumbfounded when a staff member in the doctor's office told Ann, "If you are having a miscarriage, there is nothing we can do to stop it. You will have to sit out here and wait for the doctor." I was shocked by her detachment. I wanted to scream, "Put her in a room right now! Give her space to grieve! Why keep her in the waiting room, surrounded by women with smiling faces and swollen bellies?" How could these people be so insensitive? I tried to be strong and find the "right" thing to say to her. I remember how relieved she was—how relieved we were—when her husband arrived. I wanted to offer support to her, but I felt ill-equipped to help.

Later, her husband divulged, "Everything I have ever wanted in my life, I have always gotten. Until now." I remember thinking there was nothing I could do to ensure that he and Ann would become parents, but that I could do something to be sure that I knew how to support others struggling with the same hurt. Although I had never experienced a miscarriage firsthand, I had witnessed so many friends' experiences that I believe I gained a height-ened awareness of the grief and suffering that accompany miscarriage. I had attempted to comfort friends and felt inadequately informed about how to offer support. I have been in the uncomfortable position of wanting to help someone while fumbling for the appropriate type of support to offer. I wished I had known how to ease my friends' pain, and I wondered how many other women were in need of some supportive gesture from a friend.

Ann's miscarriage forever changed my thinking about pregnancy, fertil-ity, motherhood, and supporting women who had lived through that expe-rience. From that day on, I could not take for granted that I would "just" become pregnant because I wanted to be a mother someday. I had seen a dear, intelligent, thoughtful, kind friend who appeared to have it all, until her hopes of having a child were dashed one day. After witnessing Ann's miscarriage, I feared what might happen when I tried to get pregnant someday. Also, I worried that another friend would have a miscarriage, and I would feel just as helpless as I had with Ann.

Three years later, during my doctoral program, I enrolled in Michael's Communicating Social Support seminar. I spoke with Michael about what I perceived as my failed attempt to support Ann during her miscarriage. I also bemoaned the lack of research on communicating support in the aftermath of miscarriage. The miscarriage literature I found appeared in nursing journals, where the inquiry focused on biomedical aspects of miscarriage, not psychosocial ones. Few studies investigated the lived experience and narrative sense-making processes of women who miscarried, let alone whether others' attempts to provide support were effective.

My goal was to use the class as an outlet for investigating the topic of miscarriage. It was during a conversation with a classmate about the frustration we had felt when trying to comfort friends who had experienced miscarriage that one of us noted, "There's no Hallmark card for this." It always struck me as odd that I could walk into a store and see a card that said, "With sympathy on the loss of your pet," but there was no sympathy card that conveyed sympathy for a pregnant woman who lost her baby. The "no Hallmark card" idea led to a conference paper (Fairchild, Nickell, & Arrington, 2008); additional conversations and questions led me to my dissertation research (Fairchild, 2009; Fairchild & Arrington, 2012) for which I interviewed dozens of women who had experienced miscarriages.

Personal experiences are opportunities for research (Lindlof & Taylor, 2002). "It is not simply the fact that we experience something that matters. What matters is how we think and feel about the experience. In other words, *we problematize our experience*" (p. 73, emphasis in original). My experience with Ann set me on a quest to learn as much as I could about ways to support women after miscarriage. My primary goal was to differentiate effective support gestures from counterproductive ones.

I was honored that the women I interviewed were willing to share their stories with me. Reflecting on my experience with Ann, I remember several things that she mentioned that resonated with similar themes that I would later hear in the narratives of miscarriage survivors. Women discussed the cathartic effect of telling their stories. Many women expressed gratitude at my willingness to listen to their stories of loss because many others wanted to minimize the loss or never speak of it. Few people overtly rebuffed their attempts to share their stories, but many of the women felt discouraged from sharing their experiences and feelings. However, having seen the emotional impact of pregnancy loss on far too many friends, I never failed to thank my interviewees for sharing something so painful with me. After every interview, I returned home feeling emotionally drained. I realized that there was no "cure" for grief, nor were the acts of sharing their stories with me a panacea. While I gathered their stories, I learned about potential benefits and limits of social support. I learned pragmatic tips for things to say or do—and, equally important, things not to say or do. For example, no woman wants to hear, "You are young. At least you can try to get pregnant again," or "Heaven has another angel." And she definitely does not want to be asked (directly or indirectly), "What did you do?" as though she is not feeling guilty enough already (Fairchild, 2009).

Throughout my work, I often thought about Ann. Before my encounter with her, if I had heard that a woman had a miscarriage, I would probably remain silent, thinking it better to say nothing than to risk saying the wrong thing. Since my time with Ann and other women, though, I learned that it is better to say something. Say, "I am sorry this happened to you. You are in my thoughts." Let the woman know you care and acknowledge this as a real loss. Tell her that it is okay to grieve and that you are available if she wants to talk. With Ann, I offered instrumental support. I drove her to the doctor's office. I sat with her until her husband arrived. I did the best I could. I probably said too little to Ann, worrying that I would hurt her feelings. In hindsight, I understand it is better to acknowledge the loss.

I have never personally experienced a miscarriage. When I became pregnant in 2004, however, I often feared that I would experience a miscarriage. I am the only female in my immediate family who has not suffered through this experience. I have been the friend someone called on *as she was having a miscarriage,* the person who asked me to drive her to the doctor and comfort her in the doctor's waiting room. I remember the helplessness and hopelessness I felt.

My research interest emerged from trying to support a friend who had a miscarriage in 2003. I did not realize then, before I even began my doctoral studies, how profoundly the experience of my friend's miscarriage affected me. Looking back, I know that seeing firsthand what my friend experienced scarred me. I was hurting for my friend when she had her miscarriage, and I felt the anguish of wanting to make her pain go away. My research with other women taught me that one person cannot be responsible for erasing such pain and subsequent grief. But one person can make a difference—in the communication of support through a smile, a hug, a shoulder to cry on, or another caring gesture. And although our attempts are not perfect, we keep trying.

The responses of the women I interviewed often acknowledged gratitude for my willingness to listen to them, implying that they valued that willingness as a rare and welcome type of support—albeit one that they might have appreciated even more at the beginning of their pregnancy loss experiences. In that sense, I became a new (and, I hope, beneficial) part of their evolving narratives. If one role of our research as health communication scholars is to alleviate suffering, then giving voice to my dissertation participants was the way I performed this service.

Brody (2002) is correct: People are, essentially, collections of stories. When the women I interviewed experienced miscarriage, their stories changed in terms of their perceptions of themselves and increased uncertainty about a future they might have taken for granted. Their stories assumed a "before/after" frame, with miscarriage as the moment that irrevocably changed their lives. Old stories ended; old hopes and dreams were shattered. New stories began, stories often filled with uncertainty and anxiety. Subsequent pregnancies were tinged with hope and fear that something could go wrong, as it had before. In some cases, the desire for children led women to other ways to nurture and mentor. My experiences with the women altered my identity as well. All along, I had felt sympathy for them, along with guilt about the experience that separated us. As I spent more time with them, however, I became zealous about seeking ways to assist women in coping with prenatal loss. I left each interview knowing that my story had been changed because of the women I interviewed.

Michael: December 3, 2001

The thirty friends and colleagues who attended my dissertation defense tested the capacity of the cozy performance lab. The black walls gave the defense an air of seriousness that I might have found overwhelming were it not for the fan club sitting across the room from my lectern.

Aside from the onlookers, little about the defense distinguished it from the dozens of other such meetings I have attended over the years. I presented my work; advisors asked questions, and I provided the best answers I could. However, a single question—combined with my response—makes up a moment whose impact still lingers with me.

Having endured the queries of my committee, I exhaled—did I allow myself to smile?—before the defense chair opened the floor to questions from the audience. I fielded each question with my head held high, having endured the greatest challenge I would face that day. Or so I thought. As the clock neared the end of the two-hour meeting, my emboldened voice obscured any signs of anxiety I had shown earlier. In the back of the room, the frantic wave of a former classmate drew the audience's attention. He asked about my decision to study the cancer narratives of a group of elderly white, middle-class men whose lives were relatively free of suffering, compared to the stories of people more adversely affected by social inequities.

The beginning of my answer sprang from my lips so quickly that I later wondered whether I could have stopped myself even if I had tried. "Years ago, I heard a story about a group of school kids who went to a movie theater for a field trip. The film they saw was *Schindler's List*. Some of the kids were not pleased about the trip. They wanted to see another film—one of the *House Party* movies, I think. So some of the kids acted disrespectfully during *Schindler's List*, even laughing during some scenes. Some kids didn't laugh, however. After the movie, one of the students was asked why he didn't laugh. His answer: 'Because pain is pain.'" My desire to provide comfort to suffering people through my work was—and remains—important to me.

Michael: Fall 2006

Who booked this place? I wondered upon entering. The cavernous auditorium was not the ideal setting for an introduction. As my turn to greet the department's incoming graduate students neared, I wondered whether my voice would generate an echo. The size of the room encouraged new students to distance themselves from each other and from the faculty who would guide them through their programs of study. Thus, the orientation session presented all the anxiety of a middle school dance. I could not repress the memory of my doctoral program orientation, during which faculty and students sat (and some stood) in a room with no empty seats and no visible means of distinguishing the teachers from the soon-to-be-taught. On that day, I knew that I had chosen the right program; today, as I scanned the auditorium and studied the students' stoic countenances, I wondered what they were thinking.

Each professor delivered a brief scholarly autobiography. Senior scholars touted the schools where they had studied and scholars with whom they had worked—hoping, perhaps, to impress students with names of researchers whose books and journal articles they might have read in their previous coursework. Newer faculty members attempted to provide some levity, joking about the size of the room and overtly acknowledging the awkwardness of the surroundings.

When my turn came, I rose and faced the students, unsure of what to say. "Good morning!" I bellowed, overcompensating for the size of the room. I adjusted my volume as I mentioned my name. "I study health communication, interpersonal communication, and social support," I continued, "but I'm also interested in other topics. Recently, I've been reading studies about something that psychologists call the 'impostor phenomenon.' It's a feeling of intellectual phoniness, a tendency of high-achieving students not to attribute their academic successes to their intellectual abilities. Instead, impostors externalize the sources of their successes."

I feared that I had lost my audience, but a smirk from a student in the middle of the room encouraged me to continue.

"The research I've found so far reveals three groups of people who are susceptible to the impostor phenomenon: women working in predominantly male fields, women who are more educated than the rest of their families, and first-year graduate students." Nervous chuckles peppered the room.

"So if you're having those feelings today, you're not alone. We're glad you're here. We have read your application materials, and we're excited about the chance to work with you. So feel free to contact us if you'd like to talk about research, teaching, or anything else." I returned to my seat, silently counting the handful of smiles I saw as confirmations of my statement.

Rather than leave immediately after the meeting, I wandered around the room for several minutes. A few students stopped to speak with me. One of them was Jennifer.

Michael: February 2008

Conducting interpretive research makes me a square peg in a department full of round, objectivist holes. I am a curiosity among graduate students: the professor at the end of the hall who publishes, but not always in journals that the other professors require them to read. My students have produced solid work, including some publications. But for most of them, one course is sufficient for satisfying their curiosity about humanistic inquiry.

Jennifer was an exception. She had excelled in my Communicating Social Support seminar the past spring, demonstrating an appreciation for the potential contributions of multiple research perspectives to scholarship about support. Since then, we had run into each other occasionally, chatting about her courses, my research projects, and our lives outside of academia. I remember little of what we said, but I enjoyed our conversations and felt that our conversations included moments of genuine dialogue. I was pleased when she registered for my family communication course.

A week or two into the course, I sat in my office after class to read response papers for that week's graduate class. Jennifer's paper began,

> Last week in class, I wrote down something you said, something that gets to the heart of why I think you and I "click" so well. You may not even remember, but you said, "All of our experiences matter."

I insist that my scholars-in-training not forget to honor the perspectives of the people they study. Those people might see importance in facts and experiences that researchers overlook because of the tunnel vision that can accompany scholars' research agendas.

Students rarely linger after my evening classes to discuss the week's readings. Most students have classes to teach the next morning, so when the clock approaches 9:00, the students scatter, even after the most stimulating dialogues. Tonight seemed no different. After discussing research on social support, gender, and culture, I hurried to my office and crammed a week's worth of reading into my laptop bag, overlooking this habit of taking home more work than I could complete before sunrise. Oblivious to the person at my door, I moved a stack of ungraded exams from my inbox to my bag. The knock on my open office door elicited an involuntary gasp. "Oh. Hi, Jennifer," I stammered. "What's up?"

"Hi. I just wanted to say that I enjoyed tonight's class. And I think I have an idea for my class project. For the past few weeks, Debra Nickell and I have been talking about women we know who have experienced miscarriage—some more than once—and about how research needs to address the best ways to address the support needs of those women. We study communication, but we don't know what to say to them or do for them. Deb and I were wondering whether we could work on this topic together."

A few weeks later, in a Bible study group meeting at my church, a friend disclosed that she had experienced seven miscarriages during that past decade. To my surprise, she did not cry as she spoke. Neither did I, because I was too stunned to respond at all. Later, and often, I cried for her; later still, upon hearing the stories of the women Jennifer and Debra interviewed, I cried for them, too.

Michael's Story—and Barbara's Story: Spring 2013

Lately, whenever I fly, sitting next to a woman—especially a pretty woman—makes me uncomfortable. There, I said it. It's not an enlightened view, but it's true. They remind me that I could be home with my beautiful wife and daughters. My search for a new faculty position has required many days away from home. Instead of enjoying the company of my family, I spend stretches of days conversing with faculty members and administrators at countless universities, trying to present myself as likable, congenial, good colleague material. But the more often I interview, the more I miss my family.

I just boarded a plane from the latest midwestern stop on the least exciting world tour ever. The faculty had been cordial, yet protective of their departmental culture. After what seems like my tenth interview this year, I have grown too jaded to expect an offer. At this point, I'm just tired. All I want to do is lose myself in a Walter Mosley novella and get back home, where four wonderful people are waiting to embrace me and tell me stories about the things that matter to them: the cute boy next door who smiles whenever he walks by, a daughter's latest photography award, information about how we might help a friend in need. Home is where I remove the interview mask and play the roles that I value most: husband, father, friend, neighbor, researcher.

An attendant announced that the flight was full. As my dream of a quiet flight faded, I approached my aisle seat and saw ... let's call her Barbara. I nodded and offered a half-smile, not making eye contact long enough to see whether she reciprocated. With headphones already covering my ears, I hoped Barbara would ignore me throughout our brief non-encounter. A few hours of free time with a good book constituted a far-too-infrequent luxury during the job search. I turned on some background music and drifted into Mosley's science fiction.

My strategy worked for several pages. The preflight instructions began, and I lowered the headphones to appease the attendant. However, the voice I heard most clearly came not from the front of the plane, but from beside me. I turned to Barbara, genuinely acknowledging her presence for the first time. She was an attractive forty-something woman, pretty but not stunning, whose blouse revealed enough cleavage to make me self-conscious about being nearly a foot taller than she. Quickly averting my gaze, I focused on her short red hair, styled in a modern manner that likely turned heads of men ten years her junior. Feeling guilty for finding her attractive—even more so after noticing her wedding band and being reminded of my own—I tried to return to my book.

I was hindered, however, by what I heard. Barbara was talking to herself about the flight attendant's announcements. When the attendant mentioned the possibility of turbulence, I felt the aftershocks of my trembling neighbor in my seat. She prayed for a smooth flight. She wished aloud that she had not stowed her bag in the overhead bin, denying herself reading material that might have distracted her. I wondered whether this was her first flight and tried unsuccessfully to think of advice to alleviate her anxiety. My helplessness turned into relief when she reached for her phone. I seized the opportunity to flee to Mosley. Every few pages, I glanced her way, hoping that she was feeling better—or that I would figure out how to comfort her. She never looked my way at first, tapping away on her phone instead.

At the end of his preflight script, the attendant reminded us to turn off our phones; Barbara's anxieties reemerged, this time materializing in direct conversation. "Are you from here?" she asked, forcing a smile.

Realizing that my headphones would not deter her, I capitulated. "No. Just came here for a job interview." I feared that I had opened Pandora's box, inviting a flight-long conversation about my career, my midlife crisis, and who knows what else. Instead, we chatted intermittently between portions of Mosley's *The Gift of Fire.* We spoke about work, about places where we'd lived, about nothing. When we reached the appropriate altitude, Barbara rebooted her phone. I returned to my book.

And then I saw it. On page 85, Mosley's protagonist, a modern-day Prometheus, informs an audience that they all possess a portion of his fire and that realizing their potential requires that they

> [l]ook into each others' hearts for a light to guide you. Talk about the world and what you want and what is right. Move away from dark thoughts and fears and lies.... Sit here in this spot of green and speak and listen and feel the oneness that brings us along, that drags us kicking and screaming out from our wallowing in selfishness. (p. 85)

I was dumbstruck. I perceived an opportunity to see the light in another human being and to have my own humanity confirmed in the process of engaging that other. I composed myself, closed the book, and turned to Barbara. Before then, I had not thought to ask her why she was traveling. I asked, I listened, and I looked for her light.

Barbara was visiting her mother in New England to surprise her for her ninetieth birthday. When her response failed to explain her uneasiness from the beginning of the flight, I kept listening. She was unsure of how her mother or the rest of the family would respond to seeing her because they had not been close for decades. "All families have their issues," she claimed, "but ...." Her pause made me wonder whether Barbara was reconsidering her travel plans.

My curiosity prompted several questions. However, I sensed that she wanted to tell me stories that might not have been related to my questions. I opted to be present *with* her, to listen rather than speak, to understand before worrying about being understood.

Barbara told me about her hometown, her family, and her travels. She told me about racial tensions she had observed during her days in the Deep South. She expressed a curiosity about me, and the conversation developed into a dialogue rather than dueling concurrent monologues. We discussed our families and learned that we both had been foster parents. Around this time, Barbara mentioned having gone through "miscarriage after miscarriage after miscarriage," the rhythm of the utterance suggesting a monotony that belied the statement's gravity. Barbara's words transported me to that Bible study group, to my silent, powerless response. But before I succumbed to the helplessness, my thoughts drifted again—to one of countless conversations with Jennifer. The lessons I learned from her dissertation and our collaborative research with Debra sprang to mind. Do not refer to this as part of God's plan. Do not mention religion or spirituality unless she finds value in them. *Do not divert the conversation to the joy you found through the child you adopted. Do not dismiss her loss. Listen. Let her tell you what this loss means to her.*

When I boarded the plane an hour earlier, I never imagined that the stranger beside me had such a story to tell or that she would need to tell it to me. Barbara showed no compunction about continuing her story. She openly discussed her miscarriages, their effects on her self-esteem, and the attendant challenges to her marriage. She recounted the breaking point in her relationship with her mother, the moment when Barbara told her mother about her loss, seeking some type of support. What she received, instead, was blame: "What's wrong with you? I had six kids, and nothing like that ever happened to me." She wished that her physicians had not been so quick to pass her off to others (e.g., "Is there a preacher you could talk to about this?").

And she beamed as she talked about her ongoing path toward recovery and self-actualization. Using her phone, she showed me notes of affirmation she wrote to herself, passages from her favorite self-help author about imperfection, failure, vulnerability, and self-acceptance.

As the pilot began our descent, I thanked Barbara—repeatedly—for the gift of her story. I told her that I had been blessed by our conversation, both personally and professionally. I told her about some of my recent coauthored work on women's experiences of pregnancy loss. We agreed that our conversation need not end as we disembarked and continued toward our respective destinations.

Conclusion: Our Stories

The topics that arouse our curiosities and passions reveal themselves through interaction with our social worlds. It follows, then, that variations in our experiences will yield different types of questions and sense-making processes. The questions of women who miscarry will differ from those of friends who attempt to comfort them—or from the concerns of physicians whose training might leave them unprepared to match patients' support needs. The questions of women who experience loss differ from those of loved ones, who often do not know how to address the woman's loss—or the questions of anyone who sees a stranger in pain and wishes to offer comfort. They all might differ from the questions of a scholar who wishes to disseminate knowledge about related lived experiences to scholarly and nonscholarly audiences. We wish to publish work that contributes to scholarly conversations about illness and loss—and to our personal efforts to comfort people whose social worlds overlap with ours. Our successes and failures in these endeavors become part of the stories of who we are as teachers and scholars.

In that sense, although our stories are not the same, they all can provide valuable (albeit partial) insight into experiences and consequences of loss. While firsthand accounts are important, we need not overlook the stories of others with less direct exposure to the experience. Ann's and Barbara's stories prompt questions about women's experiences of miscarriage, including concerns about the impact of miscarriage on personal and relational identities. Into which narrative types do women frame such experiences? Do women regard their stories as quests on which they learn about themselves in ways that they otherwise could not? Do they portray themselves as powerless against the chaotic experience of prenatal loss? Do any of them craft stories of recovery from the loss? (Is that even possible?) How does the loss impact relationships with friends, relatives, and partners? Do these women regard themselves as stigmatized? Does the experience lead women to reevaluate their priorities?

Yet to exclude the perspectives of particular others is to ignore other noteworthy questions. Jennifer's perspective elicits questions about social support. Which characteristics distinguish effective support gestures from ineffective ones? How can friends and romantic partners gauge partners' support needs? Michael's account raises questions about the stigmatizing effects that follow when women do not receive adequate support. His research on illness as a "family crisis" (Laing, 1969) suggests questions about men's perspectives on pregnancy loss. The connections of our stories lie only partly in our prior teacher–student relationship. Our accounts relate most closely to each other via the synergistic sequence of events that began when the stories converged. Michael's interests in illness narratives and social support intersected with Jennifer's frustrations about comforting a suffering friend. Their graduate course provided opportunities to examine research about support, gender, and health but also yielded many unanswered questions. Those questions fueled conversations and projects that modified our personal priorities (as evidenced by Michael's conversation with Barbara) and our research agendas (evidenced by collaborative publications and presentations on prenatal loss, narrative, and social support).

In our efforts to offer comprehensive insight about why humans communicate as they do, we must acknowledge multiple standpoints. In the case of prenatal loss, the best way to honor the experiences of women who have experienced pain, stigma, and uncertainty is to look for the light within those women, to borrow a phrase from Mosley (2012). We must listen to their stories, acknowledging and valuing the commonalities and differences in our experiences. Those stories are opportunities for a larger dialogue in which we add our stories to theirs. Such an approach presents the potential to generate knowledge that comforts the suffering and equips us to support each other effectively.

4. Unscripted Loss: A Hesitant Narrative of a Reconstructed Family

Julie L. G. Walker and Benjamin M. Walker

In November 2011 we lost our first child to miscarriage. Navigating this loss required reconstructing our family identity. We had to decide how being childless parents impacted us as individuals and as a couple. We had to determine with whom we would share our miscarriage story. When we shared our story, we had to choose which details to reveal. That is what this chapter is about: rediscovering ourselves through sharing our story.

Writing this thrust us both (particularly Ben) into reflective positions about how we experienced the event. Sharing our story together meant we had to negotiate our tandem writing. Several examples of tandem writing exist. Fasset and Warren (2006) used a single narrative voice with no clear distinction between which author's life included the events described. Ellis and Bochner (1992) used separate voices to write a play. hooks (1994) "interviewed" herself to convey a nuanced understanding of her experiences. We decided to separate our voices into short, interchanging segments to simultaneously share our experiences. Specifically we wanted Ben's voice to be distinct because male voices are neither invited nor included in the majority of miscarriage narratives. Below is our story: JW represents Julie in roman font, while BW represents Ben in italics.

Our Narrative

JW: The first time I positively tested pregnant was during my second year of graduate school. Ben and I had been trying for only four months so we were surprised by our success. Our conversation about starting our family began with me suggesting we should consider trying to get pregnant and Ben responding, "Yeah, we're ready for that. What did you have for breakfast? Root beer and a popsicle?"

BW: *I remember when Julie first proposed trying to get pregnant. The two of us were lying in bed, talking about life, when she stated her genuine desire to have a baby. I knew she was serious, but we had casually entertained the idea before and had determined the logistics might be too complicated to handle while we were in graduate school. I assumed she meant we should start planning for having a baby. In an attempt to be pragmatic, I started rattling off concerns so we could tackle them head on. Julie grew quiet.*

      "What's wrong?" I asked her. Julie explained she knew we'd have to work through hurdles, but she wanted love to dictate our family, not logic. Essentially, she was acting with her heart and I was acting with my brain; we needed both. I was so obsessed with being responsible that I had forgotten how miraculous this journey might be. Kids were always in my life plan, but now the moment had arrived to start trying and I wasn't able to truly experience the joy I had always imagined. What was wrong with me?

JW: We realized we had no idea what getting pregnant would really require, so Ben consulted one of our instructors, Leah, who had already been mentoring us.

BW: *If we were going to do this, we would need to be able to manage it financially. Turns out having a baby is really expensive! Luckily, our modest insurance covered most of the potential costs of pregnancy and delivery. Focusing on this type of task made it easier for me to see this baby thing actually happening.*

JW: To get started, Leah suggested we "pull the goalie." Though not an active offensive hockey move, we were pulling down our defenses preventing pregnancy. I stopped taking my birth control pills, and we began trying to conceive.

BW: *Julie and I assumed conceiving would take some time as we had heard birth control can linger in the body and impact conception rates well after someone stops taking the pill. And besides, we weren't lucky enough to be the couple that got pregnant right away. Julie went to the dollar store and got some home pregnancy tests just in case. I just kept on doing what I'd always done. The excitement felt oddly normal. What should men do to prepare?*

JW: Whenever I planned to do activities that are bad for a pregnant woman, such as drinking, I would pee on the stick. One unassuming night, I tested positively pregnant. Time stopped. I stood frozen in the bathroom, eyes glued to the two lines clearly staring back at me from my test. I checked the box to make sure I knew what I was seeing. There was no denying the positive result staring back at me.

      I walked out of the bathroom to where Ben was sitting in the dining room. He must have seen a strange emotion on my face, which I can only imagine looked like a mixture of shock and confusion because he asked me what was wrong. Four words came out of my mouth: "I think I'm pregnant."

BW: *For fathers-to-be, so much is out of your control. Conception and pregnancy can be a giant mystery because it's all happening through your partner. So I relied on Julie to give me updates on her status vis-à-vis pregnancy, which was a great misfortune because Julie loves to trick me. Her wielding this power of knowledge over an important piece of information ended up being too much for her to resist. Julie took immense pleasure in hinting that she might be pregnant. One time we entered a restaurant and Julie told the hostess to secure a "table for three" and then rubbed her belly. So when she came out of the bathroom one evening before we were set to go to a party and declared herself pregnant, my first thought was "Bullshit."*

JW: Ben's response was not exactly what I expected. I guess I should have anticipated his disbelief given the number of times I'd joked about being pregnant since we'd been together.

BW: *Of course, I turned out to be an asshole doubting Thomas. My skepticism quickly turned into joy. This is how it was supposed to feel! Excitement! Surprise! And yes, a little bit of panic. Once Julie and I settled down, we decided to run to the store to get better (i.e., more expensive) at-home pregnancy tests.*

JW: I believe life begins at conception, so I was already carrying a tiny little person in my belly. Happiness, nervousness, satisfaction … a flood of emotions washed over me. Most of all, I eagerly anticipated our journey to parenthood and the family we'd always dreamt about.

BW: *Success! We had made a baby! The following day we shared our exciting secret with Leah. She happily congratulated us but could see the big question on our minds: now what? Julie and I breathed a sigh of relief as Leah suggested steps to take in the coming weeks. We asked her not to share the news until after the first trimester, just to make sure the baby was healthy. She agreed our decision was wise.*

JW: I was a little scared about the idea of losing the baby because some of my aunts lost pregnancies. My worries were not extreme but I shared my fears with Leah. She told me miscarriage is common, especially for first pregnancies. She advised me not to blame myself if my pregnancy did end in miscarriage because ultimately I had no control. If I did miscarry it meant genetically something must be wrong, which meant that the miscarriage was not a result of me providing a bad environment for the baby.

Listening to Leah's advice was the first time I think I really realized that having a baby might be more complicated than I'd anticipated. There are so many facets to pregnancy and delivery that just aren't talked about during most child-rearing and child-conceiving discussions. While her advice gave me a whole slew of new things to be worried about, I tried to put my concerns out of my mind. After all, my only choice was to follow whatever clues my body and my baby were giving me.

BW: *Yes, we had concerns about losing the baby … but those were natural concerns considering Julie's family history. Julie and I kept the pregnancy quiet to be cautious, but I wasn't worried about it. We started planning and prepping for our new addition.*

JW: For three weeks, Ben, Leah, and I kept our secret. Every time I was tempted to tell my mom or my sister about our pregnancy, the terrifying idea that I might have to go back and tell them I'd lost the baby kept my mouth shut. I began incorporating preparatory activities into my life. I purchased a necklace to wear throughout pregnancy that I would eventually gift to the child. Per Leah's suggestion, I checked out books on the current state of pregnancy from the library. I stopped eating my graduate student diet of discount pasta dishes and hot dogs, and I started eating better.

BW: *Preparing for our baby felt like a job for Julie, not me. She would be the one going through the intense physical changes while I was just there to offer support. Besides living vicariously through her and helping her prepare, there wasn't much I felt as though I could do to get ready. I was excited to be a daddy, but what does a father do at this point? All the attention was on Julie, even from Leah, and I began to feel a little disconnected from the entire experience. Pregnancy was wonderful, but it wasn't happening to me.*

JW: Leah offered me support throughout the pregnancy, and it became a fun secret bond. When my lunch included a hardboiled egg, she would give me an affirming smile. While walking down the hallway after a class, she would ask about my nausea and would offer solutions such as peppermint drops. Leah said she wanted to make sure even though I told no one else about my pregnancy that I was still getting all the support I would have received if I had told my best friends and colleagues.

BW: *Keeping it a secret wasn't as hard as I thought it was going to be. Julie wasn't showing yet and no one was expecting us to have a baby any time soon. What was difficult at first was coming up with ways to excuse Julie from certain things. For instance, all of a sudden, Julie couldn't drink alcohol. A little game emerged, seeing how smooth a story we could tell our friends and colleagues. Julie and I shared a secret and the process of hiding it strengthened our commitment and love toward each other and our growing family. By concealing our big news, it became that much more precious. It was something to protect, something worth waiting to share.*

About three weeks after we found out we were pregnant we flew from Minnesota to New Orleans for a national conference in which we were both presenting papers. This was the biggest conference in our discipline, where scholars from around the country gathered to share research with colleagues. This meant being far from familiar doctors and the safety of our home. Julie was only six weeks into the pregnancy, but this was our first big "test." I was nervous.

JW: We arrived safely, and I made it through the first day of the conference. I stifled a smile as one of my professors advised me to wait to have children until after I finished my doctoral work. I thought to myself, "Well, guess that ship has sailed."

BW: *As much as these conferences are about scholarly work, they are also about social-izing. Julie had to avoid alcohol without appearing out of the ordinary. That meant I needed to draw attention away from any of her drink choices by steer-ing conversations or by drinking more than I usually did. I am a well-known lightweight, and my friends and colleagues embraced the idea of Ben "letting go" a little bit. I hoped it was enough to take the focus off of Julie. It worked. No one caught on to Julie's "condition" and I got to be her hero for a bit. It was nice to be able to contribute to the pregnancy in a more active way.*

JW: I awoke the third morning of the conference. The clock read 6:15 a.m. and I was not entirely pleased by the need to pee that early in the morning. As the pressure on my bladder ceased and I completed my bathroom visit, I reached for the toilet paper. I looked down after I'd wiped and saw a bright red splotch of blood on the paper. Time stopped moving.

I remember staring with dazed disbelief at my positive pregnancy test, but at this toilet paper I stared in paralyzed emptiness. Fear and panic re-placed my feelings of contented secrecy. I'd read the sixth week was when the embryo implanted into the uterine wall, and during that implantation process many women experienced a dark-colored discharge. Bright red, the webpage instructed, was not a good sign. After putting on a panty liner I walked back to bed and lay down next to Ben. There really was no point waking Ben up to share what was happening. He would know soon enough.

Trying not to cry, I turned over and was overwhelmed with my feeling of loss. In the midst of my sadness I felt a presence sitting on the bed next to me. My dad often talked about how in times of great sadness or joy he could feel the presence of his deceased father. On the bed next to me I felt the presence of my recently deceased grandmother, Nana. She was offering me peace and holding my hand in the same way I held her hand the night before she died. I felt she was telling me that everything was going to be okay, and that she was there to be with my child as it made the transition from the world of the living to whatever lies beyond. Nana always feared dying alone, so knowing she was there with my child as it passed away offers me comfort because I know my child was taken care of. After a few minutes, I felt Nana and the spirit of my child leave. I knew in my head there was a chance I could still carry my child to its anticipated July 15th birthday, but I knew in my heart my pregnancy was over.

BW: *On the third morning of the conference, I woke up nursing a hangover, the result of my efforts to cover for the pregnancy. That was when Julie told me she thought she had lost the baby. Our worst fear had been realized. As she walked me through her experience and feelings, all I could think about was how much losing the baby must be killing her. We wanted to stop what we were doing and grieve, but we were still at the conference. The private and public worlds we had so carefully separated up to this point were now directly overlapping. The only way to maintain our privacy was to get through the rest of the conference and deal with the pain of our loss when we got home. All I wanted to do was take Julie aside, hold her, and let her know everything would be all right. Instead, we acted as though we were merely tired, and trudged our way through the last day of the conference.*

JW: I told Leah what was happening, and she reemphasized what she'd told me during our first conversation about miscarriage. It wasn't my fault. I didn't do anything wrong. Genetically there was something wrong that would have led to an unhealthy baby. I appreciated her rational thinking, but I couldn't entirely believe her. Somehow it was my fault.

      The day after we returned home, I went to work.

BW: *Julie went to the doctor's office as soon as they could schedule her to check her hormone levels. If the hormone levels were low, we'd know something was wrong.*

      She texted me to say she had to call back two hours after the test to find out her results. A number more than 2,000 meant good news.

JW: I called the nurse's station and talked with Heather, a very kind nurse. She told me my level was 55. I heard what she said, but my mind couldn't register the full implications of what that meant. Heather described potential effects I might feel from what was happening, and I listened as if she were describing treatment for a broken arm. She then said, "You will want to come in weekly to get your hormone level tested, just to make sure your pregnancy terminates properly." Her phrase "your pregnancy terminates properly" was the first time anyone actually verbalized that my pregnancy was over. The full repercussions of my blood test hit me, and I could hardly breathe. I fumbled through the final few exchanges with Heather, and I hung up the phone. In preparation for potentially bad news, I'd made the phone call in the hallway outside the service agency where I worked. My body, wracked with heaving but silent sobs and moving outside my control, somehow managed to maneuver itself to an alcove near an elevator, and I melted into a small isolated outcropping in the wall. Bent in two, I silently shook with sorrow; my pregnancy was officially over.

BW: *I was at work when I got Julie's text message: We had officially lost the baby. I knew the news was probably coming, but I felt as if a car had hit me. No, I felt as if a car had hit Julie. My involvement in the pregnancy felt secondary and so did the loss. I hurt, but I hurt more for Julie than for me. The pregnancy had yet to fully materialize as reality for me, so the news felt like a loss of something that had yet to arrive. Julie had known our baby far more intimately than I had, so I knew the miscarriage was going to hurt her more than it would me. I got through what I needed to get done at work and went home.*

JW: Speaking to anyone seemed impossible, so I texted messages. Ben offered me immediate consolation and love via text. I knew he was feeling sad, but I felt so incredibly overwhelmed with my emotions that I simply couldn't think about his feelings. Leah texted me something sympathetic and I granted her permission to share our news with another professor, Jim, with whom Ben and I share a close relationship. She texted me that Jim teared up and offered us condolences for our loss. In that moment the small amount of composure I had built was smashed to bits. Jim offering condolences meant the whole pregnancy wasn't just in my imagination. There really had been a child and that child was now gone. Consumed with guilt and sorrow and loss, I stayed in the alcove until I ran out of tears.

My short drive home seemed endless. Though I drove safely a very small part of me didn't care whether I arrived home at all. When my key finally clicked into my apartment door lock and I was closing the door behind me I was struck with a second wave of sorrow. Ben hadn't arrived home yet, so I lay down in our bed and quietly cried with myself.

BW: *When I got home, Julie was there and I just held her as she cried.*

JW: He stroked my hair, he whispered that he loved me, and together we mourned the loss of our child.

BW: *Julie needed me to be strong and take care of her. To hold her and tell her everything was going to be fine. To deflect public inquiry. To do the household chores. I needed to be her rock. I didn't know what to feel. I was sad, but not like the deep despair Julie was experiencing. I had not yet met the baby, so the miscarriage felt sad but almost unreal. Without ever being a part of the physical aspect (pregnancy and miscarriage) the death seemed distant, while Julie's pain was in the forefront. I had experienced the entire pregnancy through the filter of Julie, which somehow dulled the pain of the miscarriage as it had dulled the earlier excitement. Now with this sense of loss I had no idea how to react.*

We didn't talk about it much. Being a rock meant offering support and love. I felt as though I had to flip a switch and remove myself from the situation. I had no one to talk to about the miscarriage; talking to Julie would only reinforce her negative feelings because she blamed herself. She was burdened enough with her own emotions, so she didn't need to deal with my confusion.

JW: I felt odd and without direction. What was I supposed to feel? How long was I supposed to cry? Were there people I should be telling? We didn't have much time to mourn in solitude. The next day we headed to Indiana to be with Ben's family for Thanksgiving. We decided it was best not to tell anyone about my miscarrying. Revealing what we were losing would reveal that we were trying to conceive, but it was more than that. Doctors had told the family that Ben's grandmother's health was deteriorating rapidly, so we didn't want to distract people from focusing on her. But even if I wanted to talk about it, I didn't know where to start. I was leaning heavily on Ben for his physical and emotional support as we began our journey.

BW: *It was a long drive but we made it. Julie was still struggling with the ordeal as the miscarriage had begun only a week earlier. After consulting with Julie, I told my sister about what happened so Julie would have another person to confide in and lean on during the holiday visit. We made it through. I was glad to see family, but it felt odd not to talk about our loss with anyone.*

JW: Thanksgiving Day, roughly one week after my initial bleeding began, was the most physically challenging day of my entire miscarriage. That was the day I shed the majority of my uterine lining and experienced the worst cramps I'd ever felt. The sickening part was being able to feel the pregnancy falling out of me. At one point I felt a huge surge of blood flow, so I went to the restroom to check my pad. Into the toilet fell a long, thin strip of tissue. I cleaned myself up and turned to look at the tissue. Standing there next to the toilet I had trouble convincing myself to flush. One of the last remnants of my child was sitting there in that toilet bowl. What kind of mother flushes her child down the toilet? Eventually I was able to reason that there was nothing I could do, and I depressed the handle. I watched blankly as the water refilled the bowl, leaving no trace of what I just experienced.

BW: *In the end what made the experience most difficult for me was not being able to talk about it because turning to anyone for emotional support just felt weak, like an unwarranted cry for attention. No one knew we even had a baby to start with, so we had no idea how to go about telling people we had lost it. Uncertainty led to feelings of isolation. Our marriage was all right because there was this silent, shared experience that acted as a bond. However, it was hard to know what to do and how to feel without being able to talk about the miscarriage. There was a silence that hovered around our loss. I was cut off from the world and didn't know whom I could turn to. I did not know any fathers who had lost a baby like this, and I felt as if no one could understand my complex and confusing feelings.*

JW: The thing I was least prepared for was how long losing the pregnancy took. I always envisioned a miscarriage to be a quick event where blood would splash out swiftly and painlessly ending your pregnancy. For two weeks

I felt my pregnancy drip from between my thighs. It took two weeks for the connection to my first child to dissipate. I felt isolated. I withdrew interpersonally from my relationships. The end of the semester was quickly approaching so everyone's focus on finals week meant my withdrawal went nearly unnoticed.

BW: *To this day, I sometimes feel as if I have nothing to say. At the time, it was as though I was a teenager again, overcome with emotions that no words could describe. And now I look back and think maybe I was a secondary character in this story of mother and child.*

JW: I picture conception as a romantic event with a flash of light and the beautiful music of our bodies celebrating a new life. My child's life began with its conception; its life ended when I miscarried it. I have trouble not blaming myself; maybe if I had created a better environment my child could have lived? Sometimes I feel as though I didn't really experience the loss, as though my memory is just a bad dream. Artifacts such as the necklace I wore are difficult to possess because they are tangible reminders that I was pregnant and our child did not survive. What do I do with the necklace now?

   I'm enthusiastic for pregnancy to happen again, but I fear I'll be one of those women who experiences multiple miscarriages and is never able to carry a baby to term.

BW: *We were parents, yet childless. We were ready, but got burned. There is no baby, no memorial, no family remembrance. But it did happen. We did have a baby.*

   When we try again, the specter of our first pregnancy will hang over us. Getting excited will be that much more difficult, now knowing that it all could end suddenly. Even though we did nothing wrong the first time, our next time will be filled with cautious optimism. Next time, I want to make sure we do everything we can to protect our child and ourselves. Next time, I want to see our baby.

Resisting Silence: Scripting Theory and Narrative Practice

Writing our narrative was challenging to say the least. Julie drafted the first version of the events, and Ben inserted his experiences and thoughts into the timeline set by Julie. This method produced a truer selves-portrayal because much of what Ben experienced was controlled by and focused on Julie and her body's process. Ben's narrative stemmed from Julie's, which was the reason we visually portrayed his story in italics (to convey the secondary nature of his experience). The actual process of writing and editing our narrative required us to share things we hadn't shared previously, particularly for Ben. Julie, for instance, didn't realize how much Ben suppressed his emotions to protect her until she read his narrative.

In writing our narrative, we each remembered times when we weren't actively reflecting, but now could do so to tell a more complete story. We fought with the notion that our new insights may seem disingenuous. Ben reflected that if we'd written our narrative as the miscarriage took place, he probably would've said merely that he felt sad and confused. Through writing he could elaborate on his confusion rather than simply providing reactionary commentary. More than anything we became aware of how few *scripts* are available for people experiencing a miscarriage.

Script theory (Tompkins, 1979) explains how we observe cultural experiences and create unconscious behavioral models for specific situations. Abelson (1981) defines a script as a "cognitive structure that when activated organizes comprehension of event-based situations" (p. 717). Scripts provide us with a secure sense of order, and scripts help us decide appropriate behaviors given the situational factors. Nathanson (1996) interprets Tompkins's work and suggests that through "systems of scripts … all life is managed [and] no scene can be understood … until it has been recognized … and placed in the context of the specific script with which it resonates" (p. 4). In a sense, we don't have to think about how we are going to act in most situations because we've unconsciously developed sets of expectations for how things will happen; those expectations are our scripts. We do not, however, have to follow the scripts we've developed. The way a script is performed may differ from the script's directions, and through "mindful" (Abelson, 1981, p. 723) performances or nonperformances of scripts we demonstrate our individuality.

In the case of miscarriage, few scripts exist. Movies and books describe the processes of falling in love or getting married, but there are few mainstream media images describing or even referring to the process of losing a child; none that we have seen comes close to what we experienced. Abelson (1981) suggested we regress to *maladaptivity*, or an inability to adjust behaviors to a particular situation when no script is available. Julie experienced maladaptivity when she came home from work to her empty apartment and didn't know how to behave. Ben's maladaptivity was rooted on the emotional level as he was unsure of what he should be feeling, leading to a lack of verbal grieving. Without a script, knowing what to do and say was difficult because we had no example on which we could base our actions.

More than a year after the miscarriage, Julie shared with the majority of our family and friends via a social networking site that we had experienced a miscarriage. Previously, we had shared it only with our few closest friends and our families. We found friends and acquaintances only revealed their own miscarriage experiences after Julie shared our loss. However, even after Julie's public announcement no one has shared their experiences with Ben, nor have they asked Ben about his feelings. Most stories shared with Julie omit the intimate physical and social aspects of pregnancy loss. We also know that several of our family members haven't shared their miscarriage experiences with us, despite having learned of our miscarriage. The problem isn't a lack of miscarriage stories to share; the problem is that we don't share them. The power of personal narratives may be the key to helping future couples and individuals through their miscarriages.

Personal narratives are the "stories we tell ourselves and others about our histories and ourselves" (Swan & Benack, 2012, p. 50). Pecchioni (2012) describes personal narratives as representing "the lived experience of a particular individual" (p. 762) and suggests that narratives "reveal individuals' inner lives as they explain and justify their actions while also creating and reflecting their social relationships" (p. 762). Langellier (1999) explains narratives contribute not only to an individual's sense of identity, but also to how individual narratives overlap to create "a narrative bricolage into which we are recruited by virtue of membership in communities" (p. 139). She suggests the individual reflexivity of personal narratives examines the "cultural production and reproduction of identities and experiences" (p. 128). Essentially, Langellier's assertions combined with script theory suggest personal narratives overlap to create the scripts we use to make sense of and have certainty during our experiences.

Had we "experienced others' experiences" (Ellis & Bochner, 1992), that is, heard others' miscarriage stories, we would have unconsciously developed more accurate expectations for what a miscarriage might be like. When Julie's miscarriage began, she would still have felt sorrow for the loss, but she would not have felt as uncertain about how to behave or what to expect physically. Both of us might have felt more certain about how and when to talk about our experiences. Julie would have felt less uncomfortable describing the parts of the story that took place in the bathroom, because she would have heard others describe it first. Ben would have felt less uncomfortable voicing his confusion and emotion. We would have chosen how to label our loss based on the perspectives others shared; we still struggle over whether to call it losing a pregnancy or losing a child.

When we share our experiences of miscarriage with others we provide them the material needed to create scripts, thereby decreasing the uncertainty and silence veiling miscarriage experiences. The lack of scripts and narratives regarding miscarriages misrepresented how common miscarriages are, and left us feeling alone. Frost, Bradley, Levitas, Smith, and Garcia (2007) describe the experience of a miscarriage as "a unique type of loss because of the many ambiguities surrounding the event [and the] silence, isolation, and uncertainty combine to augment the suffering" (p. 1004). We have a responsibility to share our personal narratives about our miscarriage experiences.

Langellier (1999) explains how "personal narrative performance constitutes identities and experience … where the social is articulated, structured, and struggled over" (p. 128). As we struggle through creating narratives of our lived experiences, we can both reduce the uncertainty of others, and we can renegotiate our own identities. Langellier continues by describing how "personal narrative performance is especially crucial to those communities left out of the privileges of dominant culture" (p. 129). We can recognize patterns in our scripts that may help us renegotiate the social, cultural, and gender norms present in our experiences. Gender norms are particularly interesting considering our narrative style.

With an increased societal expectation for both parents to be involved in childbirth and parenthood (Murphy, 1998) we cannot ignore men in miscarriage narratives. Men often experience what Ben calls a counterscript, an adapted script that performs against the person's best interest to fill the situational void where no script exists. Since men are expected to ignore their personal feelings in times of grief, stoicism and distance become the harmful counterscript. In the case of miscarriage, the mother physically lost the baby, so the focus is primarily on her. The father may focus his support on the mother at the expense of grieving the loss of what was his child, too. Ben survived by using his counterscript, but it was ultimately against his best interests because he avoided reflection and self-consideration. As a scholar who regularly examines his feelings, Ben was able to partially grieve through the narrative process. Those men who continue to be constrained by traditional masculine ideals may struggle to face their emotions regarding their miscarriage experiences, which is why it is especially important for men to be included in the conversations and narratives we exchange about miscarriage.

We encourage anyone who has endured a miscarriage to openly share their stories with others when they are ready. The limited portrayals of miscarriage in popular media are mangled, but few people share details of their miscarriage experiences, meaning misconceptions are not corrected by anecdotal evidence. Even if we are still working through what we think or feel, we need to talk about what we are experiencing. Our story describes a heterosexual marriage and biological conception, but other parenting units such as same-sex couples or couples whose pregnancy depends on a surrogate mother can experience a miscarriage loss as well. Miscarrying a child transforms a hopeful beginning to a desolate and lonely time. To help those who have experienced a miscarriage (physically or vicariously) we must share the stories we have to create the narrative bricolage necessary to create miscarriage scripts.

Nothing can take away the pain of a lost pregnancy, but sharing our narratives provides others a foundation needed to build their own miscarriage scripts as well as the opportunity to renegotiate our own identities. Our pain is difficult. It is real. It does not go away quickly. Sharing our stories provides us the opportunities to decipher how our identities have been changed by our experiences, and it could help those we care about make sense of their own future experience.

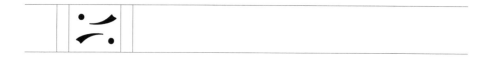

Section 2: When the Personal Is Professional

5. A Story We Can Live With: The Role of the Medical Sonographer in the Diagnosis of Fetal Demise

ELISSA FOSTER AND JODI MCGIVERN

Impending loss of a pregnancy may be signaled by a variety of noticeable symptoms including bleeding, loss of fetal movement, or cramping; in many cases, however, "embryonic demise" is diagnosed through an ultrasound procedure, which may be part of a routine prenatal screening in the absence of other signs of miscarriage. Typically, in the United States the ultrasound procedure is performed by a female medical sonographer whose position, like so many of the predominantly female ancillary health professions, is relatively low on the medical hierarchy and is not authorized to deliver or discuss the diagnosis of pregnancy loss with the patient. Although scenes of such ultrasound-assisted diagnoses are available in narratives written from the perspective of the mother (Foster, 2010; Freedman, 2009; Paulsell, 2007), and are described in the medical literature (Jurkovic, Overton, & Bender-Atik, 2013), in most accounts the person operating the technology is a "flat character" and is peripheral to the point of near invisibility. Popular films on the theme of pregnancy (e.g., *Juno, Knocked Up, Nine Months, Baby Mama*) almost exclusively depict an obstetrician or family physician as operating the ultrasound equipment without the presence of a sonographer, further adding to the marginalization of the role of the sonographer in the narrative of diagnosing pregnancy loss.

Originating with the first author's reflections on her pregnancy loss story, this chapter brings together a narrative of the moment of diagnosing "fetal demise" with the second author's reflections on pregnancy loss diagnosis from the perspective of the medical sonographer. Both authors' stories are presented and synthesized using the concept of narrative ethics as an explanatory framework that delineates the complexity of the sonographer's role in many stories of pregnancy loss. The nature of this complexity is presented along with a call to consider narrative ethics as a viable approach to the training of medical sonographers as well as to the development of a professional discourse that will provide insight and guidance for physicians and others who work closely with sonographers in the diagnosis of fetal demise.

Elissa: Experiencing Diagnosis via Ultrasound Examination

In moments of great suffering, I have noticed that it is not the suffering itself that moves me most deeply; rather, in times of trauma, grief, and loss there often occur acts of human kindness and compassion, and it is those acts that bring me to tears. When I recount the story of how I learned that our first pregnancy was "no longer viable" (Foster, 2010), it is neither the memory of our long struggle to get pregnant nor the acknowledgment of the ensuing crushing grief that makes me cry afresh. Rather, my voice falters as I describe the actions of the sonographer[1] whose job it was to confirm the end of the pregnancy in the presence of my family physician. With that memory, I experience a vivid triggering of emotion that encompasses both the suffering I experienced and the compassion displayed by another person—a perfect conjoining of one's deep need and another's appropriate heartfelt response.

By all accounts, our experience of the beginning of the miscarriage was typical. At eleven weeks, I noticed some bleeding that persisted for five days. After my primary physician, Holly, could not find a heartbeat during my office visit, she walked me over to a nearby obstetrical practice for a more complete examination. Before disrobing and settling myself on the examination table, I chatted with the sonographer. Introduced by Holly as I walked to the exam room, Audrey (a pseudonym) was petite, dark-haired, and only a little older than I was, though she seemed much more mature than I felt. I recall telling Audrey that I felt a little nervous because I was an "older Mum" who had been "trying" for some years to get pregnant. Once the exam began, I recall a single swipe of the transducer across my belly—though it may have been more—before she announced that she would feel better completing the scan transvaginally. I'd never had a scan performed that way before. For our eight-week ultrasound, the transducer was pressed firmly across my belly to produce multiple images of the little being we had nicknamed the "Cheerio"—images that were carefully saved in the back of the pregnancy diary my partner and I were keeping. At the announcement of the transvaginal scan, I must have looked a little stunned because Audrey lightened the moment by referring to the phallic shape of the transducer, noting that it was not unlike what I had already experienced. I recall chuckling, seeing her raised eyebrow, and being surprised that she did not join me in a laugh. In light of what happened next,

I now feel certain that she already knew that our baby was no longer alive, and she realized her role was to reveal that death in its most tangible visibility.

A few seconds later, the screen on the wall above me depicted an image that was too similar to the one over which my partner and I had marveled a month earlier, now preserved in the pregnancy diary—too small for the expected eleven and a half weeks of growth—a delicate being once pulsing with life now suspended in a deafening silence. The click of the sonographer's keyboard punctuated my awareness through a creeping sensation of dread until Holly quietly told me to get dressed. When I returned, Holly's first words—"It's not good news"—ushered in the grief that would stay with my partner and me, in greater and lesser degrees, from that day forward. As I surrendered to the pain of loss, Audrey exited the exam room, probably to afford me some privacy with my doctor. I don't know how long she waited, but when I finally emerged, she was standing in the hallway. She embraced me and whispered three words that would sustain me in the months and years ahead, "Please don't despair." Heartfelt. Human. Perfect.

Considering the Role of the Sonographer

In the years following our pregnancy loss, I had countless opportunities to interact with obstetrical sonographers in the context of fertility treatment and, happily, during our second successful pregnancy. The professional comportment of sonographers during the ultrasound examination can vary dramatically. Because of the intimacy of the transvaginal ultrasound scan (in my estimation, second only to the annual gynecology exam in its invasiveness), I found myself actively seeking to connect with the women scanning me, wanting them to know my story, often searching their faces for clues to ascertain what they were seeing about my future in the images on the screen. Sometimes I would tell them about the sonographer who diagnosed my pregnancy loss, and they would respond in various ways. Some felt free to discuss the emotionality of their job and the difficulty of seeing a devastating diagnosis but being barred from speaking to the patient. Some sonographers fear litigation as a result of communication surrounding a fetal demise or diagnosis of fetal anomaly. Some practices, most likely because of similar fears, simply do not permit sonographers to communicate with patients—even to offer comfort—when there is a negative outcome. One sonographer told me she loved her job but that she was simply afraid to show any emotion or discuss anything with her patients because she feared being summarily dismissed. Yet another sonographer responded to my story by admonishing the actions of her colleague, declaring, "That was so unprofessional. She should never have spoken to you like that—that's the doctor's role." I did not hesitate to tell her that her colleague's words and embrace were a source of profound comfort to me during the darkest moment in my life.

It occurred to me that the role of the sonographer is characterized by contradictions; they are highly skilled anatomists (DuBose, 2006) whose quality of work depends on their ability to diagnose patients' conditions, yet they are forbidden by law to "diagnose"; they conduct intimate, hands-on examinations of patients and yet they are depicted in medical accounts of sonography as impersonal, interchangeable technicians; they are committed to a code of ethics (Society of Diagnostic Medical Sonographers, 2006) that is intended to guide their professional conduct, and yet their patients' situations are so varied that the code provides little practical guidance. For example, among its twenty-five items, the code of ethics advises the sonographer to "be truthful and promote appropriate communications with patients and colleagues," "collaborate with professional colleagues to create an environment that promotes communication and respect," and "communicate and collaborate with others to promote ethical practice." The role of such codes is to provide global guidelines and, although their meaning seems self-evident in the abstract, when faced with the specifics of a particular case, the sonographer must rely on her own judgment concerning what is best for the patient. Further, because many outpatient obstetrical practices now have their own sonographers, hospital-based sonographers may have little experience scanning the pregnant patient and be particularly ill-equipped to respond when faced with a fetal demise or other devastating diagnosis. Finding nothing in the medical literature to help me grasp the experience and understand the responses of the sonographer in the moment of diagnosing pregnancy loss, I needed an expert to partner with me in inquiry. Jodi McGivern is that partner. To prepare this chapter I interviewed Jodi and asked her to share her experiences and perspectives on diagnosing pregnancy loss (fetal demise) in the course of her thirty-year career in medical sonography.

After completing her training in radiography in the early 1980s, Jodi fell in love with the new field of medical sonography and joined one of the first programs at the University of Iowa. After graduating, she was in a position to educate the physicians with whom she worked who had not yet seen ultrasound technologies and images. Her experience with obstetrical sonography began with her program at the University of Iowa at a time when there was no separate perinatology program; the sonographers in Jodi's program conducted all of the high-risk and abnormal ultrasound scans across the state of Iowa and in neighboring states. In the course of her career, 60% of her experience has been with obstetrical ultrasound and it remains an aspect of her work that she thoroughly enjoys. Fifteen years ago, she became the director of a professional sonography training program in which she is able to share her experiences and perspectives with the newest generation of aspiring sonographers.

Jodi: Patients Respond in So Many Different Ways

When I went through my sonography training, there was no separate course in counseling per se; it was more a case of learning by observing and my teachers were always ready to answer our questions. I had the opportunity to learn from some really great people; they were compassionate, they were honest, they were calming and very straightforward when they interacted with patients. In those teachers, I saw what I didn't want to be and I saw what I did want to be for my own patients. I knew that I wanted to provide some form of comfort in moments when there was a difficult diagnosis. And also, while I was in training, I saw my sister lose a full-term pregnancy that greatly impacted me. To see what she went through—she had no answers, no plan—I just knew that as a provider of care I never wanted to be what her provider had been, so brusque and dismissive.

Sometimes, though, it can be difficult to know how to respond to patients. For example, once when I was in training, a woman came in and we identified that her baby had anencephaly (a condition in which major portions of the brain, skull, and scalp are missing). It is not a survivable condition. Because she was a practicing Catholic, termination was not an option for her, and she was in denial for the entire pregnancy. Each time she came in to be scanned she would say, "Show me the baby's head. Show me the baby's head," and we would have to say, "Remember, it's not there. That portion of the skull is missing," and consistently remind her of her baby's condition. That was a very extreme case. More often, it is in early pregnancy when the patient asks the question "Is there a heartbeat?" In those situations, we offer the explanation and say, "It may be that it's too early, but at this stage we should be seeing it and we are not. Let's scan you again in three or four days." If I have a patient who asks me, "Do you see a heartbeat?" I don't believe in saying, "I can't answer that question." I'm more comfortable with saying, "I'm sorry. I don't. But let's go get a physician to take a second look and get some answers for you." I don't ever want to mislead a patient or give a patient false hope. I also don't want to leave a patient with fears and questions.

When teaching my students, I emphasize that there is not one way to handle the breaking of bad news. Every single patient is different. But I am a firm believer that these are not patients whom you just let go and call in a report to the doctor. To me, they deserve the doctor to come back right away and give them an answer. If it's an on-call situation and the physician is not readily available, then I'm on the phone to the physician, asking, "How do you want me to handle this? Are you coming in? Do you want me to send the patient right over to you?" We have called OB and had a nurse come down to the sonography office. If it's not a question that I can answer, then I'll do what I can to get a patient's questions answered right away, particularly when she is waiting to know whether it is a demise.[2]

Whether they are in a hospital or in a private office, the sonographer and the physician should work very much as a team; if we miss something, they miss something. If we don't document something, they are not going to see it. They are not in the room scanning with us. They rely heavily on our perception of what the patient needs at the time and most of our physicians are great about coming in and confirming, for example, "No, I don't see a heartbeat. Let's get hold of your physician and let's get a plan together." We work with some really good physicians; I know it's not that way everywhere.

Patients also respond to the news of a fetal demise with a gamut of emotions—some are angry, some are inconsolable. The hardest ones for me are the patients who are just silent, as if by not acknowledging it, it's not true. Some of them blame themselves and have so many questions: "Did I do something wrong? What could I have done to prevent this?" So many questions. And then there are those who experience a rejection response, as if they just can't deal with it, and they demand, "Get it out of me now." I think you have to handle each one of those situations differently, but they all warrant an answer.

The worst thing you can say is, "You can always have another child." Even if that's true, it doesn't just replace the child they've lost.

Responding to the Patient Whose Child has Genetic Anomalies

As sonographers, we also identify genetic anomalies—including structural defects such as spina bifida and anencephaly (which are neural tube defects), gastrointestinal and kidney problems, cleft lip or palate, and heart defects—and must respond appropriately to the patient in those cases. In the program in which I now teach, one patient and her partner came to the ultrasound lab as volunteers to work with the students. The minute the student put the probe on the patient's stomach the scan revealed an image of the baby's head and you could see severe hydrocephalus where the brain was filled with cerebral spinal fluid instead of brain tissue. And then as we started scanning further, the heart was abnormal, there were some odd contractures of the joints—babies tend to constantly clench and unclench their fists and move their arms and legs around, and this baby had its arms fixed at a 90-degree angle with its hands splayed open, which is not typical. But the images from the scan were absolutely beautiful—very clear and, sadly, unambiguous. So then we were faced with the dilemma—do we stop the scan immediately and say, "We see some abnormalities. We want you to go to your physician's office," or do we continue the scan, show the parents what we are seeing, talk about it, and then call the physician?

At the time, because we were an hour away from their physician's office, I made the call to finish the scan. I could not, in good conscience, send them away to drive an hour before getting any answers. We showed them pictures of their baby and printed images of their baby. I told them that we needed to get a better look at the baby's heart and a better look at the baby's brain and I was going to call their physician's office so they could go back that day for a second scan and a consultation. The parents accepted the information calmly and did not ask many questions. The mother told me later that she worried there was a problem with the baby, but she understood our dilemma—we were not supposed to give her the diagnosis and make a plan for her.

She called me about a year later after she had delivered her child—a son. Obviously, he has some cardiac anomalies and some brain anomalies. He is very developmentally delayed, but he is progressing. She sent me pictures of the baby and copies of the scans that were taken at the perinatal center because she thought it would be a great learning experience for the students. And she thanked me for allowing her to bond with her child and for handling the circumstances of her initial scan calmly and professionally. She said I would never know how much she appreciated that I didn't treat her fetus as if he didn't exist just because he had abnormalities.

I always ask the patient whether she would like a picture if there is something that we can scan.[3] I've had multiple patients start crying when I offer them a picture and thank me because, to them, that's still their child and they still want that connection with the child—and, if it's a demise, those pictures can be very important later on or with a second pregnancy. So, I think what is important is that we acknowledge the situation from the patient's perspective—this was a living child who was important to them and we must acknowledge that for our patients. Sometimes, when offered the picture, they say, "No, I don't want to see it. I don't want to look at it." Others say it's the only good thing that happened to them in the whole experience of losing their baby.

Diagnosing Fetal Demise

One case that stands out in my mind actually concerned a coworker and his wife. This was, if I recall correctly, their third pregnancy and they had been trying for a while. They came in to the office with a nine- to ten-week demise. It was after hours so we had no physician radiologist there, and when they asked, "Do you see a heartbeat?" I had to say, "No. I don't, but let me call the radiologist and see what she wants to do." The radiologist did come in to the office to confirm. I probably spent an hour and a half with the couple getting them ready to leave, and called a family member to come and get them. I talked with them at length to reassure them: "No, you did nothing wrong. Sometimes we can't explain why this happens." I gave them time and space to be together, to comfort each other. I provided what comfort I could—got them drinks and tissues. Afterward, I got the nicest letter from them about how much easier I made the experience for them by being calm and comforting and providing them with the time to talk about it and deal with their emotions without being rushed out the door and left to deal with it on their own. Just that little bit of extra kindness and comfort really made a difference to them. I can think of hundreds of cases in which I've gone the extra mile for a patient, and for me that means having empathy, giving them time, showing them that I care.

I've shed tears with patients—sometimes it just happens. You've scanned someone three or four times in a pregnancy and you get a bad outcome. Or you've scanned them through three or four pregnancies and you get to see their kids as they grow up .... I recall one patient who came in and it was her fourth pregnancy. She brought her twelve-year-old son with her for the scan and I remembered scanning him when she was first pregnant. When she came in for the appointment she asked about my family and I asked her about hers. It was just a really lovely conversation as she got ready for the scan, catching me up with what was going on with her kids. This was her first dating ultrasound, so she was eight or nine weeks along in the pregnancy.

She knew me well enough and she'd been through enough ultrasounds to know that as soon as I began the scan and confirmed the heartbeat I would be chatting and pointing things out, what's happening with the baby's growth and so on. So when I did not find a heartbeat immediately, she knew that my interaction with her wasn't "normal." So she questioned it right away; I told her, "No, I don't see a heartbeat right now," and then got the radiologist, who confirmed the demise. She sat there for a while and I called her husband, who came in and they sat there together. We talked through their disappointment and she thanked me for being honest with her.

I won't say that I think of them as friends, but with some patients you do form stronger relationships over time. The first-time mom coming in for a scan is no less heartbreaking but it is less personal … maybe. Even when I've seen someone over the years with successful pregnancies, when diagnosing a demise, it's the first time I'm interacting with them in a moment of distress. But, in this case, because I'd cared for her over the years and seen her at the other end of the spectrum of emotion with her successful pregnancies, I felt more comfortable responding to her in that distress.

Even after thirty-two years, that moment of diagnosis is still a gut-wrenching moment for me, every single time. If I ever get to the point at which my heart is not breaking for that patient, then I'll know it's time to retire. It doesn't get easier—I've gotten better at responding to it, but it's not easier.

Acknowledging a Common Humanity

I think that acknowledgment of loss is important for the grief process, too. When someone dies, no one wants to talk about it, but, in my mind, that's what we need the most. In my sister's situation, after thirty-six hours of labor she had a C-section and she delivered a dead child. Hospital protocols and instructions from her physician meant that she was not allowed to see the baby. Because of her own physical condition, she was not allowed to leave the hospital to go to the funeral. She did not visit the cemetery for twenty years until our father passed away. She never dealt with the loss. When I look back, her experience should have been handled differently. To never see your full-term child? It was almost as though Andrea (the baby) didn't exist to the people at the hospital—as though she could just be delivered and then forgotten. And I think my sister's process of grieving and coming to terms with her loss would have been completely different if she had had that opportunity to see Andrea and have the death acknowledged.

Having this loss occur so early in my training impacted my approach to my work. We are a very close family; I have one sister and one brother, and we were very close to our parents. This was a first grandchild and a first niece. It was a big source of excitement for our family. The loss was devastating. And for anyone to just say, "We've buried her, now let's move on. Let's not talk about it" makes no sense. Nobody helped my sister deal with that loss; I look back now and it horrifies me. It really informs how I want to treat my patients.

I said this to my students yesterday: "You always have to remember that this may be the thousandth scan for you, but this is likely the first time that the patient's been scanned. This may be the tenth baby you've scanned today, but it's the patient's first scan of the day, and it may be the first time they've seen their baby." And I remind myself of that as often as I can because there is a danger that we can become immune to the perspective of the patient.

The late-term losses really distress me, but even with those early pregnancy losses, it still makes me heartsick every time it happens. Although professionally I might know that most of those losses occur because of anomalies and perhaps it's for the best, that doesn't make it easier and it doesn't make it any less traumatic for the patient. A loss is a loss. Obviously, you can't fall apart in front of the patient every time it happens, but there's nothing wrong with feeling bad with your patient and showing some emotion. We're human, and if we lose that sense of our humanity, then I think it's time to get out of the field.

A Story We Can Live With

Something I want patients to know is that there are laws limiting what we can say. Sometimes sonographers may seem aloof or evasive and they may just not know what they are legally allowed to say. I don't think it comes from a place of not caring for their patients ... although there are some exceptions to that statement. Some sonographers may be awkward and not know how to respond to a grieving family. We do walk a fine line between what we are legally allowed to do and what morally and ethically we *want* to do.

At our national conventions, we discuss our code of ethics and point out that it provides no guidelines to help us in real situations. We really are flying by the seat of our pants when it comes to deciding what is best for our patients and what is the right thing to do. So I tell my students this: "I can go to sleep at night after getting a reprimand, even getting chewed out a bit by a physician or maybe an administrator for overstepping my bounds if I know I did the right thing for the patient. I can live with myself if I did what the patient needed; what I can't live with is feeling like I didn't do everything I could do. It is our responsibility to go above and beyond for our patients— they pay for our time, they pay for our expertise, but they also deserve our compassion." I try to instill that passion for the profession in my students. After thirty-two years, I still would never want to do anything else.

Elissa: Narrative Ethics and the Sonographer's Role

Narrative is a mode of representation and a means through which we make sense of events and relationships (Richardson, 1990). Narrative in both these senses has had an essential presence in the delivery of health care throughout history in patients' illness stories (Brody, 2002; Kleinman, 1988), physicians' stories (Coles, 1989; Selzer, 1989), and in the practice of narrative medicine that aims to make sense of both perspectives (Charon, 2006). Narratives are also cultural artifacts insofar as we have certain stories available to us, and in our narrative sense-making we are informed by cultural values. As Adams

(2008) points out, the narrative perspective is inherently "saturated with ethical qualities" (p. 177).

The concept of narrative ethics suggests that the "rightness" or "wrongness" of a given act can be judged only within the broader context of the narrative situation within which the act occurs. For the sonographer, embracing narrative ethics means that responding "rightly" (from the perspective of the patient, not the confines of legal and professional dictates) to the loss of a patient's pregnancy or the identification of a child's physical anomaly means being as attuned as possible to the patient's story even as it unfolds in the examination room. The prospect of tuning one's responses and adapting to an infinite array of subtle differences among patients is far more challenging than the prospect of learning one set of behaviors that will be "right" for everyone. However, as demonstrated by Jodi's account of a career in medical sonography, there is no universal response to loss among patients and therefore narrative ethics make infinitely more sense and are more practical than deductive, abstract ethical principles.

Thompson (2009) raises an important caveat to the promotion of narrative ethics as a practice among clinicians when she argues that empathy—specifically, a predisposition to care about the fate of another—is an essential precondition for the application of narrative ethics and that clinicians vary greatly in their capacity to experience and demonstrate empathy. Charon's (2006) model of narrative medicine does much to develop skills related to empathy—skills of listening, of reading between the lines, of being sensitive to metaphor and its conveyed emotion—and yet Thompson worries, quite legitimately, that an essential component may be missing in the clinician whose capacity for empathy is undeveloped. She suggests that for such clinicians, more prescriptive and less interpretive models of ethical conduct may be the answer.

As I listened to Jodi's stories and her descriptions of her own training, her practice as a sonographer, and the training she now provides for others, in addition to seeing evidence of her well-developed sense of empathy I noticed a consistent theme of modeling practice. As a trainee, she learned how to be with patients from others whom she sought to emulate and now she models compassionate communication for her students. Within Jodi's story are also prescriptions for how sonographers ought to respond to the suffering of patients; this is part of what I understand to be the "equipment for living" that Burke (1973) references as a functional element of stories—they help us to know what to do. As Jodi presented her values such as "I never want to leave a patient without answers," "I will always err on the side of offering comfort," and "the worst thing you can say is 'You can always have another baby,'" I can imagine others (even the least empathetic sonographer) adopting and performing such responses if they are modeled and depicted regularly in narratives of exemplary sonographic practice.

Although I agree with Thompson's (2009) concerns regarding some clinicians' lack of empathy and their subsequent inability to benefit from the subtle and nuanced demands of narrative ethics, Jodi described that she is guided by a sense of what actions will permit her to sleep at night, and she also acknowledged that there may be others in her profession who may be able to sleep just fine after carelessly disconfirming a family in distress. For those who require a more prescriptive approach to knowing how to respond to patients with compassion, narratives can be of considerable value. Reflecting on the narratives presented in this chapter, there are obviously lessons to be learned and specific actions that constitute more positive and supportive responses to families. If such narratives could be shared openly and consistently supported within the profession and across the medical contexts in which sonography is practiced, my sense is that the culture of sonography would be strengthened in ways that reflect the ethic of care exhibited by Jodi McGivern and others of her caliber. Even the least empathetic character would then be encouraged to act in ways consistent with the professional culture and avoid behaviors that constitute acts of emotional and psychic harm against patients.

Here's the rub. Currently, the sonographer's position in the medical hierarchy and the culture of litigation in the United States means that an almost untenable degree of uncertainty surrounds the communication between sonographers and patients. Furthermore, the cultural meaning of the OB ultrasound appointment has changed dramatically from the early days of sonography when it was viewed as primarily a diagnostic or screening examination. Although its medical function remains, the contemporary emphasis on seeing "the baby" and receiving the first "baby pictures" (ultrasound images) adds an air of entertainment to a clinical interaction whose outcomes, in reality, are always uncertain. Barad (2007) offers a degree of insight into the fetal ultrasound as a cultural phenomenon when she describes the extent to which visual images in our society are privileged as representations of reality. Rather than perceiving the ultrasound image as a product of the technology and the skill of its operator (the sonographer), we respond to the image as if it were, in fact, "the baby." Thus, the heightened expectations of family members around the ultrasound appointment add a significant degree of stress to the sonographer as she performs her work.

The implicit narrative in the medical literature casts the sonographer as a silent extension of the technology she wields in the service of the physician's elevated role. In reality, particularly in the case of fetal demise, the sonographer is intimately involved with the patient's story, with her body, and the loss of a child. By rendering the sonographers' stories invisible and, further, when sonographers work in a climate of fear in which they may not respond openly to patients' questions and concerns, sonographers may rightly struggle to know how to perform when faced with a patient's moment of crisis and trauma. They are literally left without their necessary "equipment for living."

A number of important outcomes of sharing sonographers' patient care narratives may be realized. First, practicing sonographers and those in training might discover many more options for offering positive and supportive responses to patients within the legal limits of their scope of practice. Second, the profession of medical sonography may find the narrative approach to ethics a useful and generative tool in the development of professional sonographic practice. And third, by having access to stories of clinical practice told from the sonographer's point of view, patients and fellow clinicians may have a more accurate and more nuanced understanding of the sonographer's role in the care of the pregnant patient. This chapter constitutes a starting point and an invitation for more voices to bring stories of both the rewards and the heartbreak of a career in medical sonography. If the potential of a narrative approach is realized, they will be stories that we all—patients and clinicians alike—can live with.

Notes

1. Prior to conducting research for this chapter, I used the common parlance for the profession that I learned as a patient, specifically, "ultrasound tech." From Jodi I learned that the correct title for the profession is "medical sonographer." The term "ultrasound tech" is strongly reflective of a medical hierarchy that undervalues the training and skill that are required to contribute to the diagnosis and care of the patient (DuBose, 2006).
2. The terms "fetal demise" and "embryonic demise" reflect the language of the medical context in which sonographers work. The meaning of the terms can be limited to describing the medical event that is the death of the fetus; it does not necessarily reflect the sonographer's attitude toward the patient or the baby who was lost.
3. Sometimes, by the time of the ultrasound, the tissue of the fetus has degraded to the point that there is no clear image to offer to the parents.

6. Searching for Grace

KRISTANN HEINZ AND ELISSA FOSTER

How does it start? Or, more to the point, when does it start?

An awkward silence filled with a sense of duty far beyond the expected makes me think that some experiences are only holograms of the past. Was the veil of responsibility projected forward in this case so that it now clouded my professional judgment? Could it be that evening twenty-four years ago? Did it start then, as I emerged from the coffee shop into that snowy afternoon?

I don't remember much about the conversation. I only know for sure I was left alone with a heavy heart and an accusation as a storm came in over Boston. I cannot even be certain that she said what I think she said, but there was a feeling of being blamed. I felt she believed it was my fault: I felt some power of mine had caused her miscarriage, or maybe could have prevented it from happening. Had I had personally taken away her dream? Maybe my young mind could have rationalized the event. Maybe it could have been dismissed if it hadn't been for one fact: The accusation came from my aunt.

My aunt, who had never had children by choice, had become a mother figure during my teenage years. And I, in turn, became the child she never had.

My aunt who was told after receiving chemotherapy for cancer that she could never get pregnant.

My aunt, who then by a miracle, conceived.

My aunt, who then had a miscarriage and lost the baby.

My aunt, who then had a talk with me in a coffee shop many years ago.

I did try to rationalize the experience. I recognized that the miscarriage had nothing to do with me, but somehow in that moment I offered the perfect channel for her despair. I think she tried to get pregnant again, but that never happened. And as time passed, the pain and confusion were healed, love prevailed, and our relationship mended. Life was accepted for what it offered. We all felt blessed and I believed we moved on.

* * *

But, right now, I wonder whether that sense of responsibility followed me into my present life as a family doctor, some twenty-four years later, as I call Grace for the third time this week. Grace was a patient who came to my office with concerns about infertility. I feel again the knot of anticipation in my stomach and hope to set things right, as if somehow this is all my responsibility. "Please pick up the phone. Let it not be too late," I silently plead with each ring. Once again I am met by her automated voicemail and I leave a message telling her that I have thought of something else that we could try, that we have not run out of options, there is still hope, and to please call me at the office to discuss it.

* * *

That was the last time I called, out of respect for her. I had seen her pain, and although I wanted to step in, it was her decision to stop treatment.

She never called back, despite my attempts. When I saw her name on my work schedule after that, it showed up with a line through it, indicating that she had previously cancelled her appointment. She never came back to the office. "Lost to follow-up" is the phrase we use in the medical world when the patient stops communicating with the practitioner. In the medical community we often seek to identify reasons that patients are "lost to follow-up." Did they move, were they unable to get to their appointments, did they lose phone service or transportation? As practitioners, we rarely ask what we might have done to contribute to our patients "getting lost."

My desire to become a family doctor came out of my public health experiences working in Maternal and Child Health. I was always drawn to pregnant women and babies. I can remember being in my late teens and thinking that surely I would have children in my early twenties, and lots of them. My major in college was nutrition, and by nineteen years of age I was running a Women, Infant and Children's (WIC) Food Program in a community center nestled in a public housing facility in Boston. It was not unusual to see me talking to a mother or mother-to-be with a child attached to my hip as I rocked the fussy infant and taught about the health advantages of good nutrition for mother and child alike. It was this love of families and nutritional prevention that led me to pursue a degree in medicine with a specialty in Family Medicine and Integrative Holistic Medicine.

When Grace came to our Integrative Family Medicine office she was looking for answers, as most patients are. Our tagline is "A Healthy Alternative in an Unhealthy World" and patients often turn to us when they have exhausted most conventional options. Many of our patients come to us carting reams of medical documents, including multiple studies and tests from many specialists. Often our patients were deemed "normal" by these institutions. They were told that "nothing is wrong" or, in many instances, they were told that the symptoms are "all in your head" and referred to psychiatry. As integrated and holistic medicine specialists, the doctors in our practice are left to read between the lines and behind the standard allopathic scene. We are expected to find the underlying cause of physiological dysfunction, which is most likely not taught in standard medical education, and ultimately to restore physical balance and health. Often we do just that. But make no mistake, we are mostly seen as a "medical outpost" in the allopathic community. Frequently, a medical consult with us is the last step in a patient's attempt to find answers and regain health. Grace was no different from the rest. Despite a complete and normal infertility workup for both Grace and her husband, they were unable to conceive after years of trying both natural conception augmented with hormonal support and in vitro fertilization. Grace arrived at our "outpost" with her family dream shattered, physically and emotionally drained.

The initial workup at our clinic involves a review of previous medical records and labs, which in Grace's case were all normal by my quick assessment prior to walking into the exam room. Upon entering, I was struck by Grace's quiet and innocent presence. She appeared in her early thirties looking like a "Snow-White Princess"—slender build, medium height, clear pearly skin, and straight dark hair. As it was fall, I remember thinking that it would be a Halloween-costume problem easily solved this year. She proceeded to tell me her story, ending with the fact that she had been told by her previous doctors that she was in perfect health, meaning that she did not have any ongoing medical problems, and she had normal lab chemistry and hormone levels. In the workup, we also evaluate the nutritional factors that influence health and, particularly in this case, conception. This involves looking at her dietary intake and running a nutritional blood and urine panel. I was feeling fairly confident the standard initial integrated medicine workup would go a long way to help rebalance her body and prepare her for conception. Providing dietary education and evaluating toxic environmental exposure form a big part of my initial visit. Grace and I spent a great deal of time talking about healthful organic eating, most of which she was already doing. We discussed how to reduce her exposure to environmental toxins, which may have hormonal disrupters. All in all, the visit went well and I was confident that I could help her.

The second visit was during winter, when we reviewed her nutritional screening panel. Vitamin C and essential fatty acids stood out as deficient. Since nutritional data indicate that these deficiencies can contribute greatly to infertility I was optimistic that we had identified at least one source of her difficulty conceiving. It seemed only a matter of time until Grace's family dream came true. I sent her on her way with a follow-up in a few months.

A few months came and went and by now it was spring, the perfect time for starting anew, but I could tell when I entered the room that nothing had changed. She was religiously taking the supplements and feeling better, stronger, and more energetic but not pregnant. Eating organic foods and still not pregnant. Avoiding toxins in plastics, cleaning supplies, cooking ware, clothing, and living spaces and still not pregnant. Decreasing cell phone radiation and still not pregnant. Doing everything right and still not pregnant. So I dug into the possibility of stress—was an emotional component contributing to infertility? Nothing emerged. Grace works as a homemaker, she loves her husband, she loves her family who is local and actively involved in her life, she had an easy upbringing, and she does some form of yoga or exercise daily. "There is no stress," she tells me. "Okay, what about a different kind of test of your hormones to see whether that gives us any other information?" I suggest. In integrative medicine we like to test salivary hormone levels in addition to blood levels. Maybe there would be an answer there. I also recommended acupuncture. Grace was up for more testing and acupuncture.

After this last visit, I did not see Grace during the rest of the spring and summer. I had a phone consult with her in the interim to discuss the results of her salivary test, which showed a low progesterone level. This hormone is very important for supporting a pregnancy, so we started her on transdermal progesterone cream. I was sure the fulfillment of her dream was around the corner—I had at this point covered all the bases of pre-conception care I could imagine. Nutritionally she was adequate, her hormones were appropriate and supported, stress and emotional health were addressed, and her toxic burden was decreased. This was the case for both Grace and her husband who, although we did not see him, had joined the program once it was implemented at home.

All the components for fertility were in place and, in my mind, it was just a matter of time. The fall came, marking a year from the day Grace and I had met. When I entered the exam room, I could see instantly her spirits were down. There was a heaviness in the room. Her eyes were cast down as she spoke. I sensed a deep disappointment with both the situation and also, perhaps, with me. I am not actually sure how the visit went. I don't remember what I said, or what she said. Our exchange was short and largely non-verbal. I was out of options and she knew it. I had done all that I was trained to do and she was left with the same result: infertility. The outpost had failed her and she left more alone and with an even deeper sadness, it seemed, than when she came to us.

After her appointment, I was left with a sense of despair and a longing to help. If I did not have the answer, perhaps I knew who would. That evening, I approached my mentor, a well-respected family medicine doctor with an uncanny capacity for information retrieval of integrative medicine facts who had been practicing this type of medicine for more than twenty years. His thought was that I should try a more energetic approach—homeopathy. Based on her case, I researched her constitutional remedy and was ready to prescribe but needed a bit more information from her. This is what prompted the first call, and then the second, and the third. But she never called back to see what I had to offer. She never came back. Grace was "lost to follow-up." But, in retrospect, maybe during that last visit, as I replayed it in my mind, in my desire to set things right, I was really lost to her.

All I can recall from my last appointment with Grace are my own feelings of not knowing what else to do or where else to turn, and I now can see how those feelings cut me off from her need. Physicians' feelings of responsibility come with taking care of all patients who come to us for help. Our success is based on our outcomes, which we usually define as fixing the patient's primary complaint. We doctors approach this request with our studies, our treatments, our interventions, and our education, and when they fail to heal, we are left feeling vulnerable. Without our typical doctoring tools (both integrative and allopathic), all we have left to offer is ourselves. However, in truth, this may be the most important thing we can give. What we can offer at that point is our presence; our ability to bear witness; our capacity to hold the space for disappointment, blame, and grief as they move into acceptance and grace.

I was not able to do that for Grace when she needed it. I was as disappointed and uncomfortable as she was and it is this feeling that causes me to wonder what part of my own experience with fertility and grief came up again to be reexamined. Did my past project a hologram of blame and responsibility that clouded my ability to be professionally available to Grace? Her disappointment indicted me; I couldn't make space for her heartbreak because it meant my failure—my failure now and in the past. I took refuge from her despair by grasping for the next plan. If I could just get it right, she could have what she wanted. I could set the record straight. I too sought something to blame—nutrition, hormones, environmental toxins, stressors—anything to make sense of her thwarted dream and give her hope that it might yet be realized. Yet in my struggle to solve the problem and resolve my past, I lost sight of Grace. Perhaps all Grace brought with her to that last visit was grief, perhaps acceptance that she would never give birth to the baby she longed for. I will never know. What I do know now is that had I let go of the efforts to shield myself from disappointment and blame, I would have been left more fully open to be in her experience and perhaps, through that, we both would have found grace.

* * *

December 2013

Ah Kristann, my friend,

I just finished reading the latest draft of your story and I feel compelled to respond. My original thought was to provide a theoretical perspective on this "case" in an objective academic voice—but of course that is not appropriate. My heart aches for Grace and, like you, I worry and wonder what happened. I am also very moved by the depth of reflection and the degree of accountability that you engage in as a practitioner. I believe you are correct when you note that few physicians ask how they might have contributed to a patient being "lost to follow-up." Regarding your own state of mind during your last visit with Grace, I think you are right when you suggest that it foreclosed other possibilities for your continued care of her … and, as your friend, I feel an urge to reassure you and comfort you, wanting you to be a little gentler on yourself.

As you described your approach to patient care, I remembered our conversation from two years ago, when my daughter was eighteen months old and had been prescribed surgery to treat her chronic ear infections. Her father and I could not abide the idea of putting our baby under a general anesthetic and sending her alone into an operating theater. We also could not understand why she was continually suffering. You gently offered us a more holistic perspective that addressed the source of the problem. Under your guidance, we removed dairy from her diet and provided supplements to boost her immune system. Our little girl's infections disappeared virtually overnight. In one meeting, you changed our story. I remember the genuine pleasure you expressed when six months went by without a single infection. I think, "What a powerful gift you have!" In light of that gift, how difficult it must be to accept the limitations of your power when presented with a need as profound as Grace's.

I also recall how much I identified with you as another mother and I could see how you bring the qualities of your mothering to your relationships with patients—energy, strength, compassion, and a certain degree of protectiveness. When I revealed my fears for my little one, you did not try to appease me but rather affirmed my own protective instincts as a fellow-mother. As you tell the story of your interactions with Grace, I perceive a similar desire to respond to her as a fellow-mother. I have come to believe that for many of us the mother identity precedes pregnancy and the birth of a child (Foster, 2005), and your response to Grace was to affirm and protect her "family dream" because you understood it so well.

When I imagine that the success with our daughter's ear infections must be replicated many times over in your practice, I think it must be natural to see all patients' stories following this same trajectory. You listen to the patient, you find a different path, and a sense of wholeness, of being in right balance, is achieved for you and for them. By helping Grace to realize her dream of having a child, all the pieces of her story can fall into place—the mystery is solved, the longing is fulfilled, the goal is attained, and all the struggle and pain of the journey are "worth it" because of the outcome. The narrative concept for this is "coherence"—and it all depends on how we are able to tell the story.

Fisher (1987) describes coherence as a feature of narrative fidelity—the extent to which stories satisfy the "criteria of the logic of good reasons, which is attentive to reason and values" (p. 10). It is not enough that we can identify an understandable set of reasons within the sequence of action in a given story (rationality), but that those reasons align with what we perceive to be good, just, and right. Despite some scholars' attempts to boil it down to a simple equation (Baesler, 1995), I am more inclined to agree that there is "no simple or unitary answer to the question of what constitutes narrative coherence" (Nicolopulou, 2008, p. 300). Rather, there is a reflexive relationship between our capacity to make sense of our experiences and our capacity to tell a coherent story—one that helps us to make sense of those experiences within the context of a greater life story (Burnell, Hunt, & Coleman, 2009; Pennebaker & Seagal, 1999). As someone who has experienced infertility both before and after the birth of my daughter, I can feel acutely the struggle to achieve any kind of narrative coherence both in the midst of the journey to "achieve pregnancy" (as the fertility specialists put it), and in the aftermath of the decision to stop trying.

Because we were eventually blessed with a child, I really cannot compare my experience with Grace's because our *narrative coherence* was accomplished with birth. "Look, we struggled for all those years and we were rewarded with this child." And yet, like so many others, our "family dream" was to have another. First we tried without medication because we heard so often the story, "Sometimes all it takes is for the body to learn how to get pregnant, and then the second child comes easily." Then we engaged in increasing levels of medical intervention for another year until it was time to stop—time to stop trying, to stop the cycle of hope and despair, to stop the injections, the blood work, the ultrasounds, and procedures. Time to "accept life for what it offered," as you put it regarding reaching reconciliation with your aunt. For us, the struggle remains to reconcile the unattained dream with the new story that we will be a family with one child. Not so bad, really, in light of Grace's story and those of so many others.

The decision to "stop trying" was painful and I was more than surprised when the nurse practitioner who had been overseeing my fertility treatments responded by saying, "Well, if you ever change your mind, just let us know." I was mystified by her parting comment. It was not until I read your story that I realized the nurse practitioner was probably responding to our disappointment by not wanting the story to end; she wanted to keep hope alive when we had already started to let it go. What angered me about the nurse practitioner's response was that she seemed to suggest that our decision to stop trying was a mere "choice"—a concept that does not fit within the paradigm of (in)fertility (Foster, 2010). The decision to stop certainly did not feel like a choice; rather, it became unbearable to live with an incoherent story and, without the "achievement of pregnancy," the story could never resolve. In my case, the decision to stop trying did not bring with it a new, complete, and fully coherent story; rather, it was the beginning of a new narrative whose coherence will be achieved over time.

As I imagine Grace meeting with you for the last time, eyes downcast, air heavy with the weight of unspoken thoughts and unexpressed feelings, I imagine her in the act of turning toward an unfamiliar and unwanted path—one that she imagines walking without the company of a beloved child. The feeling of inevitability that accompanies such a turn conflicts sharply with the deeply visceral conviction that something else was supposed to happen. Although I might know that I must accept that I won't ever be pregnant, I can still feel the ache in my empty arms. In that moment, I imagine Grace at the heart of an incoherent narrative, unable to tell her story, existing in a lonely place. I imagine you, following your deep instincts to support and protect, also faced with incoherence—your care was supposed to work, there was supposed to be a happy ending. Because Grace's relationship with you centered on the achievement of her family dream, I imagine that her need to turn toward another path necessitated a turning away from you—and this was not your failure so much as a natural consequence of narratives falling apart.

Thank you for sharing this story with me; I hope these ideas have been helpful.

Warmly,
Elissa

7. When the Professional Is Personal: Case Studies of Pregnancy Loss, My Story of Pregnancy Loss

LISA JO SCHILLING AND RACHEL E. SILVERMAN

My body is not working the way it is supposed to. My husband and I have been trying to have a child since January 2012. Our first infertility appointment was the following August. As of this writing, we have had four failed attempts at IVF and one more frozen embryo awaits our next step. After that, we have no more money to spend. Our infertility is female infertility; my husband is "just fine." Infertility feels like my body is betraying me, and no matter the amount of self-hatred and loathing, prayers, begging, hope, and bartering, there is nothing I can do about wanting a child. There is nothing I can do about the people who surround me who have children. I work as a pediatric nurse practitioner in primary care pediatrics. Just today, a mother of two whose son had strep throat complained to me about the impending arrival of her third boy. As we reviewed the diagnosis, she rattled on about wanting a girl, unaware of the blessings of having children. I can't escape it; it's every day and when I least expect it. Compassion and hope are what I stress most to my patients. Patience and determination are what I tell myself.

There is a variety of emotions that come with any sort of pregnancy loss. Each loss is unique to the person and the couple. The loss of a pregnancy may be from a miscarriage, elective abortion, adoption, surrogacy, or infertility. As no two people experience infertility—or any pregnancy loss, for that matter—in the same way, no one can fully know what anyone else is feeling or going through. Those who have had this gut-wrenching experience with pregnancy loss have some idea, but because each case is different there are often thoughts of jealousy, ideas that my situation is worse than someone else's situation. Sometimes I am jealous of people with children and I get angry with people who don't appreciate their kids or abuse them. I know what a wonder each child is and I want to help children in any way that I can. This sentiment then brings feelings of guilt. I feel guilt because I am not understanding enough of the people around me, or guilt because I am angry at my patients for their successful pregnancies. On any given day, I can have any and all emotions. And the hormones I take each day only seem to heighten my emotions.

Some days are better than others, and some patient case stories are better than others. The stories shared here are of adoption and infertility. The stories explore my perspective as a health professional and as a woman currently undergoing infertility treatment. The stories that follow are about people who have helped me become a better health care professional and, more important, a better person. Through my work, I have become a more compassionate person. When I am working and having a bad day, or thinking about all the charts I am behind on, I realize that paperwork doesn't matter. Only the patients matter. My personal stress has no bearing and takes a back seat while I care for the patients who have entrusted their lives to me. The trust, at times, is bittersweet. While it is an honor and privilege to help patients, the care I provide allows me many opportunities to question the fairness of life. The conflicts I feel at work create a split personality.

A few months ago, I was angry, jealous, and resentful of one of my patients. Frustrated with our infertility and the unfairness of life, I had difficulty finding compassion. Christine is a Caucasian female, sixteen years old, and pregnant. She is following in her mother's footsteps, as her mother had her at the same age. She came into the office less than a month after our third failed attempt at IVF. I wished with every ounce of my being that she would ask me how she could give her baby up for adoption and I would have volunteered my husband and me. "I'd take your baby in a heartbeat" was the thought that kept running through my mind as I worked with her throughout the day.

I did not cry until the next day, when I was working on Christine's chart. She had been my second patient of the day and we are a busy practice. I had no time to reflect on her and how her pregnancy made me feel until the following day. When I was finishing her chart, I cried and cried. I was jealous. I couldn't stop thinking about how unfair the situation was. Why does she get to have a baby and I don't? She spent the entire office visit in shock, unaware of the obstacles she is about to face, whereas I have been trying for years, waiting patiently and planning for what came to her by mistake, without notice. After crying, I felt disappointment with myself for having feelings of jealously. My thoughts were selfish and ugly. I thought, she doesn't deserve to be a mom and I do.

I have grown mad at myself for working in a profession with kids. When I started my nursing career, I had no idea I would be infertile. Parenthood is completely out of my hands and there's nothing I can do about it. It doesn't do any good to be jealous and mad at this young mother-to-be. All I can do is look forward to having her child as a patient next year and hope that someday I will get to have a successful pregnancy of my own with a healthy child at the end.

Ever since starting fertility treatments, patients like Christine make me want to change my nursing focus. It is too devastating to help other women have babies when I cannot. Only my husband knows I have threatened to change my specialty. On really bad days, when I am physically tired and emotionally drained from congratulating parents on another pregnancy, I come home and tell my husband I need to stop working with children. Only once have I researched the amount of additional education it would require for me to become a certified registered nurse anesthetist (CRNA). That specialty is my threat of career change, because interacting with patients will not be the primary focus, although, with my luck, I'd probably end up administering epidurals to women in labor. My threat, of course, is not realistic. Anyone who knows me is aware that my passion is children. I'm a big kid myself, and not working with kids would break my heart almost as much as not having one of my own.

Christine had a miscarriage the following month as a result of her drug abuse before and during pregnancy.

Only a few weeks later, another case brought out the split between my professional and personal lives. This example is one of the most unsuccessful adoption stories I have ever seen. A heterosexual married Hispanic couple in their late thirties has endured a decade of infertility diagnoses, has attempted IVF multiple times, and is well into the process of adoption. Adoption, for them, is their best and last hope to have a family.

Adoption is, in fact, quite a difficult process. I both laugh and shudder when people tell me "just adopt" when they learn of our infertility. Most people don't understand how difficult it is to adopt a healthy infant. A two-year waiting list is the norm, along with extensive interviews including character references from friends and family, a home inspection, and, of course, money. There are no guarantees with adoption. The birth mother has the right to change her mind at any time. Adoption leaves the desiring parents at the mercy of someone else's decision. It's a decision about who can give the child a better life. It's a decision that saves lives.

During the couple's first adoption attempt, they paid $30,000 to a pregnant teenager. Three days prior to her due date, the nursery is ready, the car seat and diaper bag are at the door, and the couple is ready for the telephone call letting them know "it's time." Instead they get a call informing them the grandmother of the birth father, who is also a teenager, wants the child. Yet another pregnancy loss for this couple. None of the money spent on medical and legal fees or maternity clothes was returned to them.

Their second adoption attempt is bittersweet and still ongoing. After recovering emotionally and saving financially, the couple adopted a six-month-old infant. Six months later, their lawyer called. The maternal grandmother wants custody of the child and is suing. The child and parents have bonded. They are forced to borrow more money for the additional legal fees to keep their child. I struggle to offer them hope. As an infertile person, I am jealous that at least they got to be parent for six months. As a professional and a caring person, I would not wish their journey on anyone. When I tell them I too know what it is like to want a baby and not have the opportunity to be a parent, I see a wave of relief wash over them. There is a shared bond we feel in this experience of loss.

Whether I share personal details or not, I am a much better provider for having to cope with my own health struggles. I do not share sympathy, only empathy, for all my patients. One patient, a woman in her late thirties and a survivor of breast cancer, thanked me for my honesty. When I told her about my infertility, her anger momentarily subsided. I didn't pretend to know how she feels; however, I understand the hope and devastation IVF brings. Even though we are both IVF patients, our journeys are different.

My efforts for coping with infertility and loss are ongoing. The feelings and training of a nurse and now nurse practitioner are always first and foremost when I assist a patient. My ability to help patients is stronger because of my own infertility. Because I know the pain of infertility, I know I can offer a type of empathy to my patients that can come only from experience. As a woman battling my own infertility, my heart breaks because I comprehend the pain of their loss. I know the indescribable hollowness and constant flow of tears. I know exactly where I was each and every time I was notified that the IVF cycle was unsuccessful. I know what it is like to receive a phone call that changes your life.

Years ago, during nursing school, I was privileged to be a part of an adoption that I will never forget. A nineteen-year-old Caucasian female, Helena, delivered a healthy infant who was the product of rape. Helena didn't want to look at the child; she didn't want to hold the child. The adopted mom was worried that Helena's decision would haunt her and make her question the adoption. It was easy then and it remains easy to understand both of their perspectives. Who can blame someone for not wanting to hold a reminder of the trauma of rape? Who can question the desperate hope of an adoptive mom in fear of having her child taken from her?

Moments before discharge the birth mother changed her mind and asked to hold the child. I still remember the room number, how she sat on the bed, the patience and understanding of the adoptive parents, and that Helena whispered something to the baby. No one knows what she whispered to the child. She thanked the adoptive parents and relief was evident in their eyes as she handed the child to the mom.

Per hospital protocol, the new mom—the adoptive mom—and her child were taken downstairs via wheelchair. I always love how people stare at new moms and babies. No one would ever know this child was adopted. All people saw was a new mom crying while she held her baby and a dad walking alongside. As the new family packed up the car and prepared to leave, the dad told me, "This is the most important ride of my life." At the time, I had no idea I would someday too hope to adopt. I was happy and proud to know this couple was going to love their baby. I will never forget that moment, standing just outside the hospital as they pulled away; it was a warm spring day with the breeze blowing and the sun shining. I smiled as I went back upstairs.

Discharging Helena took a little longer, and I did not have the same feelings of contentment. She cried uncontrollably in the elevator and I cried with her. I didn't know what to say to her. I thought to myself, "I don't know what to say; I'm not an RN yet." I stopped the elevator for privacy and she stood so I could hug her. I still regret that all I could do was hold her and cry with her. She told me giving her child away was the hardest thing she had ever done and that she knew it was for the best. I think of her often. I like to think her decision to give her child up for adoption has helped her to heal or at least live with what she endured.

I worry that my professional life is negatively impacting my personal life. I am fairly confident my personal life is making me a better professional. When yet another IVF attempt is unsuccessful for us, I cry uncontrollably for a few days. I do not sleep and I function on autopilot at work. I am two different people: At work I am happy, but when I get in my car and am alone, I sob the entire way home. I feel like a zombie. My husband holds me and lets me cry those first few days, then I stop talking to him for a few days, as though he is the reason we are not successful and he deserves my anger. Then I convince myself that I don't want kids. After that, I block all of my feelings. Then I have hope for the next cycle. I worry about my husband because he shows no emotions. I know he will do anything for us to get pregnant and faces his own demons for not getting us pregnant the natural way. At least I have a range of emotions, I think to myself; he cries the first day and then shows nothing. Instead, he attends to my every need. I need to work more on attending to his needs.

I am finally at the point at which I know that if we do not parent, my life will not end. There were a few times when suicide felt like the right choice for me. I remember the anguish of the crying hollowing my core. I felt empty inside and didn't know how to breathe. Suicide felt like my only option—why should I live when I can't live my dream? I always thought I would parent. It was supposed to be automatic: Grow up, get married, and have kids. I always said I wanted four children. Now, I'd do just about anything to have one. It took a while before I was able to share my thoughts with my husband and later my mom and sister. My husband was incredibly upset when I told him. He understood my feelings. He asked me, "What am I supposed to do if you do that? I can't live without you" and I realized there was more to life than parenting. I will always be sad and jealous of parents; I will also continue to find ways to make a difference in the lives of my patients. Life is not over for me if I do not become a mom, it is just a different life from the one I expected. I credit time and Harold S. Kushner's book *When Bad Things Happen to Good People* for helping me realize suicide is not the answer.

Almost every Sunday, I witness the love and joy of family. There is a young family of five that typically runs late for Mass. They always sit with their parents and grandparents. Each week, witnessing the joy on the grandmother's face when the grandchildren arrive at the pew is indescribable. The love is indescribable. The grandmother's face lights up. I look forward to that look on the grandmother's face each week. I want each and every person to have and feel that pure joy of love. Unconditional love is what parenthood is.

I have an unconditional love for working with kids and their parents. I love teaching the nursing students in their pediatric clinical rotations in the hospital. I love all the hugs the kids give me every day. No matter what happens with my personal journey with parenthood, I hope and pray I've made a difference for my patients. They have made a difference in my life. I wouldn't want any other job in the world.

8. *Infertility, Professional Identity, and Consciousness-Raising*[1]

Caryn E. Medved

The home I grew up in was not particularly filled with stories, tall tales, or accounts of the past. My family culture is full of unspoken love, perhaps best described as self-effacing. You stick to the facts. You don't call attention to yourself. You don't dwell in setbacks; instead you make concrete plans for the future. When my family gets together, the narrative impulse only makes a short-lived, primarily comedic appearance and often requires the aid of at least two margaritas. My experiences growing up and certainly other dispositions have led me to hold on to the private, to sequester it willingly in deference to the professional. I have tremendous respect for those who skillfully make use of the personal as a means to the theoretical; even so, my career until now has not taken that path.

Thus, not surprisingly, I'm a bit baffled at my want (even impulse) to tell the following story. All I can surmise is that I need to compose as a way of writing myself into a new subplot, if not a fresh scholarly direction. Writing it for myself, and publishing it as a story for you to read, admittedly, are two different concerns. I was astutely reminded of this distinction by a close friend a few months ago on a road trip through the Midwest. Yet let's start with the telling and then we'll circle back around to its public narration. And allow me to say up front that I'm only telling you the story I want to tell, I'm willing to tell; it's unavoidably a personal story but my purpose is primarily professional as eventually you'll see.

First, visit my office. It's dimly lit by my $10 Salvation Army lamp and, by Manhattan standards, surprisingly large. Plants are crowded into the oddly shaped rectangular windowsill. On my desk sits a small dancing elephant-headed Ganesh statue; he is the god of intellect and wisdom as well as protector against obstacles. He is my writing partner and guardian. Turn around and scan my wall of bookshelves. You'll read the following titles imprinted on the spines of the books: *The Mommy Wars, Opting Out? Why Women Really Quit Careers and Head Home, The Mommy Myth, Perfect Madness: Motherhood in the Age of Anxiety.* Move a shelf or two over to the right and you'll see *The Work and Family Handbook, The Handbook of Work and Family Integration*, and *Multi-Disciplinary Perspectives on Work and Family Life.* And, now once more, inch to your left, you'll find *Constructing Fatherhood* and *The Package Deal: Marriage, Work and Fatherhood in Men's Lives.* One or two other subjects are addressed in the volumes nestled into this hulking drab gray metal structure, including much on feminist and discourse theories. Still, there is no need to state the obvious. While I'm not destined to be a research fellow celebrated for my prolific curriculum vitae, I have managed a fairly accomplished career writing about communication at the intersections of our work and family lives.

I envision some former dissertation committee member remarking over a glass of wine at a conference: "Nice job developing a tightly focused re-search agenda" or "Good. Good. Your career focuses on an identifiable line of research." This is what we're supposed to do as scholars, right? I don't remember the means of its indoctrination. Still I absorbed this career logic at an early point in my doctoral education, for right or wrong. A line of research. A continuation. A professional self comes to be identified with the public pro-duction of a line of thought. I do, however, vividly recall the moment a fellow communication professor said to me, "Well, you've been successful because you don't have kids." [Pause: I'll give you a minute to process that one.] Yes, someone said this to me years ago waiting in an airport for a flight back from a conference. Child rearing, I inferred from her ensuing commentary, had derailed her career. What naturally must have been *my choice* not to have chil-dren, along with my preponderance of extra time to write, clearly led to my modicum of success. Now that we're on the subject: Someone else also once asked me, with a confused tone of voice, "Do you even *like* kids?" [Emphasis in original.] I was flummoxed; I cannot recall a single word from my meek response. But true to my family socialization, I held my emotions inside. This particular colleague had recently taken a leave to have her third child. At the time this particular question was posed to me, I was in my early thirties and recently prescribed Clomid. For the uninitiated, Clomid stimulates the re-lease of hormones needed to cause ovulation, that is, it's medication for those having difficulty conceiving.

Nevertheless, before my memories wander too far afield, let's rewind a few years so that you can see how my personal and professional storylines col-lided and subsequently ensnared. Or, rather, let's take a step backward so that you can understand why I am currently striving to disentangle and recompose these storylines. Let me be clear up front. This is not a story of a "lesser life," even if moments of loss punctuate my narrative as they also inevitably mark your story, even if in different ways. With gratitude to Mary Catherine Bateson (2001), this rendering is simply the continuation of composing a life, a moment in its creation. It is my story, even though, for me, infertility treatments were experienced side by side with Joe, my fearless and loving life partner of now eighteen years. I cannot speak for him; he has his own story.

My first idea for a research project as a graduate student at the University of Kansas in the late 1990s was to explore how married, heterosexual women negotiated returning (or not) to paid work after having children. One of my close friends from my undergraduate days was pregnant at the time with her first child; she recently had quit her job and announced to me, "I don't see myself ever going back to work." Okay. The option of not making a living, married or single, had never been presented to me so I was a bit puzzled but supportive. I knew I'd have children. It was part of the vision of my life. While I looked forward to motherhood, I was focused at the time on taking classes, performing my role as teaching assistant, and running a residence hall to avoid some post-Ph.D. debt. I was in my late twenties, newly married and trying to establish an ounce of financial and professional security.

This idea for an early career research project—the initial and furtive consorting between my (anticipated) family life and my (nascent) line of research—was full of promise. I would interview women resembling my college friend. I would ask about how they negotiated the meaning of their choices regarding childbearing and paid work. Critiquing the master narrative of heterosexual, pronatal femininity implicated in this project was not a part of my consciousness at that time. Eager to share this idea, I met with my adviser over coffee at our local Wheatfield's bakery. Kathy thought my outline for the project was intriguing and novel in the field of Communication Studies pre-Y2K. We fleshed out the ideas as we sipped our lattes. I spent that summer conducting interviews there in Lawrence, Kansas.

> "Do you have children?" often these women would ask at some point during the interview.
> "No, not yet. [I'd smile.] I'm just trying to first finish school."
> "Oh, yes, of course! Good idea," they'd say, and nod approvingly.

Insights from this pilot study never appeared in any journal, but its conceptual seeds generated a fifteen-year scholarly agenda and scholar's identity. This agenda also led to unanticipated complications, pain, and loss as well as, today, the inklings of new beginnings.

★ ★ ★

A few years later, my professional and personal storylines continue to coexist in relative congruence. I'm an assistant professor at Ohio University and Joe is a corporate recruiter for Abercrombie & Fitch. We live in Columbus, Ohio. Joe drives thirty minutes north of the city. I drive an hour and forty-five minutes south to Athens, Ohio. Sometimes I sleep on friends' couches or stay at a local hotel if I get tired of the drive. Eventually, I rent an apartment and live in Athens, Ohio, three days a week. Jobs are fulfilling. We are a daughter and a son, a sister and a brother, Aunt Caryn and "crazy" Uncle Joe. Yes, the commute gets exhausting. I manage. "An hour and forty-five minute commute? It's really good you don't have children," said one seemingly relieved non-traditional student after class. Looking back, I now realize that I felt entitled to have children. It was my right somehow, if not an obligation. If I felt I had a choice it was to decide *not* to become pregnant before I was supposedly ready to have children. We assumed it would *naturally* happen.

Nose to the grindstone: Finally, hard work comes to fruition and I publish articles with titles including "The Everyday Accomplishment of Work and Family" (Medved, 2004); "Family CEOs: An Analysis of Corporate Mothering Discourse" (Medved & Kirby, 2005); "Work and Family Socializing Communication: Messages, Gender & Ideological Implications" (Medved et al., 2006). I continue to drink in readings on mothering and feminism as I develop a deeper interest in the negotiation of caregiving and paid labor. One author leads to another and opens up interconnected areas of scholarship. We are leery of starting a family given the distance between home and work. One fix for this *problem* was to move to a different city, one that would eliminate the commute. I get interviews at a few universities in cities where both of us can make careers, but no offers. We press on with the everyday; we are young, we do not panic but stop the Pill regardless of our geographic challenges.

Around the same time, I decide to teach in Bangkok for a semester. That fall Joe takes time off to visit and maybe we conceive in Bangkok? We laugh and I enjoy the four-month adventure. Upon returning, a friend gives me a *New Yorker* cartoon. A couple is visiting the fertility specialist. Caption: "You know that you have to be in the same city to get pregnant." The following summer I was still not pregnant. Recall the Clomid? This medication eventually was prescribed for me to help with conception. My body didn't like it; the doctor neglected to tell me that in addition to stimulating the ovaries, it jacks up your entire body. Oversight. I am a naturally high-energy person, to say the least. But Clomid ramped up my whole system and made me feel agitated, irritable, and restless. When I mentioned these symptoms to my doctor, she replied indifferent: "Yes, Clomid can do that." Thank you for warning me.

I also recall a forty-something single graduate student who did not have children coming into my office at this time. She closed the door. A female faculty member haughtily said to her, "You'll never know love if you don't have children." She was dumbfounded. Frustrated, I apologetically remarked that people just don't think. Motherhood and marriage are taken-for-granted (and assumed *available* and desirable) choices for all women. I was sure that in my past I had unwittingly said something insensitive or indifferent to a colleague. We are all human. Yet some individuals seem unusually unaware, or simply uninterested in the ways their words can affect others' feelings. I wish I had known at that time to also say that we live in a culture fixated on women's (not men's) alleged decisions about childbearing. People don't think before they talk partly because becoming a parent isn't always a conscious choice, unless, of course, you experience difficulty. These choices are often less autonomous and more culturally determined than portrayed in the media and in personal interactions (Myers, 2001). However, I wasn't quite "there" yet to convey this level of reflexivity.

Returning to my own story: I celebrate birthdays thirty-four, thirty-five, and thirty-six with family and friends. I'd be lying to you (and myself) if I said my infertility at this time wasn't troubling, wasn't producing moments of pain. Yet I also consciously wouldn't let it be the only issue defining my life. I simply wouldn't let it be. I was feeling more competent as a scholar and teacher. I had a wonderful partner in my life, family, and friends all around me. I had a family, despite the nagging inquiry, "Do you have a family?" as if only children constituted its existence. Study after study I read included future directions for research extolling the need to redefine or to broaden the definition of "family." And some research moved in this direction by investigating (as examples) the work–life challenges for gay fathers (Galvin & Patrick, 2009) or single employees (Casper, Weltman, & Kwesiga, 2007). Yet in everyday practice, the question "Do you have a family?" primarily implies "Do you have children?" In the context of work–family (or work–*life*) research, "family" is code for children. Yes. Eldercare does get some intellectual play. However, eldercare becomes urgent in the context of the "sandwich generation," that is, working full-time while caring for both children and elderly parents (Zal, 2001).

Finally exhausted from commuting between Columbus and Athens as well as itching for something new, we packed up and moved to Manhattan. Joe moved with his job at Abercrombie & Fitch. I got a job offer at Baruch College with the City University of New York. Urban life was calling. It was time for us to live and work in the same city; perhaps, I thought, this move would be a good choice for finally starting a family. After all, there weren't any medically diagnosed reasons for my infertility. It simply hadn't happened yet. I was (and remain) grateful to teach with and learn from an amazingly international student population. I also knew that many scholars and institutes that focused on work–life studies were located in New York City and at many other East Coast universities.

We begin to visit the NYU fertility clinic. IUI. IVF. IVF. I woke up for 7 a.m. blood monitoring three times a week during each IVF cycle during the course of three years. Still no children at thirty-seven, thirty-eight, thirty-nine. I taught late mornings; continued my research. I received a Sloan Foundation grant to study couples in which wives are primary breadwinners and husbands stay-at-home fathers. During the coming years and with the help of two research assistants, we conducted eighty-eight interviews with forty-four couples discussing their work and family choices. This new research project provided enriching yet increasingly conflicted and at times painful experiences. My research and my visits to the fertility clinic emotionally intertwined. During most interviews, again, the inescapable question was posed to me:

> "So, do you have children?"
> "No … [pause] not yet," I replied with varying levels of uncertainty in my voice.

The question now felt different from the way it did in graduate school. I didn't know whether I would ever have children. The statistics were not good, despite the empathetic smiles from the nurses at the clinic. I recall a new colleague asking me, "So, do you have children?" When I responded with "Not yet," she smirked oddly and seemed a bit put off by my response. Should I explain to her that I went into the NYU fertility clinic that very morning for blood monitoring? I still had the piece of gauze on my arm from the needle and the bruises from the countless needles that came before.

I successfully hid a few emotionally challenging moments during research interviews for this new project. Being authentic while conducting interviews is important to my feminist approach to research. Even so, my fertility struggles did not seem an appropriate topic of conversation. Nevertheless, when once again a participant in Colorado asked me, "Do you have kids?" I responded with something like, "That hasn't worked out for us." I cannot explain why that response came out of my mouth on that particular day. Unintentionally, the physical and emotional difficulties of infertility leaked out into the professional. She compassionately shifted gears and told me about a book on natural fertility that her friend found helpful. On that day, I appreciated the kindness in her face and her advice. I blinked away the tears welling up in my eyes and regrouped by simply asking the next question on my list. Through moments like this one, my life and IVF treatments, as well as my line of research, continued to press forward and coexist, yet in a more troubled and complicated fashion.

Another participant, for instance, who had her first child at age forty, joyfully remarked, "It was amazingly easy for me to get pregnant at forty. We couldn't believe it!" I remember the joy on her face. I do not recall infertility issues entering into my conversations with these couples; if they had faced challenges conceiving, such experiences did not creep into their narratives. And I certainly didn't ask. Frequently, these couples shared that the most important thing they can ever do in their lives is to rear their children; kids put *everything* into perspective. Am I out of perspective? One mother cried during a phone interview, so happy her husband convinced her to have children when she was hesitant to do so. One stay-at-home father, I recall, struggled to articulate his thoughts during the interview. He stopped, and by way of rumination, asked, "Do you have children?" I responded with some sort of vague, slightly evasive, "Ah … no, no we don't." He continued, "Well [pause] people who have kids would understand this but...." After fifteen years of studying work and family issues, I am now positioned as not being able to understand something in the context of my own work because I am not a parent. Outsider. The personal disables the professional.

There also were things he couldn't understand, things I certainly didn't share. I'd recently had what is called a "chemical pregnancy." For the infertility novice, your body starts to produce low levels of pregnancy hormones but you can't sustain the pregnancy. At the same time, my hormone levels didn't go down and my doctor was worried. The so-called treatment for this condition is a lovely shot of chemicals in the ass, something similar to chemotherapy that kills off the remaining cells. I remember leaving the clinic afterward feeling physically and emotionally wiped out. We were flying home to Michigan that day for my fortieth birthday. It was wonderful to be with family and friends, although physically I wasn't my best. My body was sore and overweight from the years of IVF hormone injections. The shot was making me feel queasy. While at home, we went to a local summer festival. My niece and I went on a carnival ride. I threw up afterward. Yep. Right there on the grass. Apparently, the chemotherapy shot was working.

Back at work, I gradually started feeling a bit lost in my research. I didn't know why I felt this way. It crept in slowly, almost imperceptibly; I was not as motivated as I had been to read and reread transcripts. I was not as inspired to hear about other people's joys and challenges with balancing diapers and paychecks. At times, there was an avoidance of research. I had all of these data yet I was frustrated (I still am) with my lack of productive writing as a result of this project. I was hitting an intellectual wall as my emotional and productive energies drained. I was losing my voice. Yes. Bodies need voices, but voices are dependent on bodies and mine doesn't work in the reproductive sense. No medical explanation was ever offered. Nothing could be "fixed." Unexplained infertility. There enters (and, quite honestly, still remains at times) an oblique sense of discomfort writing and thinking about a life that is not my own.

At the same time, I continued to teach seminars at the graduate and undergraduate levels on work–life communication. And every semester a student asks, "You have kids, right?" One time a few years ago an especially uninhibited student further probed. "So why don't you have kids?" Visualize the scene. Small windowless classroom with a large whiteboard and twenty-five or so students tightly packed into 1970s-ish metal chairs. I'm in the middle of infertility treatments and all of these students are waiting for my response; it's quiet. It pains me in the pit of my stomach, but I briskly respond with a wink and an attempted smile, "Too personal. Let's move on." We continued our infertility treatments. IVF. IVF. Infertility? Remaining option? Donor egg.

Next, we sift through dossiers of women willing to donate their eggs (for money) to help women like me have a child with my husband's sperm. And, while a critical analysis of the commodification of reproduction is not the focus of this chapter, it's a surreal experience to say the least. But it was the next step. Well, let me clarify: It's the next medically assisted step for fortunate couples or individuals with the economic means to consider this option. We are shocked at the exorbitant price tag. Like so many women in my situation, not trying every available medically assisted option feels unthinkable, almost immoral. We attend the required counseling session for the NYU donor egg program. We both felt bizarrely conflicted about the counselor's encouragement to choose a donor that physically resembled me: blondish, curly hair, blue eyes. All of this experience felt very Orwellian, but it constituted one last hope. It was coercive hope, perhaps? Healthy embryos. Transfer. No pregnancy.

To top it off, it's a painful requirement that I go into the clinic for one more blood test just to confirm that I'm *not* pregnant after the donor egg transfer. I quietly plead with the nurse, "Do you really need me to come in one more time?" Yes. After we verify the cruel news in person at the clinic, one nurse says that she can put us on the donor egg waiting list again. Could we really go through this procedure multiple times? Choose donors until a miracle happens, if it does? And for how long? Or do we choose childlessness without ever having chosen infertility?

Nancy, the more empathetic nurse at the clinic, gently asks, "So what's your next step?" I respond slowly, "I think this is it." While I could not exercise agency in relation to my ability to have a biological child, I can take control of when to stop this medically assisted pursuit. I remember uneasily a friend's random remark. She said, "People mortgage their houses to have children." That's the standard? That's proof you've tried hard enough with today's technology? In my heart, I know it's time to stop. Must we reach emotional, relational, and financial bankruptcy to justify *not* trying again? With the support of Joe and a few close friends and the unspoken acceptance of my family, we do not return to the NYU fertility clinic. Joe too expresses his emotional exhaustion. He says that he can't keep "living like this" in a constant state of emotional turmoil. We focus on being grateful for all we have. We have each other. Joe and I attend a few adoption seminars; we decide not to follow this path. I wasn't emotionally able to begin another roller coaster. Adoption for us did not seem like the "cure" or panacea for infertility. And, while this chapter could end along with my infertility treatments, the storyline(s) continue. Life goes on. That's the obvious but ultimately curious point of interest here. After we choose not to continue to pursue motherhood, how do we compose a different way of envisioning the future in a parenthood-soaked world?

And I'm simultaneously at a loss on the professional side. Return to the books in my office, stacks of syllabi, and my vitae; all remain filled with research, theories, and publications about work–family balance. While the treatments are over, their intellectual vestiges remain. After going through years of infertility procedures, can I really continue to study how language and social interaction shape work and family conflict, choices, and identities? It's what I know professionally; it's what I'm known for professionally. Yet I didn't anticipate studying work and family communication and not being able to have a family (read: children). Am I somehow displaced out of my own research agenda? I feel discontent, moments of pain, and confusion as I read transcripts and theorize about discourses of parenting and work. Will I simply "get through" this discomfort? Or does my research focus need to change for intellectual and personal survival? Give me something here, I sigh, as I again gaze at my bookshelves. You've heard the backward-looking story and now I need to write forward.

* * *

As feminist scholars, we are supposed to learn from our lives. I see others studying, writing, and speaking their experiences. I am grateful for their offerings. Feminist research, perhaps ideologically, compels a focus on the personal, to take it into account. To continue my research agenda, is my only option to study "the social construction of infertility"? Must I excavate my personal experience for professional ends? Is it worth it? My (non) parental status does not define me, yet it is a part of me just like my professional identity as a work–family scholar. What happens to the continuation? The line of research? Disruption. I'm left searching for a way to reposition myself within my work. Or am I left searching for a way to reposition my work within my own consciousness? And does infertility raise consciousness? Undoubtedly.

Here is one example of my shifting consciousness. I'm beginning to realize that pronatalism is deeply entrenched in work–life studies. Pronatalism. It's not a commonly used word, but one that refers to "any attitude or policy that is 'pro-birth,' that encourages reproduction, that exalts the role of parenthood" (Peck & Senderowitz, 1974, p. 1). That is, being a parent is culturally prized above all other adult roles, particularly for women in the United States. Parenting (like marriage) is the focus of most important adult rituals and supposedly marks maturity. Parenting is also the primary focus of so much feminist work–family research, the goal of which is to create social change so that parents can fully participate in both their reproductive and productive lives. It is a goal I wholeheartedly support. Yet it's omnipresence as a theoretical, epistemological, and pragmatic filter marginalizes the life experiences of a group of women, of scholars, of women (and men) who are scholars and not parents by chance and by choice. I begin to wonder, *To what extent have my own identity struggles and research embodied pronatalism? And, if so, can the experience of infertility serve as a form of consciousness-raising?* Pronatalism allowed me to take motherhood for granted in my own life. I felt entitled to motherhood; thus, a loss was experienced with its denial. And I'm only beginning to realize how my worldview is changing as a result of my experiences with unsuccessful infertility treatments. Did I also view my research agenda through a pronatalist perspective? The personal is the professional. The personal is the political. A second realization starts to take form.

Last summer, I'm at the Work and Family Research Network (WFRN) conference at the Millennium Hilton in midtown Manhattan. There are probably thirty people in the room—pens poised, name badges strung around necks, conference bags on laps. The first presenter begins her talk on Canadian at-home fathers with pictures of her husband and son on a bike. Boom. Personal credibility and professional credibility. The next presenter begins. Slide one: first child. Slide two: second child. Slide three: third child. Hint: Mormon. The audience is laughing and gasping until we reach nine kids and he reveals a photo that looks like a class reunion. Yo. Street cred, 'nough said. While I admit I felt uneasy watching the family slide shows, I consciously tell myself not to let feelings of personal loss diminish my sense of professional competence. Finally, it is my turn. I begin. No pictures of children or personal parenting anecdotes frame my presentation. For once, my self-help strategy worked. I kicked some intellectual ass. I notice at that moment, as an outsider-within, how the overlap between the personal and professional is used to construct scholarly credibility in work–life studies.

Let me explain. I've come to wonder whether there is something oblig-atory, perhaps unconsciously so, about scholars dropping in their personal stories to authenticate their work–family research. For example, in a recent op-ed in the *Daily Beast*, Ellen Galinsky, cofounder of the Families and Work Institute and ever-present media expert, noted that she was taking care of her grandchild while writing this particular op-ed. Her decades-long astonishing career should speak for itself. Yet her grandchild says something different, something more. So, here I am. How do I compose a new professional story in a voice of empowerment, joy, and conviction? To fashion this promising counternarrative, I take stock of the roles available to me at the nexus of varying cultural scripts (Lindemann-Nelson, 2001). "Mother" is not a role in which I am cast, but other supporting roles remain viable, perhaps? Let's review the options:

First, I'm not the intellectual rock star who ostensibly "gave it all up" for her career. Nor do I see my work identity as my only identity. The all-consuming "career woman" role (myth?) doesn't fit. I don't want my life only to be my work, but I respect those who do embrace this identity. Don't misunderstand. I love my students and the hunt of intellectual pursuits. And my work as a scholar and teacher of work and family communication does provide happiness, even if it is unsettling at times. But I wasn't so busy with work that I unintentionally bumped up against the biological clock.

Second, I'm not the childless-by-choice woman who knew she didn't want to have children (Myers, 2001). I did not plan my life in this manner, even as I unequivocally respect those who make this choice. I am childless by chance and *also by choice* in that I exercised agency not to continue to pursue medically assisted motherhood at all costs or through adoption. And I now also see how our reproductive-centered culture and infertility mega-business-es prey on women, and couples, who may feel pressure or desire to pursue every available option until their mid-forties to have a biological child. I also get why people relentlessly pursue this option. I see high school classmates from the graduating class of 1987 having children and posting pictures on social media. I read articles in magazines debunking age-related infertility myths and saying "it's okay" to wait to have children later in life as well as articles promoting early childbearing. Yet none of these articles acknowledges that, for some people, successful reproduction isn't just a matter of timing; it's simply not a biological possibility.

Third, I also am not the typecast female crushed, demoralized by infertility. I am not living a "lesser life" as written by Sylvia Ann Hewlett (1986). I am writing the final edits of this chapter on sabbatical in Paris, France. I have rented an apartment here for four months. I look forward to visits from family and friends; I've renewed my love of studying the French language and presented some research in French at the University of Nantes. I do not allow *not having* children to define my identity or my path, yet it is a part of my story. And it cannot help but be an important chapter of my life story. I try to be conscious of my own reactions as former students and colleagues frequently announce impending births. I deal with inappropriate remarks from others such as reminders that my pursuits are not of equal value to parenting obligations. A colleague who is also a parent saw me studying French before I left on sabbatical and sarcastically remarked, "Who has time for that?" And, strangers or new acquaintances still regularly ask, "Do you have children?" And I continue to try out ways to respond:

> "No, not yet." [Nope. This no longer works as an authentic retort.]

> "No, I/we couldn't have kids." [This response at least clues you in to the perils of asking this question. Yet it also seems to demand further explanation on my part.]

> "No, I don't have children but I'm the world's best aunt." [Wait. This feels contrived; an attempt to perform the obligatory female role of caregiving.]

> Or, if I'm feeling a little ill spirited, I could pipe back with, "Yes, I have a daughter named Winnie. Would you like to see her picture?" [FYI: Winnie is a yellow Labrador.]

> Can a simple "No, I don't" suffice? [Hmmm... . Yet I don't want you to think, like my former colleague, that "I don't *like* children." ...]

> "No, I don't."

I am an aunt, daughter, sister, wife, friend, scholar, teacher, and mentor. I simply am a human being who deeply cares about others; I am a woman who has experienced joy and loss. I embrace all of these roles, yet I'm conscious that these are the only ones culturally available to me. Admittedly, my options are made possible by my privileged white, middle-class professional life. I can spend a semester in France, writing, regrouping, and traveling. I recognize this class privilege. I can ruminate on infertility rather than worrying about a roof over my head, steady employment, surviving war or rape, or finding clean drinking water and food. Privilege does not make my pain less real, but it must put it in perspective.

In closing, these moments of consciousness made possible through my infertility bring me full circle in this chapter. I return to my road trip through the Midwest last summer with my friend Devika. We were on our annual pilgrimage to a qualitative research conference at the University of Illinois. Devika, well versed in the scholarship of performance and narrative, poignantly asked me why I wanted to publish this story. She said, only half joking, "Look Medved, I teach this stuff. It's important to think about this." I honestly told her I didn't know why I wanted to publish it. I protested, driving through Indiana, that we don't always know our motivations before we act. I needed to trust my desire to share and allow the story of my story a life of its own. As I finish final edits on this chapter, I get her question. Committing this story to publication was *not* a means of ensuring that I would arrive at some simple resolution or newfangled scholarly agenda and identity. That hasn't happened. Publication won't make that happen.

Throughout the writing process, however, I have found a modicum of inner strength along with renewed gratitude and appreciation. I also have become even more aware of the hegemony of pronatalism in work–life research as well as in its scholarly performance. I am now also more mindful of the influence of pronatalism on my own experiences of loss. And the urgency to call out this hegemony, in my own life and for the benefit of others, has become my rationale for publicly talking about these issues. If we cannot discuss these issues, we are trapped—all of us—in our current ways of understanding ourselves, our research endeavors, and our public dialogues about contemporary work and life. It's not a new issue, but it's now my issue. As I move forward, I resolve for myself, perhaps now a better self, to continue my intellectual pursuits as a work and life communication scholar as well as allow myself to pursue new questions. Allow and embrace discontinuity. I also resolve to challenge, when I feel called to do so, pronatalist practices and discourses in work and life research and our daily language and social interactions.

Note

1. This chapter is dedicated to the memory of my mother, Mary Catherine Euting, who passed away before she got the opportunity to read my story. She provided me the love and strength to get me through all of life's challenges and joys.

9. *Hidden in Plain Sight: Mystoriography, Melancholic Mourning, and the Poetics of [My Pregnancy] Loss*

REBECCA KENNERLY

> The object that is "invested" with vision will be an object in which she is deeply invested. (Schneider, 1997, p. 184)

In this chapter, in the fashion of my previous work (Kennerly, 2002, 2008, 2009), I use the mystory, a method of research and writing that Denzin situated in/as "a genre within ethnography" (1997, p. 91) that presents partial explanations of cultural phenomenon which includes and interrogates the standpoint of the researcher in/as a member of the culture under investigation. Borrowing from Ulmer's (1989) "mystory" experiment (p. 209), which shows us "how to articulate the private, public, and learned spheres of culture" (p. 118), and Bowman and Bowman's "Performing the Mystory," which compares the neologism *mystory* with a similar neologism, *herstory*, which brings to light "the collective story of women suppressed in patriarchal history" (2002, p. 164), I take up the challenge to put into conversation a sampling of my field research, writing, and performance with and about roadside shrines to take a closer look at my personal investment in the search for the meaning of these shrines.

The patterning of this conversation is likened to Benjamin's "constellation of ideas" (in Schleifer, 2009, pp. 314–315), "one that avoids the seamless and finalized representation of death and memory and is, following Sontag (2003) an appropriate and ethical response to the textual and visual images representing, among other things, the suffering of singular and collective others" (Kennerly, 2009, p. 6). Now, here, I grant myself the same grace (and penetrating vision) that I have with others' suffering.

The primary question that calls me to take this journey in this chapter is *where*, where in space, place, memory, and story can I locate my child, and where have I already marked the loss of my child? On this journey, I retrace the research and writing I have previously conducted to illuminate how memory and meaning-making often function as disjointed images and sounds, what Denzin calls "epiphanies" (1997, p. 221) and Ulmer calls "eureka anecdotes" (1994, p. 7): moments of insight which serve to disturb the often taken-for-granted systems related to women's health and well-being that silence my and perhaps others' stories of pregnancy loss.

This time around the bend, I introduce my increasingly difficult struggle to keep the story of my pregnancy and the death of my baby under wraps. I attend to the unbidden images that come of late, find my swollen, no longer silent tongue, and temporarily configure here a mosaic of memory, shimmering with reflective bits of broken mirror and shards of glass, held together with mud and blades of grass. I revisit my own cultural performance with and about roadside shrines, I interrupt my journey with bits of discovery, of vision: narrative chunks about how I became pregnant, about the night I lost my baby, and how it is I find myself standing on the side of the road, having written myself *elsewhere*. Finally I pose a series of questions that this journey begs me to ask regarding the specific set of circumstances surrounding my pregnancy and the loss of my child in the context of women's health and well-being, provide provisional responses to a few of those questions, and conclude with my argument that there are many paths, processes, time frames, and patterns through the maze of grief and mourning, especially for non-Christian women whose pregnancy and loss are experienced within the context of serial traumatic loss and lack of appropriate health care.

Since You Asked

This is a story about my struggle to remember that I was a mother and that my baby died, and my struggle to come to terms with this loss by immersing myself in the study of others' mourning practices, although images of my pregnancy loss have eked out onto the page before I knew what was happening. Indeed, in 1999 I wrote about and later published my insistent search for Matthew's Cross, a roadside shrine marking the site where a little boy's body was found days after he went missing ("Matthew Populis' Mother Arrested," 1995). I conclude the section about my failed search for Matthew thus: "Roadside shrines and the artifacts that adorn them cleave open a gap, exposing the raw, excessive, messy body, pulsing with life, not yet dead, not yet to blame, not yet made heroic."

> Like a momma dog whose teats are full,
> frantically searching for pups who have been taken away too early.
> Nothing she can do will locate her young,
> But she searches until she is exhausted just the same.
> If she is lucky, during her search
> she will happen upon a hungry batch of pups to feed,
> temporary surrogates for temporarily relief.
> But soon enough (too soon) she is left on her own
> to ease the swelling of her breasts,
> licking them like wounds to release the milk.
> The milk seeps out slowly, like tears. (Kennerly, 2002, p. 249)

Crying in the Cat Box

For years now, whenever a television show features a pregnant woman, I weep if the mother loses the baby, and sob if the baby comes. The sound of the baby's first cry breaks my heart. But I don't talk about it. Richard, my husband, knows I lost a baby when I was young, but not the whole story. I'm not sure I know the whole story.

I know as an adult I have always struggled in the company of pregnant women: Having no positive personal story to tell, I find myself mute. I make excuses for not attending baby showers. When asked whether I have children, I glaze over and just say, "No."

More recently I found myself in brave new territory looking for a baby shower card. Our daughter-in-law and my stepson were expecting their first child, and I was thrilled at the opportunity to be a grandmother! I found a cute fuzzy-bear card that I thought was just right, not too mushy, and definitely not religious (we're not a church-going bunch). Then I found myself browsing the "new parents" cards, and I bought one of those too: I just couldn't put it down. The card is blue and cream colored with silver lattice trim. On the cover are tiny blue booties, and a tiny blue teddy bear with a golden chest and an itty-bitty red heart. Inside the tiny teddy bear dances in the top right corner, floats in a small constellation of pale silver-blue sparkles above "Congratulations on your new baby boy. So Happy for You!" When I showed the card to Richard, he said it was too sentimental and I sobbed, clutched the card to my breast, ran to my office, and tucked the card into the folder labeled "Pregnancy Loss Chapter." I tucked it there to keep it safe, knowing it was too early to buy such a thing, so much can go wrong.

Earlier, in the mid-nineties, I found myself sobbing while I scooped cat shit and clumps of pee out of the litter box. My sweet golden kitty-girl Josie was very sick: Her kidneys were failing but she was hanging in there. She hung out with me in my study, curled up on my desk no matter how late into the night I worked, struggling to finish my master's degree. She allowed me to hold her in my arms like a baby while I fed her with an eyedropper, purring between swallows. So I was cleaning the cat box thinking of Josie, and then realized that I was never going to have children. I was in the early stages of menopause, so no "Becky's babies" I thought as I cried and scooped. And then I laughed, thinking that "Crying in the Cat Box" would one day make a good chapter title in my autobiography. Soon after I packed up, labeled those boxes "next chapter," and headed for graduate school at Louisiana State University.

On my way, driving the back roads from Michigan to Louisiana, I noticed crosses and wreathes on the side of the road in every state. By the time I had my first meeting with my graduate advisor, I knew I wanted to research and write about "those things" on the side of the road for my dissertation. And so I started driving, marking the shrines on my map, and learned how to write using Bowman and Bowman's (2002) *mystory* performance method that complements how I like to work (close to the ground), and how my mind works (images and insights that come in flashes, in fragments). Eventually these fragments came together so I could draw some partial conclusion about how it is that people express unspeakable loss by placing a shrine on the side of the road, often parents of children who died in some terrible auto incident,[1] sometimes members of the local community who mourn a murdered child.[2] These sites usually mark the place where a person died, the circumstances of that death made fairly clear: a dark, poorly marked road, a curve, a hill taken too fast, sometimes involving too much alcohol. But sometimes the circumstance of that death remains a mystery, and requires some detective work.

Dancing With the Dead

I have driven more than seven thousand miles, documented more than three hundred roadside shrines in twenty-six states, and published and performed much of what I have learned along the way.[3] In the field, on the page, and on the stage I employed Bowman and Bowman's (2002) mystory method to "track down and interrogate" (p. 164) institutional and popular cultural discourse and practice that propelled my interest in and interpretation of these sites of death "in order to generate new texts or stories out of bits and pieces of research material" (Kennerly, 2009, pp. 5–6). I thought I had learned all I could from the shrines and the complex cultural performance of mourning and meaning-making happening there. However, I didn't understand that the shrines were not done with me, that there were moments of discovery that exceed description, time, and space and yet are grounded in the material world, moments of *ecstasy* born of tension, stillness, and memory.

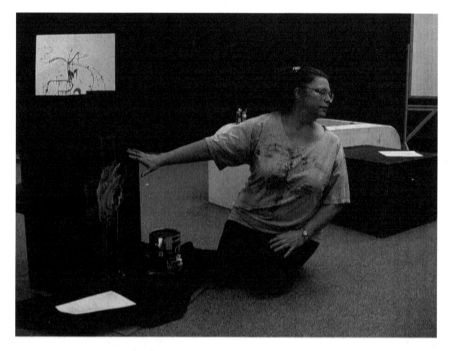

Second performance of "Getting Messy With Roadside Shrines," Black Box Theatre, Georgia Southern University, 2003.

Remembering Mother's Day, 1999

One Sunday, at the end of my first year of graduate school in Louisiana, I found myself *agitated*, so I drove out to an old cemetery I had passed on previous shrine-spotting excursions. As I have written previously (Kennerly, 2009), I had thought that the cemetery was abandoned because the yard was overgrown with weeds, and many of the markers were broken and/or sinking into the ground. However, that Sunday I found lots of people tending the graves, painting, planting, and cutting the grass. As I walked around the perimeter of the graveyard the local funeral director, Lonnie White, approached and asked whether I was looking for someone. "No," I said, "my people are elsewhere." Then he told me that the one-hundred-fifty-year-old Scotlandville Cemetery was a "Black" cemetery, which explained why there was no upkeep except by the family members of the dead. He showed me his mother's crypt, recently painted white and upon which rested a fresh bouquet of flowers. He remembered what I had forgotten; it was Mother's Day, a Cemetery Day.

Mr. White went on to explain that right down the street there is a "Private" cemetery, which also means the "White" cemetery. I went there but I didn't find whatever it was I was looking for, so returned to the Scotlandville Cemetery and sat and watched, and for reasons that escaped me at the time, I began to feel like "something other than a stranger, perhaps less of an out-sider" (Kennerly, 2009, p. 8) in the midst of this community. While revisiting my field notes and photographs of that day and subsequent days, I discovered that I was sitting and watching from the place where I felt most comfortable, a place that I returned to again and again: the stillborn section where the tiny graves have a single date.

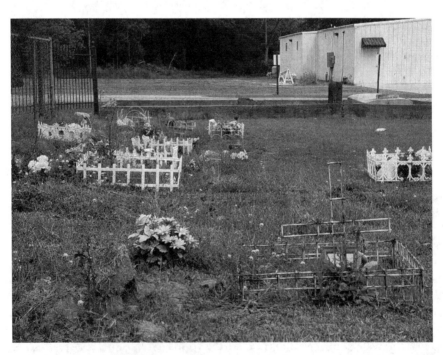

Stillborn Section, Scotlandville Cemetery, 1999.

At one time Cemetery Day practices were common in the South and oc-curred on major holidays and special occasions. These practices, thought to be dying out (Jeane, 1989; Milbauer, 1989), are very much alive in Scotlandville. In addition to local conditions that contribute to the continuance of long-standing traditions at the cemetery, I surmise that President Reagan's 1988 Proclamation 5890, declaring October as "National Observance of Pregnancy and Infant Loss Awareness Month," may have contributed to the relatively recent dates in the stillborn section of the old cemetery. Indeed, Proclamation 5890 (Reagan, 1988) calls "upon the people of the United States to observe this month with appropriate programs, ceremonies, and activities" (para. 5) to "meet the needs of bereaved parents" whose pregnancy resulted in "miscarriage, stillbirth, or the death of the newborn" (para. 1). Unfortunately, the proclamation goes on to link other forms of pregnancy loss to abortion and to offer encouragement and "friendship and temporal support" to women who give their children up for adoption (para. 3), creating an open invitation for Christian conservative groups to get involved in commemorative activities, further complicating my search for a place to mark the loss of my child. Several organizations such as the Footprints Ministry (2006) and the American Pregnancy Association (2013) offer processes and products, and links to web sites for more products, to help me through the stages of grief so I can move on with life (but never forget)—books, pins and poems featuring angels in heaven, candles, christen-ing gowns, baptism certificates, caskets, and passages from the Bible carved in stone—none of which reflects my experience or worldview.

A Gift

In the summer of 1979 I got pregnant. Here's how I remember it. I had been casually seeing a man, Abu,[4] for a couple of months, when he informed me that he needed to get to Washington, D.C., for a hearing at Veterans Affairs. I offered to drive him there. He was a Vietnam War veteran who sought, without success it turned out, along with many other African American vets suffering from post-traumatic stress disorder (PTSD),[5] to have his discharge status changed. I knew Abu had problems, but when we crossed the state line the real trouble started. He tried to control my every movement: how to look out the window, when and how to bathe, what to wear, what to eat. I almost left him several times: at the hotel, at the restaurant, on the side of the road when he jumped out of the car on the interstate. The trip went on like this for a week until I didn't have enough money to get home on my own. By the time we got to D.C. I was numb, unable to make decisions for fear of being berated. And I was ovulating. Abu refused to use any kind of birth control and I couldn't take the Pill on the sly because my health insurance wouldn't cover it, so it was the rhythm method or nothing. I tried to opt for nothing, but he dragged me from the tub and forced me to have sex in front of a full-length mirror, the look in my eyes dark and hollow. I prayed to get back to Michigan in one piece. As it turned out, I came back with more.

My plans to cut Abu loose failed when he guessed I was pregnant; in fact, he became more attached and more controlling. Although most of my friends thought I should end my pregnancy, and I believed in women's choice and celebrated the Supreme Court's 1973 *Roe v. Wade* decision, I could not abort the child in my womb. In previous years I had experienced a series of devastating losses of family members: first my stepsister and her daughter in a car crash, then my siblings, mother, and stepfather in a house fire. This child would be my family, and I would not refuse such a gift. I did, however, tell Abu that I did not want to make a life with him. He was very angry, and then he calmed down and asked me to drive him home. As we neared his neighborhood, he told me to turn down a side street and stop the car. He got out of the passenger seat, came around to the driver's side, and asked me to roll down the window. Then Abu reached through the window and grabbed for the car keys, trying to pull them out of the ignition. We fought physically; he ripped my blouse, bruised my face, and while I screamed he grabbed my tongue and tried to rip it out of my head. Then he suddenly stopped. And I drove away.

Abu began to call me at home at all hours, threatening me. I was terrified. I contacted my uncle who was a police detective in Los Angeles, thinking he and his family would take me in and protect me and my baby. But I had no idea how deep racist attitudes went in my family. I was told that I deserved whatever happened to me; I had asked for it by getting involved with a crazy black man. Stunned, I remember driving to and from work (or any damn place), caressing my belly and crying, "I'm sorry baby, I am so sorry." Then in January of 1980 I delivered a child at seven and a half months who was dead. When Abu showed up on my doorstep in early January of the next year I didn't have a clue how he found me (I had moved to a new town) or why he might be there. He looked so sad. It was the anniversary of the baby's death, and I had forgotten.

Momma Loves You

The only roadside shrine that made me cry is one that I have never written about. But there it is, in the archives of my memory, and in the photo albums of shrines located in Georgia. Here's how I remember it.

Sunday, March 3, 2003. The day was overcast. On U.S. 80 just around the bend past River Road I was surprised by a new shrine. It was so *pretty*. It was a large three-foot wreath on a four-foot wire stand in a scrubby field near a telephone pole. The wreath was heart shaped, bordered by a pink-and-white lace ruffle, filled with white fabric flowers, pale pink roses, and a large pink satin bow. A wide white satin ribbon with gold glittery letters was entwined into the folds of the bow. I rarely disturb the sites but this time I reached into the bow and unraveled the ribbon to read "Momma Loves You."

A sharp intake of breath, of shock, of pain, like a shard of something broken coming home, finding flesh, piercing the shield protecting my heart. Oh god, what happened here? Relying on color schemes that mark gendered identities, I thought the author of the shrine must be a mother who lost her little girl. I rewound the ribbon and tucked it back into the wreath and turned for home. And then I forgot all about it. Revisiting the shrine in my mind's eye, in memory, I cried: a sharp intake of breath, a shock of recognition, of pain. Here, in this writing, I pull the shard. I remember.

Pink or Blue

At five in the morning, January 5, 1980, standing in the hallway at the bottom of the stairs, I called up to my cousin, "Tom, it's time to go. Tom, wake up, my water broke. The baby's coming. Hurry." "But it's too early," he says, coming down the steps two and three at a time. "You've still got six weeks to go!" "I know," I said, holding up my now low-slung belly.

Earlier that evening I had fought with Abu. I had tried to stay calm in my dealings with him but that night I'd finally had enough. I had been at the kitchen sink washing dishes and looking out of the window when he came up behind me and started rubbing on me. I saw our reflection in the glass and that was it, no more. I wanted him out of my life but that wasn't going to happen so I shoved him away and started moving furniture around, yelling at him to "leave me alone," and sometime after midnight he finally left.

So at five in the morning I yelled up at Tom to come, and he did. Before I got in the car I went back to my room for the blue baby blanket, part of a layette my friend at work had given me before Christmas, saying it was too early for a baby shower but she wanted me to have a little something. Before we left I must have called the doctor to tell him the baby was coming. His office was far from home but close to where I worked.

My health insurance didn't cover any medical expenses related to pregnancy. I didn't know that the Pregnancy Discrimination Act, an amendment to the 1964 Civil Rights Act, had gone into effect on October 31,

1978, a law that prohibited employers from withholding medical benefits for "pregnancy, childbirth, and related medical conditions" (U.S. Equal Employment Opportunity Commission, 1978, para. 4). My friend Patsy and her husband were self-employed, and she had an "old country" doctor, Dr. Koerner, who had delivered her baby girl in his home/office, so that's who I turned to.

We drove through the dark and forty-five minutes of the mantra "Don't push, don't push, don't push," and "God, oh god hurry." The sun was coming up when we pulled into the driveway of Dr. Koerner's. Not waiting for Tom, I opened the door and peeled myself out of the car, and the tiny blanket tumbled off my lap and onto the dirty pavement. I managed to bend over and pick up that patch of blue and held it close as I waddled, with Tom's help, to the door. The doctor wasn't ready for us yet so I lay down, sprawling across several chairs. "Don't push, don't push." No, not yet.

Dark paneling, steel table, big jars lined up along the shelves in the back. "Okay, push now," and I did. And then, silence. "The baby is dead," he said, and he laid that little person on a shelf behind him.

Tom took me to Patsy's house to recover. I lay in her bed, awake. I rolled over on to my side and felt my now empty belly and thought, free, we're free and safe now. And then I slept. A few days later, my milk came in, like tears. My friends and family offered, "Perhaps it's for the best" and in some measure it was hard to disabuse them of that sentiment.

On my final visit to the doctor's office, I asked him if it was a boy or a girl. "I don't know," he said, "I didn't want to look." "Why did the baby die?" I asked. "Hypertension," he said. Four years later, Patsy called to tell me that Dr. Koerner had been murdered in his office. Probably kids looking for drugs; finding none, they killed him. A few months after this, a detective investigating the doctor's death called me and inquired about my time as Dr. Koerner's patient. He asked what happened with the baby. "Stillborn," I said. Then the detective told me that the perpetrators had ransacked the place, smashed everything. The police found a large glass jar smashed in the field, my baby's body nearby. My baby's broken body mixed up with the mud and grass and shards of glass.

Parable: Metaphor for Method

On January 30, 2000, I wrote the following for Michael Bowman's Performative Writing course, some of which was later published. We were asked to write a parable that resonated with our preferred research and writing method. The basis for this parable is autobiographically true: On this day, when I was ten years old, I almost died.

School was out! It was a bright, cool early summer day and we were playing "mud pie" at Tony and Ruthie's house. It had rained the day before, so their driveway was squishy with mud and the surrounding grass yielded easily to our tug. Taking my time, I carefully chose a colorful mix of grasses, and kneeling here and there in the driveway, tested small handfuls of mud. The mud from the center of the driveway was slippery, the mud from the edges was gritty and rough on my palms. No good. The best mud came from the deepest pothole at the far end of the driveway where the turn-around space was: It came up thick like oatmeal, mealy and sticky and workable. Jackpot! I mixed the grasses with the mud in a gallon-sized glass Mason jar I'd discovered poking around their garden shed. I wanted to see my concoction, to show it! Besides, the glass had a faint blue-green tint, like the shattered glass of the windshield of the abandoned car we were not allowed to play in: It was so pretty and maybe a little daring. And it altered the look of the stuff inside just so, which I liked very much. It was beautiful.

Wrapping both arms around the big jar, I took my masterpiece into the house and into the bathroom. I washed my hands and then the jar. Ready to show it!

> Carefully holding the thing out in front of me now, I hurried through the screen door, shouting, "Look, look, Looooo ..." and tripped on I don't know what. The glass catapulted out of my hands and went sailing over the cement porch, landed on the sidewalk, and splintered into a million pieces. I saw all of this and, as my own body kept its forward momentum, realized that I either had to somehow throw myself backward (to avoid landing square into the center of the exploded mess), or try to leap over it. I decided to leap. I threw all of my weight on to the one last step that I had and pushed off and up. I looked down as I flew over my shattered masterpiece. Shards of bright shining blue-green glass, swaths of mud and leaves of grass all mixed up, shimmering. I felt threat and thrill at once, in the strange and dangerous and accidental beauty below me, and in the freedom and power and unaccustomed daring I felt in my body as I flew, still not sure where or how I would land. (Kennerly, 2002, p. 230)

I landed hard with one foot, and painfully, and again trusting my forward momentum, curled and tumbled yet farther toward the periphery. I sat up, dazed. A large piece of mud-and-blood-covered glass sticking out from the sole of my left foot, my blood at once both spraying and pooling, mixing with the sparkling shards, the mud, the grass. This took my breath away.

Breathtakingly beautiful and wild. The doctor said, "Just one more 'nth' and you'd be dead, bled to death before you got here."

A sharp intake of breath and a flash of recognition, a Denzin-ian epiphany, an Ulmer-esque eureka moment. Oh god. Is this what I have been looking for all along, and where I have been going? I have been trying to write myself elsewhere, landing here, this time around, up, and over. In my mind's eye, I see myself standing by the side of the road, staring into a field, someplace in Michigan that no longer exists, looking for something mixing with the sparkling shards, the mud, the grass: my baby.

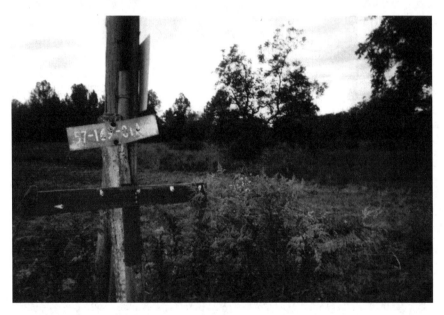

Community Post With Missing Flyer: "Have You Seen Me"? Alabama, U.S. 80, 2001.

New Questions, Partial Responses

Having worked through a process Pollock (2006) calls "going under" (p. 327), which "folds back on the researcher-subject, catching her in ... processes of transformation" (p. 328), I acknowledge that I have negotiated my belonging to a certain community of parents who have lost their children and, following Pollock, ask, "What are we going to do about it?" (p. 328). Now, from this distance in time and place, I ask: How is it that I did not seek help from social services once I knew that I was in an abusive and threatening situation with Abu? Could I have not gotten a restraining order taken out against him? Were there no shelters for battered women and their children? And I imagine that I am not alone in this situation: What are the current statistics of single pregnant women in abusive relationships? How many women in trouble were told that they deserve what they get, for whatever reason? What happens to those women and their children? How many women who have miscarried or had stillborn children have been told that it was for the best, given the circumstances? How many women have been denied lawful health coverage for their pregnancies? How many of these pregnancies end with the death of a child? And then there's this: Was it my fault? When did my child die, when I shoved the furniture around, or on the long trip to the doctor's office, or weeks before? Answers to these questions are for me to pursue in another place, another time. For now, I experience a sense of freedom and power and an unaccustomed daring to even ask these questions.

I can say that at the time I did not see myself as a woman who could, should, or needed to become enmeshed in a net of social services (even though this may have been helpful, or at least would have given me options). I saw myself as alone (although I clearly was not) and able to fight my own battles. I can also say that I, like Abu, have also most likely been suffering from PTSD. According to medical professional sources related to pregnancy loss and PTSD (Lapp, Agbokou, Peretti, & Ferreri, 2010; Olde, van der Hart, Kleber, & van Son, 2006) and popular cultural web sites created by women who experience pregnancy loss (Brooks, 2001; McGuinness, 2012), women who experience such loss suffer not only from a prolonged and unresolved grief, but also from symptoms similar to my own: loss of memory, unbidden images, uncontrollable crying, and more. I offer that my situation was complicated by my experience of serial loss and I shielded myself from grief in order to survive, and in the process carved out a liminal space for myself somewhere between the land of the living and the dead, and one that, without the anticipation of the birth of my grandson to trigger these images and the generative writing practices I have learned and demonstrated here to work through these images, would remain unacknowledged in the everyday world where I struggled to function. What is more, that grief would remain unspeakable, and the joy at the birth of a new family member would remain inaccessible.[6]

Conclusion

Haney, Leimer, and Lowery (1997) write that modern society has a disenfranchised relationship with death while other, older social orders had a healthy, more intimate relationship with death, one that puts grief "in the past where it belongs" so that one can "move on with the business of life" (Kennerly, 2002, pp. 249–250), and that resistance to this normative path of moving on constitutes a refusal of solace, what Freud called melancholia. Ramazani contends that modern elegists tend to enact "melancholic mourning" (1994, p. 4), a creative process characterized by mourning that is not so much resisted as it is *in process* and therefore *unresolved*. Melancholic mourning resists inherited practices that restrict grief to an increasingly shortened time frame and confine it increasingly to institutionalized places (Ramazani, 1994). Building and maintaining roadside shrines, I have argued, often function as a public performance of melancholic mourning, one that is always in process and unresolved (Kennerly, 2002). In this chapter I have retraced the maps I have previously drawn in my search for the meaning-making practices of others who loved and lost and refused to move on. On the way I have excavated significant chunks of my own memory and several key bits of information new to me concerning policies and practices that purport to support women's reproductive health and well-being but that in my case fell well short of doing so. In this chapter I have also interrupted the narrative flow of time and tale to illuminate how memory and meaning-making often function as disjointed images and sounds in order to resist the often taken-for-granted systems of mourning that ultimately place the experience of grief and loss in the past, often framed by Christian conservative discourse that marginalizes other worldviews and forms and processes of mourning. In the process, I have created a shrine-like mosaic of images that reflects and refracts and materializes my own performance of melancholic mourning. I appreciate the courage it takes to claim and name a lost child, and so in the company of this narrative community I take this opportunity to mark this phase, this temporary place of respite in my search for my child. Here I name and dedicate this work to:

DIARA-SHAE[7]

January 5, 1980

I could not have come so far without you

It is my hope that this use and discussion of mystoriography, and my struggle to recover the story of my pregnancy and the loss of my child in the context of specific policies and practices, will generate interest in the method as a means of helping people work through tragic events like pregnancy loss, or at least to provoke recognition and respect of this or similar methods of storytelling that do not resemble a linear narrative of grief and mourning, but rather allow for memory and meaning-making to materialize in fragments that may reveal the story of pregnancy loss bit by bit in/as a loose mosaic. Mystoriography is research and writing practice that can—as in my case—respect the depth of an individual's pain, her intellectual, psycho-emotional, and creative resources, and her ability make sense of terrible loss in her own time, on her own terms, supported by people (like you) who are willing to witness the story/fragments as they emerge, and in the process, celebrate life as it is lived: in the time of the telling.

Notes

1. See Everett (2002) and Kennerly (2002) for lengthy discussions about shrines built by parents who have lost their children in car incidents.
2. See "Matthew Populis' Mother Arrested" (1995), Polly Klaas Foundation (n.d.), and Seybert (2009) for feature stories about missing children whose bodies were found on the side of the road after having died elsewhere. Also see Winter (2012) for a short discussion and image of a recent shrine for Polly Klaas, who was abducted and murdered in 1993.
3. See Kennerly, 2002, 2008, and 2009, for published work. See Kennerly 1999, 2000, 2001, and 2003, for performance work.
4. Abu is not his real name; according to Kapoor (2013), Abu is an African name meaning "father." I have, however, used the real names of other people in this chapter.
5. According to J. Bowman (2013), veterans in the late 1960s were diagnosed with post-traumatic stress disorder (PTSD) "as part of their discharge, but were denied benefits by the Veterans Administration" (para. 2), but "when the government said PTSD was classified a mental illness many White veterans began getting benefits for treatment but because Blacks say they were denied so many times they stopped applying" (para. 9). More recently, since the Obama administration has been "pumping money into the system" (para. 3) more Black and Hispanic vets are receiving treatment.
6. I am happy to report that Theo, our beautiful grandson, was born to healthy and happy parents on July 22, 2013.
7. Both Diara and Shae mean "Gift": Diara is an African name, Shae is an English name, and both names are used for both boys and girls (SCBS Baby Club, 2010).

Section 3: Space, Time, and Pregnancy Loss

10. On the Identity Politics of Pregnancy: An Autoethnographic Journey Through/In Reproductive Time

Michaela D. E. Meyer

No light, no light in your bright blue eyes
I never knew daylight could be so violent.
A revelation in the light of day,
You can't choose what stays and what fades away.
"No Light, No Light" by Florence + the Machine (2011)

January 14, 2009. My second niece's birthday. I'd missed my period all through the holidays and I was constantly exhausted. It finally occurred to me that maybe, just maybe, I was pregnant. I woke up early, before Doug was out of bed, to take the test. *Just pee on the stick, figure out what to do from there.* Waiting, waiting. *This box says wait five minutes. What am I actually going to do if this test is positive?*

My marriage wasn't in a good place. Six months earlier, we'd had a serious talk—where is this going? We're two years in and it just doesn't seem to be working. Are we working on this? Or are we calling it quits? We agreed to work on it. We agreed to try. So, I was trying—trying to be more clear about what I wanted out of life. While we were "working" on our marriage, I hadn't thought about having children until I became an aunt. It changed the way I looked at parenthood, made me realize I wanted to be a parent someday. Someday. Once everything was settled. Prior to getting married, we'd had conversations about having children ... eventually. For me, it was always something to be tabled until I got my career settled, until we were financially stable, until we'd been married for an "appropriate" amount of time, until I could feel good about bringing a child into the world. Doug always agreed. Always supported the idea of someday.

I've been running such a long time—I've been hiding from the truth.
I've been battered, been broken, been buried, now I'm death proof, death proof.
                    "Release Me" by Jack's Mannequin (2011)

June 8, 2012. May had been a crazy month—the first-year anniversary of my second marriage, a trip to my sister's house, an amazing vacation to the ocean, a memorable birthday celebration, all while wrapping up the semester. I was exhausted. *Too much partying in May*, I told myself. Then that first Monday in June, when I was supposed to "go back to work" in my mind, I just couldn't do it. I sat on my couch and watched Netflix instead. I stumbled on to *The Rebound*, a film chronicling a relationship between an older woman and a younger man. I had a soft spot in my heart for the story, as James is almost eight years my junior. Halfway through the film, Catherine Zeta-Jones realized she was pregnant because her breasts were aching. As she walked through the story, I thought, *Huh, my boobs hurt. Yes, I'm tired too. Things smell weird to me too!*—and I made the connection, maybe, just maybe, I might be pregnant.

I can't be. I'm not going through this again. It's clearly a false alarm. I had my period at the end of April, so it wasn't unreasonable to think that I skipped the month, especially with longer cycles. *It's a fluke. I am tired because I've been too busy, having too much fun, for an entire month. Plus, my spring semester was seriously stressful—teaching four classes, two conferences, three writing deadlines, and editing a journal? That has to be the explanation. There is no way I could be pregnant.* I decided to wait until Friday. Friday the eighth. If I didn't have a period by then, I'd take a pregnancy test.

Things with James were in a wonderful place. We'd been married for a year, happily in the process of planning for our future. He desperately wanted to have kids—a family—and I was clear when we started our relationship that it might not happen. He was supportive. He said he'd be happy adopting or fostering. He said we could do it. And I thought, *Yes, I want this. I want to have a family, and I want to have a baby.* James said he didn't care how our story happened, just that it did—that we'd try, and if it didn't work, we'd figure it out. I said, after one year. Let's try after one year.

* * *

This chapter presents an autoethnographic narrative account of two pregnancies, existing in two different moments, at two different times—one that resulted in a miscarriage, and one that resulted in a successful birth. As an academic method, autoethnography seeks to connect lived experience to research by turning "the ethnographic gaze inward on the self (auto), while maintaining the outward gaze of ethnography, looking at the larger context wherein self experiences occur" (Denzin, 1997, p. 227). Autoethnography offers researchers the ability to "retrospectively and selectively write about epiphanies that stem from, or are made possible by, being part of a culture and/or by possessing a particular cultural identity" (Ellis, Adams, & Bochner, 2011, para. 8) and provides a way of chronicling and critiquing past experience to make better, hopeful experiences possible (Adams, 2009). It is particularly useful in analyzing intrapersonal issues such as grief and loss where social stigma may be involved (Arrington, 2000). It makes possible conceptualizing "remembrance" as "the act through which interpersonal meaning is rendered" (Meyer, 2007, p. 29).

This narrative journey makes two important contributions to communication scholarship. First, it situates and interrogates the idea of reproductive time through personal narrative, illustrating how pregnancy narratives are spatiotemporally located within identity and/or body politics. To do so, I unpack cultural conceptualizations of reproductive time tied to dominant medical and social discourses of the experience of pregnancy. Second, this chapter illustrates how identity politics matter as part of communication. Examining stories occurring at two times, under two sets of circumstances, troubles the possibility of understanding identity in a strictly linear fashion. Thus, time is a disjointed and fragmented part of identity construction, one that—while it can be written about in linear ways—cannot be understood in simple "historical" conceptualizations of "clock" time, when past, present, and future exist simultaneously.

* * *

Five minutes. *Nothing. It's supposed to make a plus sign, and it's still a negative sign. So* … no pregnancy. I put the stick down on the counter and took a deep breath, but I didn't believe it. Something felt different. I'd skipped periods before, been late, never had it felt different, like anything other than stress delaying the inevitable. I made a cup of tea. I watched some TV I'd recorded. I checked my email. An hour later when I had to pee again, I walked back into the bathroom. I glanced at the stick. Sometime in that hour, it turned positive.

Positive! Positive! I had to sit down to process everything I was feeling—this was what I'd been waiting for. A baby! I was excited about the possibilities. I could barely contain my joy. I was going to be a mother. That was a game-changer. Whatever problems Doug and I were having, we'd figure it out because now we were going to be a family. *A baby! I'm having a baby!*

* * *

Friday was the day. The eighth. And still no period. I woke up early, while James was still asleep. My hands were shaking as I took out the test. *Just do it, I thought, just pee on the damn stick and get it over with. Five minutes, right? Let's just see what happens.* So I peed on the stick. It didn't take five minutes. It immediately turned positive.

Positive. Holy crap. Positive. Well, that doesn't mean anything. I will not get my hopes up. I will not be excited about this. I can't. We'll have to wait to see what the doctor says. All kinds of things go wrong in the first trimester. This is not a baby yet, I reminded myself. *You can't get too attached this early.*

* * *

Pregnancy narratives in contemporary culture are dependent on a normative formation of time. We communicate about pregnancy primarily through increments of time—biological clocks, family planning (for the right "time"), gestational age, weeks of pregnancy, fetal development milestones—but rarely do we challenge the cultural norms associated with this demarcation. Halberstam (2005) explains that the "time of reproduction" is culturally regulated by "bourgeois rules of respectability and scheduling for married couples," and regardless of an individual's (or a couple's) desire (or ability) to adhere to this timeline, "many and possibly most people believe that the scheduling of repro-time is natural and desirable" (p. 5). Pregnancy stories often follow this culturally desired relationship to time, and as a result, miscarriage narratives are frequently silenced in favor of upholding this cultural orientation to conception and birth. Miscarriage is a traumatic experience precisely because it deviates from the normative conceptualization of pregnancy—a woman becomes pregnant, the baby grows and is ultimately born (relatively easily and quickly) healthy and happy. This cultural narrative of "happy endings" for pregnancy "exacerbates the experience of those whose pregnancies do not end happily" (Layne, 2003b, p. 1881).

* * *

I spent the rest of the morning in my own head. *How do I break this to Doug? I should let him sleep. I'll tell him later. After work. After dinner. Once we've had some time to relax from the day. I should make something great for dinner—what do I have on hand? I'll run by the store. Maybe lamb. Lamb is one of his favorites. And I'll call the doctor's office to make an official appointment. We'll need that. But, I should tell my sister, and my sister-in-law, and my mother. They will be so excited!*

Dinner that night was perfect and afterward, I broke the news—"I'm pregnant. And I'm very excited about it." Doug looked at me, "That's …

new. Okay. So, what are we doing?" I hesitated, then replied, "I already made an appointment with the doctor, so they'll check it out here in a few weeks." Pause. *Oh crap*, I thought, *This is too complicated. He's going to lose it.* He drank more wine. "Well, I guess we'll see what they say, but for now, I guess that's exciting." *He said exciting—he's excited about being in this!* I felt better than I ever had about our relationship.

* * *

"Okay, you have to wake up now," I said, rousing James out of sleep.

"What? Did you take the test? What did it say?" he said sleepily.

"It's positive," I said. He nearly jumped out of the bed.

"That's so great! That's so awesome! I can't wait to tell everyone! We're having a baby! I'm gonna be a daddy!"

I took a breath, "Calm down, seriously—you can't tell anyone." He looked at me quizzically. "You can't tell anyone because this is not a thing yet. This is just one phase—you get the positive test and you have to check it with the doctor. You can't tell anyone until we get an all clear from the doctor, do you understand me? I'm not going through this again. Look, I'll call the doctor and set up the appointment to check it out, but it's not a big deal yet. No reason to get excited."

He sighed, "You can be happy, you know. This might work." But I couldn't be happy. His excitement was too much pressure because he didn't know the opposite—the pain that was too much when your child was lost.

* * *

Miscarriage narratives belong to a "politics of imperceptibility," or a non-normative approach to time "which is unleashed by the force of events, by unexpected impacts, surprising encounters" (Grosz, 2005, p. 194). Discovering that a pregnancy is unlikely to be successful is difficult to reconcile, particularly within a pronatalist cultural context that prefers a medicalized/technologized view of the body in conjunction with emotional detachment. Foucault (1977) observes that medical discourses are often communicated as objective facts, and that these "facts" govern the body politics of human experience. Miscarriage is a particularly tricky discourse for a number of reasons. First, very few women are ever offered a solid medical explanation for miscarriage. Instead, miscarriage is seen as something that "just happens," an insignificant, routine event governed by the body (Moulder, 1999). The inability of the woman's body to produce the child is largely explained by timing, not specialized medical knowledge. Second, the institutionalization of medical discourse positions women's experiences of grief after miscarriage as "unhelpful," a series of emotions that would best be "managed through processes of rationalization" (McCreight, 2008, p. 7). Thus, many women seek meaning by framing their miscarriage experience(s) through "the right time in terms of lifestyle and life stage" (Simmons, Singh, Maconochie, Doyle, & Green, 2006, p. 1940). This logic suggests that once a woman adheres to normative notions of preparedness for motherhood, a child will appear. Thus, our cultural demarcation of grief over miscarriage as "unhelpful" serves to regulate women's experiences and emotions by offering "the right time" as the rational solution. Ultimately, women desiring children are left waiting for that "right time."

* * *

Doug came with me to the first doctor's appointment. I'd read up on what to expect. This was when we should hear a heartbeat. The doctor came in, set up the ultrasound, and ... nothing. Pictures, no sound. *This must be normal*, I thought. *This must be what usually happens.*

"It looks like you have a molar pregnancy," the doctor said, somewhat coldly. "You should consider terminating it immediately."

What? What is a molar pregnancy? I tried to ask, but was speechless. *Terminating? I don't want to do that. Maybe the timing is wrong.* I looked to Doug for support, but his face was stony and blank. Finding my voice, I said, "I read somewhere that babies develop in different stages. Could it just be a timing thing? I mean, maybe we are too early for this appointment in the baby's development?"

"The fetus is not viable," the doctor said.

"But what does that mean? Clearly there is a baby on the screen there?" I asked. "It's not a baby," the doctor said, "You will need to terminate this pregnancy. The sooner, the better." I looked back to Doug to gauge his reaction to the news. Between his face and the doctor's words, it became clear to me that I was the only one invested in this pregnancy. I was the only one in the room who believed my *fetus* was a *child*.

On the way home, I said, "I want to wait."

"You heard the doctor," Doug replied. "This is not going to work out. We should figure out the next steps."

I cannot accept this. This is not how it works. Women get pregnant and then they have babies. That's how it works. "I'm going to get a second opinion from a different doctor. That was terrible, and I'm never going back to that OB/GYN again." Doug sighed, and resigned himself to my decision.

Needing affirmation, I called a close friend and recounted the experience to her. I asked whether she thought I should get a second opinion before making a decision, and she recommended seeing her obstetrician. I scheduled an appointment for two weeks later. *The first doctor was wrong*, I told myself. *The baby just needed another couple of weeks to get situated. This appointment will be fine.* Doug chose not to come with me. Again, the same ultrasound.

"I know this is not what you were hoping for," the doctor said, "but the baby is not developing the way it should. At this point, we should have a heartbeat beyond growth."

Yes, I think to myself, *at least you think it's a baby*!

"But, it's growing?" I asked. "So that's a good thing? Right?" The doctor paused, and pointed to the picture.

"Yes, and no. The growth at this point is not a good thing. Do you see here? Your baby decided to attach very close to your fallopian tube. A centimeter this direction," she pointed, "and it would have been an ectopic pregnancy requiring surgery. With this, we can do a regular D&C and prevent any damage to your reproductive system."

It took me a moment to process. "So, you're saying I have to abort this pregnancy."

The doctor was careful in responding, "In my medical opinion, this baby will not develop to term, and given where it has attached and how far along you are at this point, waiting for a natural miscarriage could cause hemorrhaging and damage to your system that would make it more difficult for you to bear future children."

I am heartbroken. But finally something makes sense. At least the doctor is able to explain, partially, why this is happening.

* * *

"Are you sure you don't want me to call out of work?" James asked.

When I'd called to schedule our first appointment, the only time that was available was right in the middle of James's work day. Although I wanted support, I also didn't want him to come. It seemed easier to face without him, and if the pregnancy wasn't viable, I could spare him the pain of seeing it.

"It's fine. Lauren is coming with me, so I won't be alone. It's really nothing. They are just going to check whether I am able to have the baby or not. There are lots more appointments later that you can go to if it works out."

He stared at me for a moment, paused, and then said, "If you're sure."

"I'm sure," I said. "Don't call off work for this. We need you to have this job. That is more important. I'll let you know how things go. I promise I'll call you as soon as I know anything." He sighed and agreed, but he clearly wanted to be there.

Lauren drove me to the appointment and sat with me while I stressed out about the ultrasound. Having survived the stillbirth of her second-born child, Lauren understood. Listened. Held my hand. When they did the ultrasound, I saw the picture—the same baby I'd seen before, but this time there was noise. A loud, strong heartbeat.

"This is a strong one!" the doctor said.

I couldn't believe it. "Wait, so everything is fine? That's my baby? It's okay? It's doing well?" I asked.

"Yes," the doctor said. "Everything looks perfect here—the attachment is solid, strong heartbeat and vitals, progressing fine. You are in good shape."

"But," I said, in shock, "there are still things that could go wrong, right? I mean, it might not work, right?"

The doctor shook his head, "I wouldn't worry about that. Everything looks good here. You have a viable baby in there."

* * *

In a socially constructed hierarchy of death, miscarriage comes last. The lack of a physical body to mourn often places miscarriage outside of cultural death rituals, leaving mourning mothers and fathers with few systems of social support for their grief (McCreight, 2008). In their study of women's narratives of pregnancy loss, Fernandez, Harris, and Leschied (2011) found consistent instances of "disenfranchised grief" across stories, noting that "these women described how their losses were dismissed or silenced by acts of commission or omission either when people expressed opinions insensitively or refused to acknowledge their grief" (p. 158). This presents strong communicative challenges for women seeking to make sense of and cope with their miscarriage experience.

* * *

I accepted what the doctors said. I read up on the Internet. Everything suggested it didn't matter what choice I made. This child—Doug's and my child—was not coming into this world. I could wait for it to terminate naturally, risking hemorrhaging that could cause reproductive issues later, or I could ask for a medical intervention. Based on my last appointment, I wasn't even sure waiting was an option. I had to have an abortion—medically—otherwise I might not be able to have children in the future. Of course, they called it a D&C, not an abortion. But to a woman raised Catholic who wanted a child, the terminology made little difference. The procedure itself was the same. The difference lay only in what I imagined that child to be versus a medical reality that had to be dealt with. *Fine*, I thought. *I'll be okay with this because it's a medical necessity. I don't want this, but my body is betraying me, so fine. Let's fix it. Let's move on.*

When we went in for the procedure, Doug was there. Held my hand. Waited with me. The staleness of the waiting was palpable. In the prep room, I was bedded next to another woman, who turned to me and asked,

"Are you okay? Is this your first?"

"Yes," I said. "I've never done this before." She had two kids with her, holding her hands.

"You know it don't matter when these things happen, it's terrible."

That's the last thing I heard going into surgery.

After the procedure, I came to—barely. I was conflicted. Mad at myself and my body—its inability to produce a baby. Mad about my choice here. Maybe I should have waited. Maybe the medical advice was wrong? Frustrated spiritually that I was forced into a position of "aborting" a "baby." How could this be happening to me? All of these things I thought upon waking out of the anesthesia. When I woke, Doug was there, holding my hand.

"Hey," I said, "Is everything okay?" He looked at me, squeezed my hand and said,

"Yes, we really dodged a bullet with that one. Everything is fine."

Fine? I thought. Really? This is not fine. I am not fine. My life is not fine. I just lost my—our—child and apparently, you don't care.

★ ★ ★

A substantial body of research suggests that miscarriage is one of the most traumatic experiences in a woman's life (Brier, 2004; Hutchon, 1998), often producing symptoms similar to post-traumatic stress disorder (Engelhard, van den Hout, & Arntz, 2001; Hale, 2007). In this sense, the miscarriage creates trauma that is continually managed over time. Social expectations of women post-pregnancy loss are predicated on modern notions of "appropriate" grief work (Silverman & Klass, 1996) in which the "working through" process is valorized (Neria & Litz, 2004) and periods of "re-grief" are seen as weaknesses in an individual's ability to relinquish bonds with the deceased (Volkan, 1975). But we can rarely ever return to what we were before these tragedies occurred (Hollander, 2004). Thus, we develop communicative strategies to assist with our internal and external grief work. We manage subsequent pregnancies, anniversary dates, or other would-be milestones in the child's life as emotional spikes to be dealt with and experienced largely alone. This process is specifically linked to time, because individuals can experience a resurgence of grief at different moments throughout the life course (Peppers

& Knapp, 1980). Women working through this grief as a result of miscarriage may consciously or unconsciously withhold emotional attachment as a protective mechanism, particularly in subsequent pregnancies, compared to women who report no experience of miscarriage (O'Leary, 2004).

* * *

"Everything was fine," I told James when he came home from work.

"So, the doctor said things are okay then?" he asked.

"Yeah, I heard the heartbeat and everything," I said.

"Oh man, really? The heartbeat? I bet that was cool. Was it cool? I should have been there."

I feel guilty. I should have encouraged him to be there.

"It's fine, we have another one scheduled later and you can see it then."

We settled into a routine—lots of sleep for me, searching for a house, trying to eat right, exercise when I wasn't too tired, and writing—my typical summer retreat. After a couple of weeks, we got the call:

"Your screening came back with abnormalities, and we suggest you see a genetic counselor."

I ignored the voicemail. They called again. I ignored that voicemail. I wanted to wait. If it turned out to be bad news, I didn't want to tell James. I wanted him to have a few more days of happiness, excitement, and hope. They called again. I finally answered.

"You screened high for Down syndrome and trisomy 18. We'd like you to see a genetic counselor," the woman said. *Of course.* Given the last pregnancy, and how it ended, I assume this is yet another means of my body betraying me. I come from a long line of Catholic farm women—sturdy, fertile, except for me. Of course I have a genetic abnormality.

"Yeah, but this is optional, right? We don't have to see them, do we?" I asked.

"I'm not saying you have to get any additional tests, but their ultrasound equipment is better. If anything, we'll get a much better picture of where the baby is at in terms of development."

So we met with the genetic counselor, who walked us through the advanced ultrasound readings. I was against doing amniocentesis, but instead, she suggested a blood test that separated my blood from fetal blood by DNA and determined any chromosomal abnormalities. *It might not be covered by insurance. The co-pay may be a few hundred dollars, but we have money in the medical savings account. Nothing from the ultrasound reading is conclusive, but this test is 99.7% accurate in screening for Down syndrome and trisomy 18.* We decided to do it.

And then we waited. For three weeks. I waited through the first trimester, then waited through the second. I started having full-blown anxiety attacks, chronic insomnia. James tried to tell me things would be okay, but I didn't know how to be calm. Finally the call came:

"The test was negative. Your child has no chromosomal abnormalities …"

Finally, for the first time, I feel hopeful.

"… but we'd like to see you back in a week to check in, since the birth weight right now is very low, and we still want to check the heart development."

A couple of weeks later. They performed another ultrasound, and found another abnormality—"bright bowl." We met with the specialist again. I was sobbing, an uncontrollable mess. James tried to calm me, and asked questions that I couldn't through my tears.

"What does this test really mean? What is 'bright bowl' a symptom of really?" he asked. The counselor was kind. She offered me tissues, and said,

"This is a very common, unreliable ultrasound reading. It could be something, it could be nothing."

Choking through sobs I said, "But the woman reading the test said it was an issue."

The counselor shook her head. "Yes, it might be. But this could also be a residual effect of a common cold. You've done the genetic screening, and there were no red flags there. You can do additional tests at this point, which would help us know more about the health of the baby." We paused.

"What about the weight, and the heart?" James asked. "That's what you wanted to look at."

She smiled, and said, "Those look pretty good."

I am focused on breathing. Making sure that I am taking one breath in, one breath out. James took my hand, and said,

"I'm sorry, but we're done. My wife has been put through enough. We did the routine tests. We did the additional tests. And what you have is basically another 'maybe'? We know that already. This whole pregnancy has been 'maybe' from the beginning. We are done with testing, and we're not coming back." He helped me stand, and walked me out of the hospital. I was still crying.

"Maybe we should go back. Maybe we should do more tests," I said as we were walking away.

"We're done with tests," he said firmly. "I don't like what it's doing to you. We will deal with whatever happens. At this point, we are having a baby, and everything is going to be fine."

* * *

"Fine," of course, means many things, depending on context, relationships, and time. My first marriage ended shortly after my miscarriage, which is not uncommon (Shreffler, Hill, & Cacciatore, 2012). Relational dissolution can happen for a number of reasons, but in my case, the first pregnancy made clear that Doug and I did not share the idea of "someday." The pregnancy made "someday" a reality, and when faced with that reality, it became clear we wanted different things out of life. In my second marriage, "fine" means something different. Prior to getting pregnant, James and I talked at length about the "reality" of a baby—coming up with options and plans should biology, time, or economics prove uncooperative. We had contingency plans, working to make "someday" a reality jointly within our relationship. In other words, my two pregnancies happened in completely different relational circumstances, in separate emotional moments, under the care of different medical staff, with vastly different outcomes. In the first, I lost a child, my primary relationship, and a good deal of economic stability. In the second, I gave birth to a healthy, vibrant son, in a loving, stable partnership with far better economic stability.

Given these differences, it is tempting to separate these narratives as each happening in its own time, for its own reason. This cultural logic—right time, right place—is offered to many women who miscarry. But this preference for time as an explanatory force rendering interpersonal meaning denies women's fundamental experience of miscarriage. As Berry and Warren (2009) observe, experience is "spatiotemporally rooted in (or informed by) given locations (physical, emotional, thoughtful contexts), subject to divergent meanings, and is necessarily subject to change over time as reflection (and further reflection) changes what happened" (p. 601). Women do not experience miscarriage in a linear way, contrary to medical explanations and terminology. Culturally, we are encouraged to see each pregnancy differently—each as an individual story, as diverse as the genetic possibilities for each individual fetus, as unique as each individual child that results from conception. But instead, perhaps pregnancy—and procreation more generally—is a larger narrative, one that includes pieces of prior experience in a search for reproductive meaning and identity.

In that way, reproductive time becomes an important concept to interrogate. For me, as it is for many women, the miscarriage experience was isolating. Everything about the "time" seemed right—I had just gone up for tenure, was in a relationship that had lasted eight years, and had recently turned thirty. After the miscarriage, explanations from well-meaning people close to me about how this "wasn't your time" only made it worse. I expected my first pregnancy to live up to our cultural conception of birth stories—to be part of that narrative of reproductive time. In my large Catholic family, there was no discussion of unsuccessful pregnancy, only birth stories (usually specific to individual children). I have more than one hundred cousins. The world I grew up in did not account for miscarriage. That made it all the more difficult coming to terms with the outcome of my first pregnancy. It was a foreign experience for my immediate family, and for many of my close friends who had very little trouble getting pregnant (and often their pregnancies were conceived while on various forms of birth control). I found a support network in places I didn't know existed prior to my loss—grief share support groups, acquaintances who suddenly became close friends because they risked telling me their own miscarriage narratives, Internet support sites where women from all walks of life shared their stories. Suddenly, it wasn't an isolating event that I was experiencing alone, but part of a larger, silent cultural narrative—a narrative that was only rendered visible when I became a part of it.

That experience also impacted the birth story of my son. All of the joy, excitement, and hopefulness during that pregnancy was lost on me. I assumed the worst. I spent a good deal of time withholding emotional investment in the outcome of the pregnancy. The first experience was so isolating, I found it difficult to imagine anything beyond the day-to-day changes in my body. I equated being pregnant to the scene from *Alien*, unsure of what would appear at the end of the nine-month stretch. And the "time" was more tenuous—having been married for only a year, to a much younger partner. Suddenly, reproductive time meant something different. Despite the possibility of a successful birth, the romanticized cultural narrative of pregnancy would never again be part of my conceptualization of reproductive time. And in many ways, my partner was robbed of that joy—his experience silenced by the persistent tendrils of my own grief that I simply could not (and in many ways still cannot) let go. I cannot imagine a birth story untouched by one of the darkest periods of my life.

Yet, the interplay of my miscarriage and my son's birth produces a paradox of sorts—I grieve the loss of my first child, imaging what his/her future would have been like, but had that child come into the world, I would not have the life I have now with my son. I would have stayed in my marriage to Doug, or at least tried to for some indeterminate period of time, or potentially become a single mother. How can I grieve the loss of my first child without grieving the loss of my current life? How can I be thankful, recognizing that where I am now is a happier, more joyful place without being saddened by the possibility of what could have been? The relationship between time, identity, and space "leads to a *perception* and an *image* similar to what is currently being experienced, without which the present experience would have fallen apart" (Kristeva & Guberman, 1998, p. 19). Ultimately, time exists in narratives of experience as the buoy around which identity is conceptualized, negotiated, and renegotiated.

We are called to present our lives as a collection of stories that exists in time. Stories of conception, birth, and childhood become the foundation for personal and family identity. In telling these stories, we are rendered, through communication, as a life subject. The creation of a "*community* of language as a universal and unifying tool, one which totalizes and equalizes" is the crux of understanding cultural conceptualizations of reproductive time in relation to communication (Kristeva, 1981, p. 35). Our human fascination with time is directly related to the assumption of time as historical progression, one that moves from past, to present, to future and is experienced (primarily) in the present. As a result, we have a cultural demand for "narrative accountings of 'how and why,' for self-conscious avowals of motivation, for strategic weighings of what's opened up in relation to what's shut down" (Dinshaw et al., 2007, pp. 180–181). These narrative accountings, our communication about what opens or closes, constructs our identities in a space where interpersonal meaning is rendered. Our lives are not confined to "clock" time, or to a more specific conceptualization of "reproductive" time, but are instead experienced fluidly. Instead of thinking of time as linear temporality, academicians call for a "rewiring of the senses" that expands and values a broader range of temporal experience (Alexander, 2005, p. 308). When we experience events that are considered "off time" or "out of time," these moments challenge our conceptualization of "time as project, teleology, linear and prospective unfolding; time as departure, progression, and arrival—in other words, the time of history" (Kristeva, 1981, p. 17). Our identities are never far removed from their contextualization in past experience, but our communication about identity, the community of language we develop to render visible this identity work, can transcend linear conceptualizations of time.

Therefore, given the deeply personal yet socially constructed nature of reproductive time, it becomes necessary to situate the experience of reproduction in relation to discourses of identity. Autoethnography interrogates communication and identity as both cultural and interpersonal contexts simultaneously. As a result, writing about personal experience "is risky writing" precisely because "it is difficult to write about the self and to be an escape artist from the self at the same time" (Gannon, 2006, p. 484). As my story illustrates, miscarriage produces numerous identity challenges, while at the same time invites a critique of life itself. The loss of a child calls forth the question, "What more could I have done?" Often, the answer women are given from medical staff, trusted family, and friends, even popular culture representations, is that perhaps it was the woman's "fault"—failing to attend to one's health (planning prenatal care, increasing "healthy" living/eating habits while decreasing "unhealthy" habits), failing to plan correctly (fertility charting, sex planning), failing to adjust the timing of one's life events (career stability, economics) for the impending child. These are offered up as "comfort" in the wake of miscarriage. In essence, miscarriage is an indicator that it was simply "not the right time" for that woman. But this cultural logic assumes that women can control the process of reproduction, control our bodies in a manner that will submit to our will, in a way that regulates the (un)happy outcome. The impulse to understand human experience as a larger life-story implicates storyteller as subject, necessitating that "any critique of a life *text* is simultaneously a critique of *a life*" (Adams, 2009, p. 623, emphasis added). Rendering the larger narrative of silence surrounding miscarriage experiences visible disrupts our normative understanding of miscarriage as individual, biological experience and exposes the politics involved in regulating women's bodies and experiences via medical and technological knowledge systems.

Thus, any story of miscarriage is, by implication, an identity story—a journey undertaken as part of a story of reproductive time. My miscarriage narrative is past, present, and future simultaneously. How that experience is *communicated*—whether it be met with silence, with grief, with activism, with community engagement, with relational formation and dissolution—ultimately impacts our individual, and cultural, understandings of time and human experience.

11. The Healing Journey

DELEASA RANDALL-GRIFFITHS

This is the story of a voyage, a journey not only across the continents toward the Aegean, but across a sea of loss toward happiness and healing. This narrative is nestled within other larger narratives, like nesting bowls. It is a layering of cultural values and assumptions on top of relational needs and expectations. As with any story, its beginning is an arbitrary selection and the ending a momentary pause in the stream of life's experience and perceptions.

My journey begins in 1998. I was a successful career woman in my late thirties, never married, but in a loving relationship with a man I hoped would someday be my husband. At the same time I was trying desperately to squelch a strong desire for children, a desire that had nagged me since my late twenties. In the book *Women's Ways of Knowing* Belenky et al. (1986) write, "Many women ... experience giving birth to their children as a major turning point in their lives" (p. 35). I found out that there are other turning points lurking in the shadows of women's lives. I was about to experience one of them firsthand.

When I try to remember the early events of the journey some things are strikingly clear and others are vague. I remember having what I referred to as a "month-long period" of heavy bleeding. In retrospect, I also recall a trip to New York City during which I was out of my normal routine and I absent-mindedly forgot to take my birth control pills two mornings in a row. When I discovered my error I went ahead and took both pills. I had taken my pills late before. At the time my actions seemed insignificant. I assumed it would all be okay. But in retrospect, I see they formed one of the most significant acts I would ever commit.

I made an appointment to see my primary care physician, Dr. B. The bleeding had not stopped and I was concerned by this extended menstrual flow. I went to the appointment alone, assuming nothing major would occur that day. Dr. B might have asked for a urine sample upon my arrival. I don't recall. I do remember she had blood drawn and I had to wait a long time for the results. I was confused because I came in that day for a simple appointment about my period. I never expected the appointment to take so long. I had no clue what was coming.

Most of the details are fuzzy. Dr. B. was always straightforward with her diagnoses and counsel. That day she seemed particularly detached and mechanical. I can now only assume that what I was seeing was her version of professional concern, but at the time I did not understand. I can't recall her exact words. Somehow, all in one breath, I heard the elation-worthy news I had long dreamed of: "Your pregnancy test was positive." This was quickly followed by the devastating, "But you are having a miscarriage."

I wish I had a recording of the entire day so that I could play it back again and again. It feels like some time during that day, sitting in Dr. B's office, there should have been a moment, just a brief moment, when I was actually pregnant. I know I wasn't. I know that window of opportunity had already closed. Still, I wish I could have something tangible to look back on. I think one of the worst aspects of a miscarriage is that you have nothing to hold on to.

Dr. B said something about needing more testing because of the danger of an ectopic pregnancy. I now heard the urgency in her voice. Should I be worried? My head was spinning. I knew what a miscarriage was, but I had no idea what "ectopic" meant. My mind was trying desperately to comprehend how the word "pregnancy" found its way into our discussion in the first place. I had not planned for any of this. I wasn't prepared for it. I wanted it all to go away.

Dr. B's plan of action was to send me for an ultrasound right away. The urgency in her voice told me that time was an important factor in our proceedings. She sent me up to the receptionist area of the office to wait for instructions. I vividly remember standing at the receptionist's glassed window. I was wearing a white cotton sweater. It is funny what you remember in a time of crisis. I can still see that sweater in my mind to this day. That was back when short sweaters were still in fashion. My sister had given me this sweater as a hand-me-down. It was 100% cotton and stark white, clinical white, crisp and clean. How could such a horrible thing be happening amidst all this purity? I remember staring down at the sweater. It was the only thing I could focus on that was real and known. Everything else around me was a swirl of "I can't believe this is happening to me." I felt my first sensations of shame while I was standing there. I couldn't fully comprehend it, but my entire identity had changed since I had walked through the doorway to the examination rooms. I was suddenly a woman having a miscarriage. The receptionist behind the glass was aware of my new identity, too. What did she think of me? What did

I think of me? I was not ready for this role. Everyone around me seemed oblivious to my need for support. I tried to maintain my composure, partly out of shock and partly in an attempt to comply with others' wishes. The staff around me performed the actions of their daily business mechanically, while I was slowly descending into an abyss.

A nurse walked me down the hallway to Dr. B's furthest examining room. She handed me a huge thermal container of water. I was told I needed to drink lots and lots of water. This was somehow connected to the ultrasound, but no one explained exactly how. I was told to drink as much as I could. Then I was left alone. It was just me and the water. It was cool, but not refreshing. I have been thirsty many times in my life, times I would have given almost anything for a cool drink of water. This was not one of those times. This time the water felt like an obligation. The room was quiet. Muffled voices down the hallway occasionally invaded the silence. I had way too much time to think. I was scared and confused. How in the world did I end up in a situation like this? I was a responsible modern woman who had managed to avoid unexpected pregnancy for many years. How did this happen? The missed pills in New York never entered my mind at this point. I couldn't keep any coherent thought in my mind for very long. My thoughts were jumping from place to place. My body was pulsing with nerves.

I wished I had someone with me. My boyfriend, Tom, was at work in a town twenty minutes away. My family lived five hours away. In the rush of events no one asked whether I needed to make a phone call. I sat drinking that water as if my life depended on it. The thermal mug was like my white cotton sweater; it was tangible. The coolness running down my throat was not comforting, but it was real. I could feel it inside me. In fact, it was the exact opposite of this pregnancy I had just learned of. This pregnancy was intangible, incomprehensible. Why hadn't I felt that inside me? Wasn't there some sort of maternal instinct that should have warned me about all of this? If this had been a test of women's ways of knowing, I had failed completely. I spent what felt like an eternity sitting in that room. Everything was in a fog. I finished every drop of that water, though. I was fearful of what would happen if I did not. Uncertainty was the rule of the day.

Finally a nurse came for me and escorted me out of the examining room. I left the building and drove myself to the parking lot, of the ultrasound location, two buildings down the street. I must have been moving like a zombie, without much thought beyond my white sweater and my now very full bladder, which I later learned assisted in the ultrasound imaging. I called Tom from the waiting room. His confusion and concern were both evident.

But even if he left immediately he probably couldn't get to me in time for the support I so desired. I felt alone in uncharted territory. The ultrasound was fairly uneventful. At first the technician seemed to exhibit the same air of urgency I saw at Dr. B's office. But after a few moments of moving the ultrasonic wand across my jellied stomach she seemed to relax. I was not having an ectopic pregnancy, whatever that meant. I was still confused, but felt less imminent danger.

When I finally got home I looked up "ectopic pregnancy" in my copy of *The New Our Bodies, Ourselves* (Boston Women's Health Book Collective, 1992). I read about an ectopic pregnancy's life-threatening potential and understood Dr. B's sense of alarm. I was happy not to have that drama added to the mix of emotions I was feeling. But somehow I felt that anything beyond the crisis of an ectopic pregnancy was seen by the medical community as an ordinary, run-of-the-mill miscarriage, something that has been happening to women for millennia. "One in six pregnancies ends in miscarriage, 75 percent of these before twelve weeks. Miscarriage, then, is a fairly common event" (p. 506). To me, however, there was nothing ordinary about any of it, no matter how many had occurred. This time it was personal. Tom came home and I finally received the support and comfort I had so desperately needed. We were both still in shock. Our relationship hadn't even progressed to the point of engagement rings; how were we now discussing a miscarriage? I knew I needed to take control of my health care options. I found a local obstetrician with whom I felt I might be more comfortable. We made an appointment as soon as we could.

It was a stressful time for both of us. I wanted a baby so desperately. My biological clock began ticking loudly soon after my twenty-eighth birthday. At this point I was thirty-seven and I felt that time was running out. The whole marriage and family issue was the one source of contention in our otherwise smooth relationship. He wasn't ready for marriage and I was frustrated by that fact and running out of patience. News of a miscarriage only added to this underlying tension in our relationship.

The bleeding continued; my feelings toward this "month-long period" had changed drastically. It was no longer a mere nuisance; it was a constant reminder of loss, failure, and pain. I thought back to all those weeks of heavy blood flow, of the clotted matter that I had no way of explaining. How is it possible that I lived in ignorance for so long? I asked myself a million times, "Shouldn't you have known you were pregnant?!" How did I get pregnant in the first place? I was on birth control pills. I had continued to take those birth control pills throughout the month-long period. I knew those actions, however unintentional, had contributed to this loss. Somewhere along the way I remembered the trip to New York. I felt shame, guilt, and remorse all rolled into one humongous ache in my soul. I knew there was no way to rewind the clock and take those two birth control pills on time. Nor could I forget them, try as I might.

In many ways I did not feel entitled to grief. I couldn't help placing my grief within the context of my family's grief. The loss of a first-born child is not a new story in my family. It happened to both of my grandmothers. My paternal grandmother, Georgia Crider Randall, lost her first child after only one week. More tragic still is the story of my maternal grandmother, Alma Camp Passwater, who lost her first child when he was only eight years old. So my loss was cradled in the context of their loss and it paled greatly in comparison. I hadn't even known I was pregnant. I'd had no time to dream or plan ... or fall in love with anyone or anything.

Harder still was the secrecy of it all. How does an unmarried, aging woman even begin to talk about an unexpected miscarriage? There was shame layered upon shame. There was the shame of having had premarital sex coupled with the shame of impending spinsterhood and feeling unwanted as a wife. I live and work in a conservative rural town. My story felt incongruent with the dominant cultural values surrounding me, even if it was the turn of the twentieth century. On top of that was the impact of my own upbringing. While one part of me felt like a liberated adult, free to have responsible sex any time she chooses, another part of me, deep down inside, still held on to the old beliefs: "Why buy the cow when the milk is free?" But the shame that runs deepest, that will forever haunt me, is the shame of having taken those birth control pills while a small life was trying to grow inside of me.

Even though Tom hadn't been ready to be a father, he stood by me every step of the way. It was hard for us both as we sat in the obstetrician's waiting room. We watched other parents with their tiny babies tucked safely in their carriers. I used to love seeing babies out in public. I have always been drawn to their innocence and wonder. These parents, sitting a few feet away from us and smiling down at their precious children, didn't have a clue about our story. For the past decade, however, the sight of a baby ignited a yearning for something missing in my life. I think it was a new experience for Tom, however. We exchanged glances, half-smiles, and knowing looks. There was nothing that could be said. There was nothing that could be done. Thoughts of what might have been, what was now lost, filled the space between our chairs. Occasionally, we talk about that little life to this day. Although we never knew a gender, over the years that baby has become more and more clearly male in my mind. We sometimes estimate the birth date. We calculate his age. As I write this in 2014 he would probably have just turned fourteen. He will always be an absent presence in our lives.

The new obstetrician, Dr. C, was honest with us about my situation, but she expressed her concerns with compassion and humanity. She was the opposite of Dr. B and her brusque approach. Dr. C. spent time with us, making us feel that we were the most important case she would handle all day. She told us she wanted to take the least invasive approach as possible to deal with the aftereffects of my miscarriage. She explained that blood tests could indicate the levels of human chorionic gonadotropin (HCG), a hormone secreted during pregnancy, in my system. She assured us that the human body was often capable of cleansing itself without the need for surgery. She told us that we could wait a few weeks, doing a blood test each week, to see whether my HCG levels lowered. My body might be able to handle all of this on its own. But it would take time to tell. If the HCG continued to show up in my blood tests after a few more weeks, a dilation and curettage (D&C) would be needed. Both Tom and I were in favor of this approach. We'd choose "nature" over "the knife" whenever possible. So, we left Dr. C's office feeling that we had a course of action and we trusted her to guide us along the way.

I went to the local hospital for my first blood test. I was shocked during my first visit when the woman processing my paperwork coldly referred to the reason for the blood test as "an aborted pregnancy." Bewildered, I quickly corrected her, calling it "a miscarriage." She repeated the term "aborted pregnancy" like she was saying the words "blue sky." My reaction was intense. Hearing those words attached to my situation was a kick to the stomach. I kept wondering whether this woman had any idea what I was going through or how it felt to have an emotional experience labeled in what felt like such an insensitive way. I now understand that "aborted pregnancy" is the standard medical terminology used for any miscarriage, but at the time I had no idea. Once again, I was faced with a situation in which my cultural values and assumptions collided with my lived experience. Why had I reacted so intensely? Why did those words carry such impact? Why did this hospital employee appear so unfazed by my reaction? Only in retrospect did it occur to me that the word "abortion" carries a very different meaning in everyday parlance than it does in the medical community. I am a pro-choice advocate. Abortion is one of those topics about which I am pretty certain where I stand. In my mind, however, the term "abortion" is intricately connected with the notion of "choice." In my situation I felt as though I had made no choice, at least not a conscious choice. To make a choice, you have to have time to contemplate a situation, to live with it long enough to decide. I felt like the decision was made for me before I even had a chance to weigh in on the subject. I had no choice.

By the end of March the HCG was still showing up in my blood samples. It was clear that my body was not able to cleanse itself naturally. The D&C was scheduled for a Friday in early April. It was springtime, the season for rebirth. But for me it felt like the cold depths of winter. I did very little research on the procedure. I really didn't want to know any more than I had to about the elimination of what would have been my first child. Dr. C was very supportive. She came to speak with me right before the procedure, while I waited in the OR prep room. She assured me that I would be home resting by the afternoon. Tom was my constant companion and my pillar of support. I woke up to find him right by my side in the recovery room. He pampered me all weekend, tending to my every need. We told only a few people about the procedure, family and a few close friends. I was already feeling enough shame about my situation; privacy seemed the better part of valor. My friend Tricia sent an edible arrangement of flower-shaped cookies. They were the one bit of sweetness in an otherwise sad affair.

My miscarriage was a difficult loss to grieve, mostly because it was a private affair. But that fact made it no less hollowing. When there is no body, there is no grave, no funeral, no marker of the loss. I really had no way to honor this little lost spirit. Most of the time, I felt like I did not deserve to grieve publicly. I have known women who lost young children to cancer or other illness. Their grief seemed justified. My loss seemed so trivial compared to those losses. Even women who knew about their pregnancy for weeks or months, women who had time to plan and dream, even they seemed more entitled to grief than I did. My dreams were taken away before they began. Mostly, my pain felt like a secret penance for my part in this tragic loss. If I had only known about the pregnancy I could have stopped taking those birth control pills. In my mind it could have made all the difference in the world. It could have saved that little life.

After my miscarriage I was beyond ready for family and marriage. Unfortunately, Tom, whom I loved dearly, still was not. So I focused my energies on cultivating patience and letting go my will to control every event occurring in my life. I saw a flyer for a trip to Greece called "Journeys of Discovery: Ancient Feminine Wisdom." Ever since I had read *Odyssey With the Goddess* (Christ, 1995), a memoir that chronicles a similar tour, I had dreamed of making this journey. In my journal during those months I composed the following: "I knew it was a necessary part of my healing journey. I knew I had to go." If marriage and children weren't right for me at this time, world travel was certainly in order. I am not sure Tom fully understood my need to travel, but he was supportive when he saw how excited I was to finally see Greece and the ancient sites I had only read about in books. I think he understood that this trip was not about running away from anyone or anything; it was about embracing something important and releasing the burdens of the past. The twelve-day trip was scheduled to begin at the end of May. It had only been a few months since my miscarriage, but my physical health was fine. I paid my deposit, applied for my passport, and spent the rest of the spring packing for my adventure. That moment marked the beginning of my healing process.

This trip to Greece was amazing—five women on a journey to the sacred world of the goddess. In Greece, the historical and architectural sites were certainly captivating, but the spiritual aspects of the trip were the most life changing. I had shared my story with Gayle, the leader of our tour, on the drive to the airport. She knew I was looking for closure surrounding my miscarriage and answers to my questions about what the future held. One of the hardest parts of grieving my miscarriage was the lack of ritual. Only a few people even knew about my loss. There was no place for public grief, no funeral, no time to let go. I was seeking a way to release all of my unwanted burdens and leave them somewhere in Greece.

It was at one of our first stops in Delphi, at the Sanctuary of Athena, that my healing truly began. In ancient Greece, Delphi was considered the "navel of the world." The *omphalos* (literally meaning "navel") was "symbolic of the navel's identity with the womb as the feminine center of life" (Neumann, 1991, p. 132). The site features a sacred *tholos* (round building), the circular ruins most often depicted in literature about Delphi. Our guide referred to Delphi as the "uterus of the Greek world," another symbol linked to femininity and the womb. She told us that for hundreds of years women came to the Sanctuary of Athena if they were hemorrhaging after childbirth and they were miraculously healed. I was clearly in the right place. The physical effects of my miscarriage had ceased months before, but my heart was still hemorrhaging and in need of healing. Ironically, we also learned that Georgios Papanicolaou, inventor of the modern-day Pap smear test, came from Kymi, a city located on the coast, just east of the ruins at Delphi. Maybe this really was the "uterus of the Greek world."

We were so drawn to the Sanctuary of Athena that we decided to return there later that night. My *Fodor's Greece* guidebook (Rockwood, 1997) features a description of the "Sacred Way" as a pathway leading up to the more famous Temple of Apollo. But it was the path leading down to the more feminine grounds of Athena that proved to be the more sacred way for our tour group. It was dark when we left the Hotel Amalia, perched high above the town of Delphi. A radiant moon was lighting our way as we ventured back down the hillside to spend more time in that sacred space.

Even though the Sanctuary of Athena was wide open in the daytime, the gate was locked at night—a chastity belt for this ancient ruin. Once inside, we performed a simple ritual near the center of the temple. This ritual included a sage smudging and lighting a tiny candle to mark whatever it was we brought to this night. I lit a quivering flame in honor of the child I never birthed. We each took time for private contemplation and communion with the sacred. As I sat on one of those ancient rocks, viewing the same beautiful, circular temple that women had viewed for centuries, I felt a kinship to women of all eras and all places. Streep (1994) describes this site by stating, "The ancient association of the Goddess and the circle carries with it echoes of prehistory, the concentric patterns of earlier ages, ... the roundness of the female body, the swell of pregnancy" (p. 180).

I sat there meditating on my need for healing. I wanted to let go of the burden I had been carrying. I felt so safe in that space, like it was the safest place I had ever been in my life. I felt cradled in feminine history. I decided then and there to release the spirit of my unborn child in this sanctuary, this powerful place of women's healing where he would be safely cradled, too. I would let him rest there in peace. It didn't feel as though I were abandoning him; he was in the care of the ancient ones. I felt a powerful sensation of healing and release. I felt at peace with my loss for the first time. I told myself if I were ever to have another child I would bring her to this sacred place and tell her my story ... our story.

I left Greece with fewer burdens and a clearer vision of where my future might lead. I was less focused on forcing things to happen and more focused on trusting the process of life. I now consider this trip as the fulcrum of my life's story. The following winter Tom and I bought a house together. One thing led to another and by June we were married. Our wedding date, June 3, 2000, was exactly one year after my trip to Greece. To me it was a profound affirmation of the healing that took place in Greece and my willingness to let go of the old to make room for the new. Tom still wasn't ready for children, so I bit my tongue and practiced patience. In 2002, however, we had a beautiful baby girl. We named her Faith because faith means believing. As it turns out, that baby girl had a wisdom all her own. She chose her birthday, two weeks past my due date and after three days of Pitocin. It was May 31, 2002—exactly three years to the day of my moonlight excursion to the Sanctuary of Athena in Delphi. Was it a coincidence? I'll let you decide for yourself. All I know is that so many times along the way I almost gave up on my dreams. It was a long and difficult journey, but the destination was well worth the trip.

Reflecting on the Journey

Illness narratives have the power to reveal rich context/hidden assumptions and meanings. Rita Charon, a surgeon at Columbia University, is the leading advocate for what she calls Narrative Medicine. Charon (2006) discusses how quantitative and qualitative researchers are "pitted acrimoniously" against each other in the study of health and illness (p. 29). She compares scientific knowledge's search for the universal to narrative knowledge's focus on the particular. "Narrative knowledge enables one individual to understand particular events befalling another individual not as an instance of something that is universally true but as a singular and meaningful situation." This quote reminds me of the incongruence I felt as I read the generic statistics on miscarriage in *The New Our Bodies, Ourselves* (Boston Women's Health Collective, 1992), and the feelings I was experiencing in the moment. While the universals can provide vital information in some instances, there were times when what I needed was the uniqueness of individual experience. Charon (2006) describes the purpose of narrative as "[attempting] to illuminate the universals of the human condition by revealing the particular" (p. 9).

Charon uses her training in literary analysis to describe five narrative features of medicine. The first four of these features align with Kenneth Burke's (1989) dramatistic pentad. The chart below compares both Charon's and Burke's terminologies.

	Charon	**Burke**
Context of the illness (Where and When)	Temporality	Scene
Subjects involved in the experience (Who)	Intersubjectivity	Agent
Motivations/reasons for the experience (What/Why)	Causality/Contingency	Act/ Purpose
Particulars of telling of one's unique experience (How)	Singularity	Agency

Context: The impact of context on my understanding and evaluation of events became a key aspect of analysis for this narrative. My story cannot be understood without an understanding of the larger cultural contexts in which it occurred. On a macro-level, my experiences with the insensitive and depersonalized aspects of the medical industry (my initial encounter with Dr. B or the woman filling out the forms for my blood work) highlight my frustration with medical practices in the United States that treat disease as a disembodied entity rather than one aspect of a complex human system. My own philosophical stance toward the patriarchal nature of medicine also frames my levels of trust and influences my perceptions of medical competence. The more immediate contexts of my community, my university, and my rural midwestern upbringing contribute greatly to my expectations and assumptions about social appropriateness. Until I tried to explain my experiences I was unaware of the depths of those cultural values. The context of my family's history, my grandmothers' losses, and my mother's views on medical authority impacted my feelings of entitlement to grief and my role as my own medical advocate. At the most intimate contextual level, my relationship with Tom was impacted by my past relationships and the ticking of my biological clock. The timing and location of the trip to Greece contributed to the depth of my spiritual experience. Finally, my contextual distance as I looked back more than a decade later to tell the story allowed me to reflect on the events in a more objective manner.

Subjects: All of the contextual variables are intricately connected to my sense of identity and my perceptions of those around me. Being single, unmarried, and in my late thirties at the time of my miscarriage added complex dimensions to my story and contributed greatly to my feelings of shame. My age and relationship history framed the events of the story with a particular urgency and complexity. Tom's role in this story was pivotal to the telling. His relational identity as it intertwined with mine complicated our incongruent sets of needs and desires. We were two individuals on a shared path, but our pace was not in sync much of the time. I felt an urgency he did not share. In addition, I am the central character of this story, but in terms of intersubjectivity, Charon (2006) notes, "The narratively skilled reader or listener realizes that the meaning of a narrative—a novel, a textbook, a joke—arises from and is created by the meeting between teller and listener" (p. 52). For Kenneth Burke, this dynamic incorporates the person who is telling the story with the audience to whom it is told. Charon adds a fifth feature, Ethicality, to her list of narrative features as a way to emphasize the role of "witnessing" in narrative and the co-creation of the narrative between the speaker and listener or between the writer and the reader. This book on pregnancy loss is rooted in the importance of this co-creation of understanding. My story combines with the other stories in this collection and with the reader's own story to accomplish what no quantitative analysis can, because narratives breathe life into the details of illness and give voice to our co-created and embodied experience.

Motivations: Charon's Causality/Contingency combines both of Burke's notions of Act and Purpose. For my story, the plotline of events—spanning

several years—is shaped by my need to tell this particular story in this particular manner. Only certain details were chosen to highlight my emotional and
spiritual journey. As I wrote the story, I became painfully aware of the role
my actions played in this story. I mostly felt like a passive participant in these
events while I was experiencing them. It was only in retrospect as I pieced
together the events that I understood the role my actions, or inactions, had
played in the event. The shame I still carry with me is centered on my perceptions of guilt about taking those birth control pills, both the two pills that
were taken late and the numerous pills that were taken after the fact. Getting
past that shame was part of the motivation to write this chapter. The process
of creating this version of my story, for this audience, caused me to reflect
much more deeply on many levels. I had to evaluate my attitudes toward my
culture's patriarchal worldview and how that has impacted Western medicine.
I had to reflect on my deeply seated expectations about marriage, family, and
sex. I had to examine my relationship status and the impact this miscarriage
had on my assumptions about timing and control.

Particulars: My narrative is unique to my individual experiences and is
therefore told from a singular point of view. My own personality, belief system, and biases provide the underpinning of my understanding of the events
and therefore shape the retelling. For me, this opportunity to tell this particular story in this particular collection of pregnancy loss stories forced me to
narrow my focus in important ways. There was much about my trip to Greece
that seemed pertinent to my healing, but ended up being bracketed out of
this telling. I think because we experience life as a linear conglomeration of
feelings and perceptions, it is often difficult to home in on the key aspects
of a singular narrative. That was part of my challenge in writing this version of
my tale. I kept asking these questions: "What details make my experience of
a miscarriage distinct?" and "What images and descriptions can be given to
evoke my experience in a way that is understandable?"

The retelling of my journey to healing is an attempt to offer as many
details as I can about the chronology of events. But, more important, it is an
attempt to capture the emotional essence of my experience as well. Mattingly
and Garro (2000) state, "Narrative mediates between an inner world of
thought–feeling and an outer world of observable actions and states of affair" (p. 1). Since the 1980s, alternative medical practices have allowed for
stories that "supplement the biomedical model with healing and holistic
therapies plumbing inner resources of the psyche and spirit in a mythos of
healthy-mindedness" (Langellier & Peterson, 2004, p. 189). The story of
my trip to Greece—a country credited with the creation of Western thought

and at the same time deeply imbedded in prehistoric feminine wisdom and mythology—chronicles healing that comes from outside the biomedical traditions of Western culture. Including my story in this volume of essays validates my experience in the world of narrative healing. My hope is that readers will find some personal connection—some comfort and healing—in the words on the page and the images those words create.

12. Once Upon a Time: A Tale of Infertility, In Vitro Fertilization, and (Re)Birth

LISA WECKERLE

Fairy tales have always loomed large in my imagination. I read *Grimm's Fairy Tales* at a very young age and found them to be confusing, terrifying, and fascinating. I continued to return to fairy tales by reimagining them in plays I wrote and directed. I liked turning the passive princesses into independent girls who rescued themselves. When my husband and I first started talking about having kids, I often pictured myself reading my revisionist feminist fairy tales to my spunky daughter.

When the kids didn't come and I started on my journey of infertility treatment, I found myself returning to the fairy tales again, only now I noticed different things. I was struck by how many of them include longing for a child. "Rapunzel" begins, "There were once a man and a woman who had long, in vain, wished for a child" (Grimm, 2009b, p. 36). "Thumbelina" begins, "Once upon a time there was a woman who wanted a tiny, tiny child. She had no idea how to get one, so she went to see a witch" (Andersen, 1999, p. 30). In "Kip the Enchanted Cat," the queen tells Kip, "You are luckier than I.... I may be queen, but I have no babies" (The Russian, 1999, p. 55). These fairy tales portray infertility as an unbearable longing, the beginning of a dangerous journey into the unknown, or a curse of bad luck.

Because fairy tales are one of the few kinds of literature that portray infertility at all, they shape our understanding about what it means to want a child and not be able to have one. In fairy tales, infertility functions "as a dominant motif, one that underscores the implications of childlessness in social, psychological, and religious contexts" (Beall, 2008, p. 485). We have done little in our culture to overcome the silence surrounding infertility in other forms of storytelling, such as personal narrative.

Because fairy tales communicate expectations about gender roles, fertility, and maternity, writing fairy tales into my story of infertility allows me to acknowledge and reimagine the social scripts that mediated my infertility experience. According to Harries (2004), "Fairy tales provide scripts for living, but they can also inspire resistance to those scripts, and in turn to other apparently predetermined patterns" (p. 103). My revisioning of fairy tales within my infertility story communicates both my desire to fit my story into an existing cultural narrative and the problem of defining personal experience through cultural narratives that never quite fit.

In this chapter, I will draw upon fairy tales and other forms of folklore as I share my journey from infertility to in vitro fertilization to birth. In addition to references to folklore, my story is also structured as a three-part hero's journey, indicative of the structure of fairy tales, myth, and folk tales. In his analysis of the hero's journey, Joseph Campbell (2008) noted that it was often divided into the separation, the initiation, and the return:

> [A] hero ventures forth from the world of the common day into a region of supernatural wonder: fabulous forces are there encountered … a decisive victory is won: the hero comes back from this mysterious adventure with the power to bestow boons on his fellow man. (p. 23)

I have structured my narrative into three sections, which correspond to the three phases described by Campbell. Following my narrative, I will show how Campbell's ideas about the hero's quest provide a useful framework for understanding infertility. Finally, I will explore feminist critiques of Campbell that offer alternative ways of thinking about infertility and the hero's journey (Lefkowitz, 1990; Murdock, 1990; Nicholson, 2011).

Separation

> [A] hero ventures forth from the world of the common day into a region of supernatural wonder.
>
> (Campbell, 2008, p. 23)

I don't remember when we started trying, and I don't remember when we figured out it wasn't working. We didn't know how long it would go on. We didn't know you could be infertile and never really figure out why. No observable defect other than age, no missing parts, no blocked tubes. One doctor looked at my chart and asked, "So, why are you NOT pregnant?" As if I knew and were holding out on her.

I asked one doctor whether I could move on to in vitro fertilization (IVF) since intrauterine insemination (IUI) had failed so many times before.

"I see here you've had just two rounds of IUI with the current fertility drugs," she said.

"Yes. But I had three before that."

"Well, we like to do things in threes."

What the hell kind of answer is that? "We like to do things in threes"? What is this, a fairy tale in which everything happens in threes? Were my eggs like the porridge of Goldilocks and the Three Bears—the first egg too hot, the second egg too cold, and the third egg expected to be just right? I waited for an explanation of why "we" liked to do things in threes, but the doctor just smiled as if it were settled and gave me some instructions for starting the next IUI. After that exchange, I decided I had had enough of her. I was ready to switch to another fertility specialist, my third specialist in three years. "Ha!" I thought, "We do like to do things in threes."

During my infertility treatment, I felt alienated from other people, partially because of the depression and anxiety that was a side effect of the fertility drugs. These feelings often struck me like jolts to my body—they were not reactions to outside forces, but seemingly random forces that grabbed hold of my consciousness and would not let go. I avoided social situations. I felt profoundly alone.

There is nothing that invites a story so much as telling friends and family that you are trying to get pregnant. There were two types of stories that I heard: disempowering stories told by people who did not go through infertility themselves and affirming stories told by people who were struggling with infertility. Like an urban legend, the disempowering stories were told by people who had "heard about" a case of infertility. What struck me was that most of the storytellers, although they did not experience infertility directly, considered themselves authorities on infertility. If they knew of one case of infertility, that single experience became synecdochical for all other cases of infertility. People seemed to have a strong desire to create a master narrative out of a single experience of infertility they had heard about (never directly experienced) and then subsume my story into that narrative.

In contrast, I found the stories that my "trying to conceive" friends told me to be helpful. We would swap war stories: drug side effects, stupid things people said to us, how we had to take a fertility shot in a public bathroom. Other "trying to conceive" people seemed to know how to listen without being dismissive or giving unsolicited advice. We were able to tell our stories to each other and see connections between them, without assuming our experiences were identical. There were some missteps. I told someone that the dye test would not hurt at all and her dye test was excruciating. Even I forgot that going through infertility is something that is different for everyone.

Computer-mediated message boards helped me see even more responses that people have in regard to infertility struggles. No one story could provide me with the overall picture of infertility, but by reading multiple stories I was able to see thematic connections to my own experience. Message boards (e.g., "Trying to conceive" on iVillage) also offered a patient perspective on the procedures that were previously only explained to me by doctors who had never been through them. The way all the texts interacted with each other reminded me of a concept I learned of in graduate school, intertextuality (Fiske, 2011). Long and Strine (1989) claim, "In order to know, we need more perspectives than our own, more than the monologic voices of author-ity. Intertextuality fosters a way of being in the world that assumes all of us bring something complex to our experiences, that we are capable of acting, of engaging others, including texts, and not simply reacting to them" (p. 474). I found this to be a good analogy for thinking about infertility: Each reader (or person who experiences infertility) brings to bear on his or her understanding of new texts (the experience of infertility) the sum of his or her experiences with other texts (what literature, personal experiences, and other people's stories teach us about fertility/infertility).

Initiation

Fabulous forces are there encountered, ... a decisive victory is won.
(Campbell, 2008, p. 23)

Almost as soon as I started, I found myself wanting to escape from IVF. It was as if I had stepped on to a roller coaster, ridden to the top of the first drop, and now wanted to get off but couldn't. I hated living by a clock: shots at nine o'clock every night and ultrasounds every morning. I hated the waiting: waiting in the doctor's office staring at a blank ceiling, waiting for ovulation, waiting for my eggs to ripen. I hated the removal of the human touch: instead of sex, I had vaginal ultrasounds.

I especially hated the shots: the mood swings they caused, the sting of them, and even the smell of the alcohol cleaning my skin. As I got the shots, I often thought about the things that fairy tale characters had to do to get a child, like baking a boy out of gingerbread. I wanted to trade in my needles for flour and a rolling pin. I wanted to be elbow deep in a bowl full of dough, kneading it with my own hands. That seemed so much easier, more natural somehow. I wanted to carve a boy out of wood like in Pinocchio or plant a rye seed that grew into a child like Thumbelina. The following poem reflects my desire to escape from the clinical rituals of IVF and into the magical rituals of fairy tales and folklore:

How to Make a Child

Close your eyes
Hold your breath
Make a wish

> Spread your legs
> Swallow these pills
> Stimulate the ovaries

Sometimes it happens after you see a shooting star
Or find a four-leaf clover
Or toss a lucky penny into a well

> Bleed for 3 days
> Ultrasound the follicles
> Count your eggs

You could cry and wait for your tears to grow
Or if you're handy, carve one out of wood
Or if you've a strong stomach, cut open a wolf's belly, see what comes out

> Insert needle
> Draw blood
> Take 3 shots in the belly

You could spin one out of straw
Or bake one out of gingerbread
Or just ask your fairy godmother to do the work for you

> Start the IV
> Count backwards from 100
> Harvest eggs
> Collect specimen

For most it's as easy as a careless frolic in the woods
The letting down of hair
Kissing a stranger at midnight

> Fertilize in the lab
> See how many make it
> Insert the viable ones
> Lie back
> Don't move

Sometimes it hurts
You have to spill three drops of your own blood in the snow.
Or you have to cut off a piece of yourself
A finger
An eye

> Progesterone shots
> Bed rest
> No sex
> No coffee

No wine
No chocolates
Just waiting
Be patient

Sometimes it's simple
Looking beneath the cabbage leaf
Guessing a stranger's name
Finding one in a basket on your doorstep

Insomnia, night sweats, bloating belly
Nausea, stabbing headaches
Blood tests
Shots
Bruises
Numbness

Sometimes it's dangerous
Eating from a witch's garden
Luring one into your candy house
Burn sage in moonlight
Form one from mud and bones
Find one
Buy one
Steal one

Waiting, resting, hoping, crying
Phone call
Hoping but being afraid to hope

Close your eyes
Hold your breath
Make a wish

The one thing my IVF experience had in common with the fairy tale way of getting pregnant was that breathless, repeated wishing. Every time I called in for the results of my pregnancy test, I would automatically close my eyes, stop breathing, and hope like hell that I was pregnant.

On the first IVF try, everything went smoothly. Several eggs were harvested and five days later, two exceptionally well-defined, fertilized eggs were put back in. A few days after the eggs were reinserted, I felt different to myself, transformed, as if something magical were taking place inside my body. Two weeks later, I got the call that I was not pregnant. So we began again. On the second IVF try, everything was a mess. There were fewer eggs to choose from, and once inseminated they didn't grow as large. I was sure that it wouldn't work.

Two weeks later, I got a call from the nurse. The test was positive, she said. You're kidding me, I replied. You're pregnant, she said. I was happy to be pregnant but also felt alienated from my own body, as if I had misread it and needed a medical professional to translate it for me. Not only could I not get pregnant on my own, I couldn't even tell when I was pregnant.

All in all, I was lucky. I was lucky to be able to afford the procedures. I was lucky that they worked. I was lucky that I had a partner who supported me through the process. Some of my friends got lucky too. Some of my friends are still trying. Some of my friends have stopped trying. In most fairy tales, the good characters are rewarded and the evil ones are punished. However, in infertility, becoming pregnant has absolutely nothing to do with whether you are good or evil. Thinking about pregnancy as a miracle bestowed upon those who deserve it or worked hard to get it demonizes those who don't get pregnant and idealizes those who do.

Return

> The hero comes back from the adventure with the power to bestow boons on his fellow man.
>
> (Campbell, 2008, p. 23)

Shortly after I got pregnant, my doctor told me that I would probably need a C-section. He told me my fibroids were so big that going through labor would be dangerous. It would have to be a C-section, the baby would have to be taken out early, and I was probably going to lose my uterus. My doctor told me my uterus would be impossible to put back together again. These words echoed in my mind and transformed into a well-known nursery rhyme: "All the king's horses and all the king's men, couldn't put Humpty together again." I envisioned the doctors and nurses, some on horseback, gathered around my fragile uterus hopelessly trying to fit the broken pieces back together as I bled out on the operating table. I had climbed up on a dangerous wall by undergoing IVF, and I was headed for a great fall. So, when people asked me, are you looking forward to the birth? Aren't you so excited to meet him? I smiled and said something vague. But really I was afraid I was going to die. When I appeared worried, people said, "Oh, you must be worried for the baby, but he'll be fine." No, I wanted to scream. I'm not even thinking about the baby really. I'm thinking about me. I'm thinking that I made this terrible mistake on purpose, and I should be selflessly willing to give my life to this unborn child … and I'm not. I don't want to sacrifice myself. And that's what mothers are supposed to do, right? Sacrifice.

Around this time I went on a writing retreat and we were working with poetry based on objects. We had to pick a word randomly out of a hat and write spontaneously and I wound up with the word "egg." I had a hard time starting my writing, but once the first sentence came up, the rest flowed out of me quickly.

Eggsistential Crisis

I am turning into an egg
This is not good news
Think of Humpty Dumpty.
Think of the waiting, boiling pot of water
Think of what we do to them
Think of the fragile shell
Think of a waiting pot of boiling water
Crack them
Poach them
Split them
Scramble them
Devil them
Think of your insides being all that matters

I am an egg
I am all womb
I hold a watery universe inside me
I hold the future
When it is done
I will be destroyed
It's either me or the thing I carry

This poem showed me that I was feeling objectified, consumed by the process of IVF, and terrified of the future. In fairy tales, it is a dangerous business, wrestling life into being. Sometimes the baby's life must be paid for with that of the mother. Snow White's mother wishes for a child and then pricks her finger, bleeds into the snow, and becomes pregnant, only to die in childbirth. Through the metaphor of the egg, I realized my needs, wants, and entire identity had become subsumed by those of the baby.

The night before my C-section I wanted two things: chocolate ice cream and to run away to Mexico. I don't know why I chose Mexico in particular. I think I got the idea from *Thelma and Louise*: Mexico as a place where you can escape your country's laws, escape your old self. I fantasized about climbing through the mirror of the hospital restroom like Alice in through *the Looking Glass*. Or perhaps leaning out the hospital window and catching a ride with a pointy-eared guy in tights who could take me to Neverland where boys never grow up and pregnant women never deliver. I started joking about it around the night before, and I kept bringing it up. On C-day at five in the morning on the way to the hospital, I told my husband to stop the car.

"I have an idea, we can just skip this whole C-section thing and go to Mexico," I said.

"But you're pregnant, and you'll still be pregnant ... you'll just be pregnant in Mexico," he responded.

"But I won't have to have the surgery. No doctor will make me have the surgery in Mexico. The baby can just live in there, and I can just be pregnant ... forever."

Of course my husband started the car again and drove to the hospital.

As a precaution to prevent bleeding out, I knew that I would have tubes inserted into my femoral arteries. I felt the tubes being threaded through me and had to remain completely still and straight. Then I was rolled into the operating room. My glasses were removed, turning the room into a cloud of light with blue blobs moving around in it. My husband came in. I thought he'd be beside me holding my hand, talking to me during the operation. But they quickly ushered him across the room, where he could see the birth and cut the cord. The anesthesiologist and his team were next to me, monitoring my eyes and asking me questions. He gave me an epidural and soon I felt the bottom of my body go tingly. I was afraid that I would feel it when they cut me open. I felt my body being tugged around, but it didn't hurt. There was a lot of scurrying and the room was charged with energy. After a while, a nurse told me I would feel a big push, as if an elephant were sitting on me, and that I didn't need to do anything, that it was just the doctors pulling the baby out. As I felt that push, a flood of something—joy? endorphins?—rushed through me, surprising me with its intensity. I feel something, I thought to myself. I actually felt a surge of emotion and I didn't think I would. I cried and then the baby cried and then my crying husband brought the baby to me and I saw him. I couldn't believe that we had both made it. And then my husband and the baby exited to the NICU. I was left in the operating room to be sewn up.

The operating room shifted from a party-like chaos to the feeling of cleaning up after a party. I was relieved that the baby was born, but I knew that I was not out of the woods yet. My doctor told me that the fibroids were not as bad as he had feared, which made me feel better. The nurse gave me something to calm me down and I drifted into a foggy sleep.

Considering all the risks, everything went very well. My baby had to go to the NICU for respiratory contractions, but was breathing on his own. When

I woke up and was still alive and knew that he was okay, I was profoundly relieved.

I dedicated myself to walking to the NICU and trying to breastfeed him. He did not seem at all interested. I also was instructed to pump so that my milk would start to flow. When it did, I was enormously happy. That satisfying plink as it hit the bottom of the bottle. Of course, at first it was only the tiniest little bit, not even enough to fill a syringe. At that point, it is a yellowish pre-milk called colostrum. Liquid gold, one nurse called it. It's that precious; the first few drops give the baby an immunity that no manufactured formula can. I was amazed that I could make milk. I felt like Rumpelstiltskin at his spinning wheel, turning everyday straw into reams of gold.

All of the nurses had conflicting ideas about breastfeeding. The ones in the NICU gave formula. The lactation consultant had different ideas. "Breast is best. You can't let his lips even touch a bottle nipple … What do you mean he has a pacifier in NICU? … Breast is best!" She reminded me of the Queen from *Alice in Wonderland*, red with anger and incessantly screaming, "Off with her head!"

But the worst by far was the nurse who told me I shouldn't breastfeed. I asked her to have someone in the nursery bring me my baby so I could try to nurse him. At first she said sure, but then she came back. No baby.

"I see in your chart you're on Prozac."

"Yes."

"Well, you can't breastfeed on Prozac."

I tried to explain that it was a low dose and I talked to my doctor about it, but she just kept talking about how it gets in the milk and damages the baby. She made me feel like I was trying to poison him, as if I were Snow White's stepmother tempting the innocent child with a juicy apple that was secretly deadly. Finally I gave up arguing with her. I told her I didn't feel good and I needed a doctor. When he came in I had a nervous breakdown about the breastfeeding edict. We talked a bit and then he gave me Xanax and I slept for a long time.

When I woke up, it was a different day and a different nurse and no one else gave me a hard time about breastfeeding on Prozac.

I know it was a combination of things that led to that breakdown. But it was that nurse telling me I couldn't breastfeed that sent me over the edge. As if I would have to choose. Either I could be natural and not need Prozac. Or I could be unnatural and give up breastfeeding.

What I wanted to say was: I need to try this. Through this whole process of having a baby my body has failed me. I couldn't get pregnant without a doctor putting a baby in me. And I couldn't give birth without a doctor cutting him out of me. I couldn't do any of the things that I was supposed to be able to do. So let me just pretend to be a regular mother who can do this one thing naturally. If it doesn't work out, I'll be okay. But for right now, please just let me have the experience of trying to feed him myself. Let me have the struggle of when to try and how to try. Let me have lactation consultants and doulas and sore nipples and all of it.

It was a struggle for me at first. It is for a lot of women. It doesn't work for everyone. It's not for everyone. I don't look down on mothers who choose not to do it or can't do it, but I was so happy and proud that I could do it. So much of my infertility experience was passive: lying back in the stirrups as the eggs were inserted, lying flat and motionless on the operating table as the baby was extracted. Breastfeeding was the opposite of all that. I think about the term "expressing your milk." It means to get it to flow out of you. Breastfeeding helped me not only to flow out of myself and connect with my baby, but also to flow back into myself and reconnect with my own body. I breastfed timidly at first, discreetly under a shield hiding in my car, hoping no one would see me. But after a while, I breastfed with impunity: in restaurants, at a party, and even on an airplane squished between two big burly men. I didn't care. I was the opposite of ashamed. I was no longer passive or silent or dependent. I was transformed.

My Infertility Narrative as a Hero's Journey

Joseph Campbell analyzed myths drawn from multiple cultures to develop his model of the hero's journey, which he calls the monomyth. For Campbell (2008), the hero is usually conceptualized as a man, so I will use male pronouns in my summary of Campbell's ideas. A hero begins as a man with extraordinary but unrealized abilities. He is called to adventure by some force threatening his world. The call may happen several times before the reluctant hero accepts his challenge, after which he "ventures forth from the world of the common day into a region of supernatural wonder" (p. 23). The fabulous forces include mental and physical challenges to test the hero's abilities, but they also include various helpers that guide the hero on his travels. However, for the defining challenge, the hero generally faces his challenge alone. If the hero is successful, "Often the boon is something that allows the restoration or regeneration of the life of the community" (p. 23).

While there is much to critique in Campbell's theories, I will first demonstrate how the hero's journey can be applied to my own experience of infertility. In many respects, my journey of infertility mirrors Campbell's monomyth in which the hero separates from community, endures mental and physical challenges, and returns with a boon.

Separation. Infertility represented a foreign world filled with new people, new language, and new spaces. The world of "trying to conceive" is populated with various guides—pharmacists, doctors, nurses, and genetic counselors. The jargon associated with infertility—IUI (intrauterine insemination), IVF (in vitro fertilization), TTC (trying to conceive)—reminded me of the linguistic vertigo experienced during a visit to a foreign country. The guides seemed fluent in this secret language, thereby emphasizing my outsider status and lack of competence. In terms of supernatural wonder, the ability to see my inner body projected onto a screen was surreal. Like Campbell's hero, I was venturing into a new space in my infertility journey—not just waiting rooms or doctor's offices—a new space that existed within my own body.

Initiation. I underwent various physical and mental challenges in an effort to win the boon—a baby. I had to undergo the discomfort of vaginal ultrasounds, the pinch of needles going into my belly, and the abdominal cramping that followed egg-harvesting surgeries. I had to suffer through depression and anxiety caused by hormonal infertility treatment. After five years, seven rounds of IUI, and two IVF cycles, I became pregnant.

Return. Sometimes the hero's journey back home is just as perilous as the journey away from home. There were complications that had to be monitored because of my age and IVF status. Furthermore, my fibroids would make vaginal delivery impossible and probably result in severe bleeding during the C-section. But in a hospital operating room on March 23, 2010, I gave birth to my baby, Benjamin Tobias Beyer. He was born healthy, with just a little breathing anomaly and jaundice that cleared up in two days. So, like the mythic hero, I returned from the world of infertility and pregnancy with a boon—my son. Yet, because of the dependence on others to deliver the baby, it did not feel like my victory. For me, breastfeeding my son was the part that helped me to feel like an active hero. Breastfeeding was a means for nourishing my son, and my means of reconnecting with my alienated body.

Thinking about infertility narratives within the terms of Campbell's hero's journey has several advantages. First, because a hero's journey is meant to be shared, positioning infertility narratives as heroic journeys counteracts some of the silence that surrounds the experience of infertility. Second, framing infertility narratives as heroic journeys offsets the objectification that permeates the experience of infertility. So much of fertility treatment involves being acted upon. Framing my infertility treatment as a heroic journey helped me to think of myself as a subject rather than an object.

Problems With Viewing My Infertility Narrative as a Hero's Journey

While Campbell provides a framework for viewing the journey of infertility as heroic, his theories have been critiqued by feminist scholars for framing the hero as masculine and Woman as the symbol of fertility, maternity, and goal for the heroic male (Lefkowitz, 1990; Murdock, 1990; Nicholson, 2011). Drawing on feminist critiques of Campbell, I will show how viewing infertility through the hero's journey highlights two problems: (1) viewing women as synonymous with passivity and fertility, and (2) assuming that a worthy hero always succeeds in her goal.

In contrasting the female hero's journey with the male's, Campbell et al. (1988) stated, "She becomes a woman whether she intends it or not, but the little boy has to intend to be a man. At first menstruation, the girl is a woman. The next thing she knows, she's pregnant, she's a mother" (p. 138). In this statement, Campbell claims the female *receives* her maturity from biological forces beyond her control—something that happens *to* her—while the male *achieves* his maturity through force of will—something that he *does*. In her critique of Campbell, Frontgia (1991) argued, "The actual possibility of the hero's journey, and therefore of heroism, is thus implicitly denied women, for they have supposedly reached their maturity, their developmental being, through the advent of normal reproductive function" (p. 16). While it is laudable that Campbell defines childbearing as a heroic act, it is also problematic that this is the only avenue open to female heroes.

As problematic as Campbell's definition of woman is, it also accurately encapsulates how much of contemporary culture defines and values women. There is still an assumption that a woman who does not bear a child is somehow less of a woman, that there is something wrong with her physically, psychologically, or morally. Furthermore, what about women who choose not to bear children? Or women who are forced to bear children against their will? Campbell conflates all pregnancy with a positive transformation into womanhood, regardless of circumstance or choice. Lefkowitz (1990) noted, "It is clearly the powers of the female body that Campbell wishes to celebrate, and not the force of the female will" (pp. 432–433). An essential part of the hero's journey is the hero's choice to go on the journey. If the journey is forced upon the hero, then it is a different kind of journey altogether. It is to be hoped that there is a way to honor childbirth as heroic while at the same time refusing to oversimplify it as a universal portal from childhood to womanhood.

The second problem with Campbell's model is that he defines success by the completion of a task, something tangible. This is problematic for people who set out to have a biological child, but never get pregnant. We need to re-conceptualize the hero's journey as one of transformation rather than acquisition. In studying narratives of couples that remained childless after pursuing infertility treatment, Peters, Jackson, and Rudge (2011) found that couples demonstrated resilience by redirecting their energies into new goals such as their relationship, travel, further education, and career development. These people should be considered heroes as well.

Campbell also suggests that the success of the hero's quest is wholly within the power of the hero, and that the failure of the hero to achieve her goal means she is unworthy. Lefkowitz (1990) describes Campbell as "a priest of a new and appealing hero-cult—the religion of self-development" (p. 429). Medical problems are often described as physical manifestations of psychological or moral failings. Cancer patients are told they will get better if they really want to, depressed people are told to cheer up, and infertile women are told just to relax and let nature do its thing. Obscuring complex cultural and biological reasons for infertility and emphasizing personal agency to overcome any obstacles scapegoat the infertile person as responsible for her inability to conceive.

The comments of other people during my fertility treatment demonstrate how many people think of becoming pregnant as either a sign that you have done something right or a sign of inherent worthiness. People often wanted to explain my infertility as something that could be fixed by a change in my attitude or actions: "You should just relax, you are trying too hard," or "You should tell your husband to stop wearing briefs." The other common response was the "Everything happens for a reason" response, the idea that we have absolutely no control over the situation. People advised that once we acknowledged a "greater plan" we would find peace: "Whatever is, is"; "If it's meant to be, it will happen when it's time"; or, "God works in mysterious ways." All of these responses left me feeling profoundly disempowered. If pregnancy is completely within my power, then not being pregnant is my fault. I was not trying hard enough, or trying too hard, or not trying in the right way. However, the reality of infertility treatment is that you can have the right support system, the most advanced tools, the best doctors, and still not get pregnant. Conversely, if the pregnancy were completely outside of my power, then all of my efforts were futile exercises, something to keep me busy while the universe decided whether I was allowed to get pregnant. There needs to be a space for ambiguity and integration: a way to acknowledge the agency of the person trying to get pregnant, while also acknowledging that that agency works within a constellation of other forces.

We need to find a way to define the heroic journey and infertility struggles through process, not product. Not everyone who embarks on a journey of infertility will come back with a baby, and that does not make those who get pregnant more heroic than those who remain childless. If we conceptualize the boon of the infertility journey as creative energy that can be expressed in a variety of manifestations (not just through a baby), then the hero's journey can be recuperated as a useful model for people experiencing infertility. Infertility narratives demonstrate the importance of conceiving of the hero as someone who goes through transformation, not necessarily someone who acquires a desired object or outcome. Through telling stories about infertility, we can help shift cultural perceptions of what it means to be infertile and what it means to be a hero.

13. The Empty Woman: Dealing With Sadness and Loss After a Hysterectomy

ELIZABETH ROOT

This pregnancy loss narrative is not a story of conception; it is actually a story of deception. The only conception in my life was a false conception that I definitely did not want to have children. It was not until after an elective hysterectomy to deal with problematic fibroid tumors that I became aware of how deceptive the strength of that stance was. This chapter will first chronicle how a single woman in her late thirties made the tough choice to have her uterus removed and was subsequently startled by the difficult emotions that surfaced, experiencing grief at a time when peace and healing were expected. After I share my story, aspects of Jerome Bruner's (2002, 2004) writings on narrative will be employed to analyze a time in my life when I felt defined by my emptiness, a woman without a uterus.

My Narrative of The Empty Woman

To share my experience in having a total abdominal hysterectomy, I will pres-ent specific memories organized around five themes of shame, stress, single-ness, surprised sadness, and secrecy. My narrative context is that I identify as a white, heterosexual, able-bodied, middle-class, single female who considers herself a professional career woman. The timeline of my hysterectomy takes place during my first two years as an assistant professor. The diagnosis of hav-ing significantly large fibroid tumors both in and around my uterus came a month before I began my tenure-track job. The surgery occurred a year later, six weeks before I returned to teaching fall term of my second year. My narra-tive highlights how the choice to have surgery, because it involved my uterus, represented more than a health issue; I was not able to separate the decision from other complex issues including my single status at the age of thirty-nine and my decision to abandon the possibility of bearing my own children.

Reading the Operative Report: Shame

The surgery was deliberately scheduled in mid-August, after I finished teaching intensive summer courses and exactly six weeks before fall term began. Recovery from such a major surgery was a full-time job for the first few weeks, since I ran out of energy quickly and unpredictably. One day I took my slow, calculated walk down the driveway to check the mail and discovered the operative report in my mailbox. My surgeon, aware that I was an academic, had suggested I keep a copy for my records. I quickly opened the letter, not anticipating I would find anything unusual since the surgeon had kindly debriefed me in the hospital. However, the report was formal and technical; there was one sentence that caught my attention and confused me:

> 39-year old nulligravid female with symptomatic fibroid uterus, desires definitive treatment.

The word that puzzled me was "nulligravid." Since I had no idea what that meant, I did what any academic would do and Googled it. The online definitions that surfaced for this word shocked me: a woman who has never been pregnant, a woman who has never had children. My first reaction was to be horrified that the medical establishment had such a vocabulary word to sum up my life. While this is true that I have never been pregnant, in my post-surgery state this label upset me. I felt shamed and diminished.

"Nulligravida" implies a lack of something. The root word "gravida" describes a woman who is pregnant/has had pregnancies, so the implied root condition for women is to be pregnant/have pregnancies. To be labeled as "null" is to have connotations of having no value, or being invalid. Instead of seeing the label as a necessary medical term, that specific label acted as an emotional trigger. In my mind, this term emphasized how I had not lived up to my potential for bearing children, and, perhaps even worse, made a decision to finalize my state of being "nulligravid." I received no academic satisfaction reading the operative report, but instead felt like a weakness of mine had been exposed and labeled. I stuffed the paper away and did not read anything else in the report for several years.

Deciding to Have Surgery: Stress

The decision to have surgery was not a simple act and stretched out over a year. My initial reaction to the diagnosis of problematic fibroids was to feel emotionally upset. The news was delivered over the phone by a blunt, unsympathetic doctor who acted is if, upon hearing the news, I would immediately request surgery. Instead, I attempted everything I could to avoid surgery. For several months, I tried acupuncture, visualization, and meditation. I would breathe deeply and envision the air coming inside, wrapping around and into my uterus, massaging the fibroids, and shrinking them with each breath-touch, and then I would visualize exhaling the fibroids out. I would lie under a heat lamp during acupuncture, with needles sticking out of my feet, legs, hands, and abdomen, trying to relax and hoping the treatment was working. I would take my Chinese herbs faithfully, doled out each week by my acupuncturist. These treatments, besides focusing my attention on trying to will away my tumors, also helped take my mind off my job stress as a new assistant professor.

Unfortunately, all the mental work and acupuncture treatments did not demonstrate any overt effect on the fibroids, as documented by a second ultrasound four months after the first one. At this point, I did not know what else to do, so I did nothing. I let my new job consume me, telling myself that when it was convenient, I would schedule a doctor's appointment for a second opinion. The main symptom that steadily developed during this time was an increase in emotions, including unusual bouts of crying. I could not place the exact cause of the tears; I just felt emotionally upset and found that crying was a release from the increase in emotions. Since I am not a person who cries easily, this new emergence of feeling weepy was surprising and bizarre. I had a strong sense that this was not "me." My growing fear was that I might start crying in the middle of teaching a class, for no apparent reason. I blamed my fibroids for feeling so emotional.

My logic was that the fibroids were interfering with hormone levels and were therefore the cause of this inexplicable emotional upset. I convinced myself that the only way to adequately address my feeling emotionally out of control was to directly confront the fibroids. I was aware that many women who suffer from fibroids experience discomfort, pain, and bleeding. While I did not have these strong physical symptoms, I fully believed my symptoms were mental and emotional. The knowledge of carrying around such large tumors caused mental distress, along with the uncomfortable feeling that I was losing control of both my hormonal balance and emotional stability.

Not happy with my initial gynecologist, I sought another doctor. My new gynecologist was kind and appeared understanding as he described several possible treatment options based on his analysis of my ultrasound records. Besides surgery, he also explained how I could consider managing the tumors through hormones. One option involved sending my body into a type of false menopause, since a reduction of estrogen could stop the growth of the fibroids and even possibly shrink them. I worried about having to take hormones sporadically for the next fifteen or so years until natural menopause might come, afraid the tumors might shrink for a while but grow back when the treatment ended. This doctor also addressed my concerns about hormonal imbalance, explaining it was possible that the blood flow to the uterus and surrounding areas was drastically affected by the large tumors; my ovaries might not be getting the amount or quality of blood they needed to function adequately. This information sealed the deal in my mind to go ahead with surgery, since none of the other treatment options sounded attractive. Once the hysterectomy was scheduled, I wanted to find peace and simply move forward toward recovery.

Leading Up to the Surgery: Singleness

One night, about a month before the surgery, I was alone at home, watching a romantic drama. As happens in romantic movies, there was a scene when the two leads had their first intimate experience, and as I watched the two lovers undress each other, I shocked myself by bursting into deep sobs. Suddenly I had been reminded that, without a current lover, the next time I would have a physically intimate moment such as the one being enacted on screen, I would have a large, noticeable scar on my abdomen. While I had considered many aspects of having a hysterectomy, I had not previously thought about how it might influence my love life. This movie scene caught me by surprise and forced me to realize that the upcoming surgery could become a complication for romance. My scar might need to be a topic of conversation with new potential partners; I might feel a need to describe my appearance in a sensitive area of the body. Also, I anticipated having to discuss why I might not want someone freely touching my stomach, especially if the area around my scar had become sensitive. I already did not have much success with romance; this seemed to add another obstacle to my future experiences.

My single status was an important characteristic in everything surrounding the surgery, since I was upset by the fact I was making this decision by myself. The older I became, the more I realized that while I desired companionship, this was challenging for me to achieve. I was embarrassed to admit that at thirty-nine I still had never truly figured out romance, that I still felt like I was completely alone, and that I did not know what to do about my circumstances. The decision to have a hysterectomy was a time when my singleness was amplified. I experienced anger at having to make the decision on my own, wishing I had someone to help provide perspective, someone to whom my fertility or lack thereof might matter. Watching bad romantic movies provided no comfort at all.

Watching Julie and Julia *Post-Surgery: Surprise Sadness*

My first big solo outing after the surgery was to go to a matinee. I was proud for attempting this, and I planned it considering that I would get tired, but could just relax in my theater seat. My choice of movie was *Julie and Julia*, part of which described the life of Julia Child when she was learning to cook in France. The previews made the movie look amusing. I did not know much about Julia Child's life, so I was unprepared for my reaction when the movie subtly indicated that Julia Child had trouble having children. There is a scene, early on, with a slight clue that Julia might want children but cannot have them. Later in the movie, Julia receives a letter from her sister, pregnant with her first child. In this scene, Julia reads the letter to her husband, begins to choke up when she learns about the upcoming baby, and then starts to sob, all while telling her husband how happy she is for her sister. This scene struck me as a very tender but sorrowful moment, and I sat in the dark theater and cried along with Julia Child. To my surprise, her sorrow was somehow my sorrow, too.

It was during this movie, feeling weak after surgery, surprised by deep sadness, when I had to ask myself: Did I actually want children? If I still did not want children, why did I feel so unhinged and upset after the hysterectomy? Why would I feel such a connection with Julia Child around this issue unless I also harbored deep feelings about having children, too? No one, prior to surgery, had warned me that I might need time to mourn the loss of my uterus. Without any mental preparation for this sorrow, I began to question my supposedly strong stance on childbearing, and realized there was doubt: Did I not want to have children because I really did not want to bring up kids? Or was this stance just a protective posture to draw attention away from the fact that I had never met someone with whom I wanted to have children? I could not find any easy answers to these questions; all I knew was that a sadness and feeling of emptiness engulfed me after the surgery.

Teaching Classes Post-Surgery: Secrecy

I began my second year as an assistant professor six weeks after the surgery. Six weeks is the typical recovery time slated for a total abdominal hysterectomy, and while I was capable of fulfilling my job duties, for the first few weeks of the term I also tired easily. The sofa in my office was a useful piece of furniture to help me recover between classes and meetings. I tried not to show how guarded my actions were, specifically when I had to sit down or stand up in front of people. I also bought a new work wardrobe, since no zippers, snaps, or buttons were comfortable to wear on my still-swollen abdomen. I declared it a victory when I was able to find some "fancy" sweat pants—sweats cut in a style that mimicked regular pants—and bought a few big, blousy shirts that I hoped hid both my stomach and the fact that I was teaching in sweat pants.

At a time when I still felt physically weak, I wanted to hide my recovery as much as I could. Topics related to the uterus, including menstruation, ovulation, and menopause, are usually, if not always, socially muted. If, for example, I had undergone knee surgery during the summer break, I would have spoken about this freely, even publicly announcing this in my classes. The knee is an appropriate body part to discuss socially; the uterus is not. Declaring that I had undergone a hysterectomy would have been, for me, an uncomfortable statement regarding my new empty internal space, implicating many indirect messages about my status as a woman who was not able to bear children. I could not openly discuss such a situation because I was, myself, struggling with how to accept this new existence. My summer surgery was kept as secret as possible.

These specific memories of shame, stress, singleness, sadness, and secrecy highlight crucial experiences during my decision to have a hysterectomy and the resulting recovery period. I initially made the decision to have surgery because I believed my stance on not wanting children was definite; I thought the end result would be relief and healing. However, after the surgery, I was surprised to discover sadness and doubts about the decision. To address my feelings of emptiness, the removal of my uterus was an act that needed time for mourning.

My Analysis of The Empty Woman

To analyze my experience of feeling empty, I will use excerpts from Jerome Bruner's (2002, 2004) writings on narrative. The act of storytelling is one to consider carefully because, as Bruner (2002) points out, "Stories surely are not innocent: they always have a message, most often so well concealed that even the teller knows not what ax he may be grinding" (pp. 5–6). Narrative analysis sheds light on the concealed messages contained within personal stories.

Identifying Underlying Expectations

The first step of analysis is to identify the underlying expectations hidden within a narrative, based on Bruner's (2002) description that a story does not begin until something unexpected happens: "Narrative in all its forms is a dialectic between what was expected and what came to pass. For there to be a story, something unforeseen must happen" (p. 15). All stories present ways in which people cope or come to terms with the unexpected. This subtle aspect of narrative provides insight into what was initially assumed to be the expected series of events. The story then highlights the situations in which the expected sequence of events goes awry. To apply narrative analysis to my story, I must first identify the areas of dialectical tension between what was initially assumed and then what subsequently happened.

From this first step of narrative analysis, I have identified three underlying belief systems that are concealed within my story. To more easily refer to these belief systems, I will use the term "ideology," based on the simple definition of ideology as an organizing mental framework through which to view the world. These specific ideologies are products of my greater cultural context and of my individual interpretation of these cultural messages. As Bruner (2004) specifies:

> Given their constructed nature and their dependence upon the cultural conventions and language usage, life narratives obviously reflect the prevailing theories about "possible lives" that are part of one's culture. Indeed, one important way of characterizing a culture is by the narrative models it makes available for describing the course of a life. (p. 694)

Therefore, these three ideologies not only indicate ways in which my cultural context has highlighted specific "narrative models," or belief systems, but also provide insight into how I have personally interpreted the importance of these narrative models. The following section will briefly describe each ideology as a set of expectations; my narrative was formed from the fact that my life departed somehow from each set of expectations.

Ideology of Choice

The strong belief that I should have choice in life exists throughout my narrative. Whether or not I have children should be my choice to make, independent of other life circumstances, such as infringing health issues. When I thought my fertility was fine, I was satisfied in declaring my choice not to have children. However, when there was threat to that choice, when the possibility came that my body might not allow me the choice anymore, I felt stress and sadness. It was my choice to have the hysterectomy when there were perhaps other options available, but once the surgery was over and no reversal was possible, I deeply mourned the loss of choice.

This loss of choice and control is linked to the experience of hysterectomy in a narrative study by Markovic, Manderson, and Warren (2008). One woman, even though she did not desire more children, still felt "she had lost control over her reproductive decision-making with hysterectomy"; this "undermined her own sense of embodied womanhood and femininity" (Markovic et al., 2008, p. 471). This example echoes my own despair at losing choice with regard to reproduction and illustrates how I believed I should maintain the luxury of choice throughout my experience. The ideology of choice, articulated as my belief that to have children or not should be mine to make as I deemed fit, strongly influenced my entire perspective.

Ideology of Romantic Partnership
It is also evident in my narrative that I strongly believed I should have a romantic life partner. Even though I have spent most of my adult life as a single woman, I continued to believe this was not the most optimal mode of existence. While I was satisfied to be able to work, travel, and go to graduate school freely, all of this was colored by the expectation that sometime during these experiences I would meet a life partner. I was convinced my singleness was not a permanent life-state; I never made the specific choice to be a single woman for my entire life.

This ideology has also been called the "committed relationship ideology" (Day, Kay, Holmes, & Napier, 2011) and the "ideology of marriage and family" (DePaulo & Morris, 2005). DePaulo and Morris explain this ideology by describing how certain "habits of the mind" (p. 57) have formed strong assumptions that a committed romantic relationship is the most important adult relationship. People in the United States "assume that adults who marry and have children are better people who are happier, less lonely, and more mature, and leading more meaningful and more complete lives than those who do not marry and have children" (DePaulo & Morris, 2005, p. 58). This ideology is not only deeply embedded in Western culture; I also discovered how profoundly it was embedded in me.

The ideology of romantic partnership is also connected to age. Even though I would rarely articulate this directly to myself, I believed it was acceptable to be single only until a certain age. My struggle with fibroid tumors began when I was thirty-eight; the upcoming reality of turning forty was an important factor in my decision to have the surgery and to force myself to accept the reality that I would never have children. There was something about turning forty that made me realize I was supposed to have found my romantic partner by then. One of DePaulo and Morris's (2005) early studies found that forty-year-old single people are perceived more negatively than are twenty-five-year-old singles, indicating culturally perceived age norms for the point at which people should marry and have children. In my own life, messages about single women and age have been consistently communicated through the media and also through conversations with friends and family, either subtly or overtly indicating that if I wanted to marry, sooner rather than later would be better. Turning forty and being single was not a situation I embraced at all.

While I feel ashamed to admit this, there are elements of fairy tale beliefs about romantic relationships that also inform this ideological stance. At about the same time I was beginning to be indoctrinated into the world of fairy tales, Lieberman (1972) described how the treatment of females in fairy tales reveals cultural patterns that have influenced the development of gender identities. While many of these themes focus on beauty, another important theme is how most of the heroines are passive and submissive; "the helpless, imprisoned maiden is the quintessential heroine of the fairy tale" (Lieberman, 1972, p. 389). Rodman Aronson and Schaler Buchholz (2001) echo this sentiment: "Girls are taught through fairy tales and modern media that if they look and act good, sweet, pretty, and basically passive, a male figure—the prince—will rescue them from taking care of themselves" (p. 112). I obviously accepted this theme in my own life, passively waiting and hoping somehow, at some time, to meet my romantic partner. While it was something I wanted very much, I thought all I could do was wait and hope. When it did not happen in the time frame that I wished it to, I began to lose hope that it would happen at all.

This ideology of romantic partnership also provided the overall context for having children. It was my unquestioned assumption that the decision to have children should be made within the context of a partnership. As a child, I was raised in a conservative Christian home where it was emphasized that romantic coupling should be heterosexual, that marriage is the only way to validate a romantic pairing, that bearing children should happen only within the legitimacy of marriage, and that divorce is problematic. Because of these strong messages, I did not consider it a possibility to bear and bring up children alone. Without a romantic partner, then, I did not have the valid context or opportunity to choose to have children. These messages about romantic partnerships have been so intensely rooted within that I discovered how I still interpret my life through that frame, even to the point of defining my own single existence as "lacking" somehow. Therefore, the ideology of romantic partnership influenced every aspect of my experience with fibroid tumors.

Ideology of Successful Independence
Since I was not able to achieve success under the ideology of romantic partnership, I instead strove to appear successful as an independent, single

woman. In the context of my surgery, since I was losing hope of finding a romantic partner the closer my age came to forty, and since I was making the ultimate decision not to have children, I wanted to appear as though I had my life together in every other way. This ideology of successful independence is also evident in one of DePaulo and Morris's (2005) early studies; when they asked almost one thousand college students to list characteristics of single or married people, single people were most likely to be described as independent. Both independence and commitment to a career were attributed more to single people than they were to married people. My acceptance of cultural norms about single people being strongly independent made it challenging for me to ask for help when I needed it.

Belief in this ideology made it difficult to talk honestly about my decision to have the hysterectomy. It was not easy to discuss openly how emotionally out of control I felt, or how much it upset me that I had to make this decision on my own. If I could not even admit to myself that I might want children, how could I talk about this with others? These feelings do not reflect the actual kindness of my friends and family; I never gave them the chance to respond to my true feelings. My struggle with fibroid tumors coincided with a time when I felt more lonely and isolated than ever before. I had relocated across the country for my job, and had difficulty forming a new sense of community. Most of my conversations about the surgery were long-distance phone calls, so I could hide how emotional I felt and could choose to present the situation in a confident manner. No one questioned my supposed confidence in my decision. My interpretation of this lack of questioning was that family and friends simply accepted my status as a single woman who would never have children. I did not know how to admit my discomfort with their perceptions, so I acted accepting of their unquestioning support. I did not want to appear to be a sad, desperate, single woman. This is how strongly I believed that I needed to appear successful and independent.

To summarize the first step in my narrative analysis, my decision to have the hysterectomy and the resulting recovery experiences were strongly influenced by all three ideologies. Even though each ideology is described separately, they are all intricately linked together. When faced with the diagnosis of large fibroid tumors, I acted decisively to demonstrate my acceptance and my independence in the situation. The resulting sadness post-surgery made me feel like I had completely deceived myself. Because I could not gain perspective within the situation to identify these underlying ideologies, I could not clearly see and understand all the complicated expectations connected to the symbol of my uterus.

Engaging in "Self-Making"

The second step in my narrative analysis comes from Bruner's (2002, 2004) emphasis on the role of narrative in creating our sense of self. Narrative functions inherently on two levels: (1) systemically, since cultures are shaped by dominant narratives, both in form and function; and (2) individually, since we organize our own lives and experiences in narrative form. Bruner contends that we are shaped culturally, cognitively, and linguistically in ways that directly influence how we tell our life narratives; these forces, in turn, influence how we perceive and organize our experiences: "In the end, we *become* the autobiographical narratives by which we 'tell about' our lives" (Bruner, 2004, p. 694, original emphasis).

We become our own narratives because there is no essential self for us to come to know. Instead, self-making is a constant process of constructing and reconstructing "our selves to meet the needs of the situation we encounter, and we do so with the guidance of our memories of the past and our hopes and fears for the future" (Bruner, 2002, p. 64). The second step in analysis, after identifying the underlying expectations, is to consider how these expectations shape the narrative construction of self. In the next section I will briefly describe two ways in which I narratively constructed myself within the context of the three previous ideologies.

A Marginalized Woman

When the preceding ideologies are combined, the result is an overarching narrative highlighting how I see myself in a marginalized position. I am supposed to have choice with regard to bearing children, but I do not. I am supposed to be in a romantic partnership, but I am not. I am supposed to be successfully independent, but I do not feel that way. All these failures to achieve what I should have or should be demonstrate how my narrative self-concept is that I do not fit into the dominant, "normal" trajectories for these categories.

The strength of this marginalization comes from the strength of the assumptions that marriage and motherhood define being a woman, so there are two identity categories that are troublesome. The first is that I am not married. DePaulo and Morris (2005) overtly state that "adults who are single in contemporary American society are a stigmatized group" and highlight how singles can be targets of social rejection, economic disadvantage, stereotyping, and discrimination (p. 60). In a similar manner, Letherby and Williams (1999) point out how being single increases the feeling of isolation in a couples-dominated world.

Besides my single status, the second problematic identity category is that I cannot bear children. Society simply accepts "the ideology of motherhood as the norm" (Letherby & Williams, 1999, p. 723). As Letherby (2002) explains, "Women without children still represent the 'other' in societies that value children and motherhood" (p. 10). Cultural norms in the United States prescribe procreation for all women; messages to young women indicate they cannot be fulfilled as women without children (Taylor, 2003). Gillespie (2003) also highlights how women who choose to be childfree are seen as "deviant, unfeminine," and as transgressing "traditional models of femininity" (p. 124). Navigating through these two problematic identity categories that highlight a "failed" sense of womanhood result in feelings of marginalization. In this manner, my narrative highlights my construction of self as a marginalized woman.

An Empty Woman
The second narrative construction of self in this analysis is how, for a period of time after the surgery, I defined myself based on what I was lacking: I was lacking a romantic partner, I was lacking my own children, and, most specifically, I was lacking a uterus. During the process of recovery, I learned how strongly symbolic the uterus is. When considering whether to have the hysterectomy, I wanted the decision to be relegated to issues of health—a clinical, medical choice. However, the decision to remove a uterus from a woman's body is connected to so many other elements. Undergoing a hysterectomy can cause women to consider symbolic aspects of their uterus that were previously taken for granted (Elson, 2003). Flory, Bissonnette, and Binik (2005), citing Bachmann (1990), summarize the symbolic meanings of the uterus as "femininity, childbearing, sexuality, strength, vitality, youth, attractiveness, competency, regulation of body processes, and control of the rhythm of life" (p. 126). Because of cultural assumptions about the connection between the uterus and femininity, the lack of a uterus left me, for a while, feeling like I lacked aspects of my femininity and my strength.

While I initially consider my uterus as problematic because it was the source of the tumors, once it was removed, I experienced a sense of loss and emptiness. The removal of my uterus meant a loss of possibilities. I could no longer consider how I might, one day, meet a romantic partner and bear children with him. I could no longer consider what it might be like to carry a life inside of me. I could no longer consider that one day I might feel more connected to the larger community of women by joining them in telling my own pregnancy or delivery stories; my marginalization of being a woman who would never bear children was now finalized. My pregnancy loss was a loss of possibilities before they had a chance to begin. While I initially thought I did not want children, after the surgery all I could see was the emptiness that this loss of possibilities created. In order to recover, I had to acknowledge that sense of emptiness, mourn the loss of my uterus, and dedicate energy to finding ways to redefine myself.

To summarize the second step of analysis, I combined the identification of three underlying ideological expectations to articulate how I created my sense of self as an empty, marginalized woman. Bruner (2002) describes how "the narrative gift seems to be our natural way of using language for characterizing those deviations from the expected state of things that characterize living in a human culture" (p. 85). My concept of self as an empty, marginalized woman came from my self-narratives told to describe my perception of deviating from the expected role of a woman to have children. In this sense, narrative is "irresistible as a way of making sense of human interaction" (Bruner, 2002, p. 85).

Conclusion

My purpose in sharing this difficult time in my life is threefold: first, to give voice to the struggle that one woman experienced during her process of undergoing a hysterectomy; second, to illustrate how Jerome Bruner's concept of narrative provides ways to analyze stories; and third, to provide the opportunity for others to find some aspect of resonance with their own difficult experiences. Bruner (2002) highlights how narrative has the capacity to make the "familiar and the ordinary strange again" (p. 9). Through the reliving of my experience and the resulting analysis, I have been able to identify ways in which I created my sense of self. I was convinced I did not want children, until diagnosed with problematic fibroids. After the surgery, I felt I had deceived myself because of my deep sadness around the loss of my uterus. The deception was that I had fooled myself into believing I did not want children, when actually what I wanted was to have a romantic partnership that provided the possibility to have children if my partner and I wanted them. This analysis demonstrates how much I accepted the culturally communicated ideologies, specifically of romantic partnership, and had internalized them so deeply that I was not able to see beyond their limitations.

If I end here, though, I might give the impression that I still exist in a state of sadness, which is not a proper representation of my entire experience. Even though there may be no concrete ending to my story, a current update is that as I write this chapter, I am four years post-hysterectomy. One year after the surgery, fearing that my sadness was turning into a deeper depression, I began therapy with a kind, patient counselor. While it took time before I could say aloud, "I felt so sad after my hysterectomy," I am now able to share my story. After allowing for physical recovery time, I felt my hormones shift to a better balance. I have been in a romantic relationship for two years now, with a supportive partner who accepts me as I am, with no capacity for pregnancy. I ultimately do not regret the decision to have the hysterectomy, since the resulting life journey, though difficult, allowed me to learn so much about myself and how I create self through my narratives. Bruner (2002) describes how the process of self-making through self-narrative is

> restless and endless, probably more so now than ever before. It is a dialectical process, a balancing act. And despite self-assuring homilies about people never changing, they do. They rebalance their autonomy and their commitments, usually in a way that honors what they were before. (p. 84)

My narrative began when I felt full of tumors and unstable emotions, and described how, for a while, I felt empty and sad after my hysterectomy. Currently, I am learning to fill myself in other ways with life and creativity. I am learning to enjoy this "dialectical process," this "balancing act" of self-making, in ways that honor my previous sadness as well as my hope for what is to come.

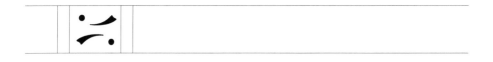

Section 4: Without the Sense of an Ending

14. Melancholy Baby: Time, Emplotment, and Other Notes on Our Miscarriage

JAY BAGLIA

> In reading the ending in the beginning and the beginning in the ending, we also learn to read time itself backwards, as the recapitulation of the initial condition of a course of action in its terminal consequences.
>
> (Ricoeur, 1984, pp. 67–68)

Time tends to be a complicating facet in all stories, whether for scholars or readers-for-pleasure, or for those who are simply entranced and confounded by the inevitabilities and idiosyncrasies of a life lived. Time moves within us and around us. We think back to the past and we think ahead to the future. In this chapter, I evoke past experiences and imagine the future before, during, and after the story of our miscarriage.

In Paul Ricoeur's (1984) ample meditation on time and narrative, he revitalizes Aristotle's concept of emplotment (*muthos*) and explores this anew as the organization of agents and acts within a temporal setting, progressing toward an end. Emplotment mediates—for the audience—between stage one (what Ricoeur calls practical experience, or pre-knowledge) and stage three (from which the recipient of the story must draw conclusions). Ricoeur refers to these three stages as mimesis$_1$, mimesis$_2$, and mimesis$_3$. Mimesis, following Aristotle, is representation. As a mimetic activity, a narrative represents a version of reality. "There is reality," writes James Carey (1989) "and, after the fact, our accounts of it" (p. 20). Because emplotment as mimesis$_2$ serves as a liminal space, what precedes it can't be fully interpreted until the story reaches its end. Ricoeur suggests that "narrative attains its full meaning when it becomes a condition of temporal existence" (p. 52). Such an explanation is surely relevant not only to fiction but also to the many forms of nonfiction (whether referred to as history, personal narrative, autoethnography, or biography). Narratives of chronic illness—and infertility is both diagnosed and treated as a chronic condition—are often absent of what most of us would consider a satisfying ending.

In the process of writing this chapter, I outlined three goals: (1) to retain some of my narrative of our miscarriage as it was originally constructed in the hours and days immediately following the miscarriage (culled from my journal and from email messages to my siblings); (2) to begin not at the beginning; and (3) to foreground my own somatic responses of what I'd like to refer to as episodes within the larger narrative. In so doing I hope to provide a pregnancy loss narrative that draws explicit attention to emplotment generally and temporality specifically.

Miscarriage had been a scholarly interest of mine even before we—that is, my partner and I—experienced it. As someone who teaches and researches health, gender, and the body, I had found miscarriage to be an area almost devoid of qualitative research that concentrated on the male perspective.[1] Once we did experience our miscarriage, I found myself uncertain about what my role was in the grief process, especially when confronted with my perceived responsibility in the arena of providing support.

Cinematically, some of my feelings were epitomized by a minor character in the feature film *Away We Go* (2009), who sees himself both as cheerleader and helpless fellow traveler. Tom (Chris Messina) is married to Munch (Melanie Lynskey); they have experienced five miscarriages without any successes. Tom admits, "People like us we wait till our thirties and then we're surprised when the babies aren't so easy to make anymore and then every day another million fourteen-year-olds get pregnant without trying. It's a terrible feeling, this helplessness, man. You just watch these babies grow and then fade. You don't know if you're supposed to name them, or bury them."

October 2010: Old Friends

We are attending a conference in St. Petersburg, Florida, with our three-month-old daughter, Aria Joy. She is named for our mothers, a combination of their middle names. We sit at the Hurricane Restaurant on Pass-a-Grille Beach, famous for its blackened grouper sandwiches. We are here with Carolyn and Joe, two friends who live in nearby Tampa who drove across the bridge to meet us for lunch. I have known Joe my entire adult life. Carolyn has gone overboard with gifts. Aria won't be able to wear most of these expensive garments for at least a year but I suspect Carolyn has enjoyed the shopping as well as the giving. I make a mental note to pick up the lunch tab. It is an absolutely breathtakingly beautiful October day on the Gulf of Mexico. We enjoy our fresh seafood and cold beer and the discussion moves easily through news about aging parents, home ownership, and future travel plans. Throughout our conversation, Aria sleeps. From inside the Hurricane come sounds of a televised college football game.

Our baby opens her eyes, smiles, and squeaks and Carolyn shifts in her seat and turns her attention to Aria. "You certainly are a pretty girl, so pleasant and good-natured." I take a sip of my beer. "We waited a long time for her," I say. "We weren't sure she'd ever come." Carolyn acknowledges the history of our efforts to have a child. "Joe told me about the miscarriage. When did it happen?" "About a year and a half before Aria was born," I reply. Carolyn turns back to Aria, "You might have had a big brother or a big sister!" I am caught off guard but delighted with Carolyn's inference. She has done what most people have refused to do. Carolyn acknowledges the significance of the loss by asking questions, but also speaks about our loss in the same way we always do about the baby that miscarried. For a time, growing in my partner's body, that baby was a member of our family. In some ways, she or he still is. Someday we will talk to Aria about that pregnancy and that loss.

Friday, September 12, 2008

This was a very sad day for us. We lost the baby at eleven weeks. Elissa had noticed some spotting for several days and had even expressed concern about this to her doctor earlier in the week. It had been an extremely busy week. We were vulnerable. *Vulnerable* has the same etymological root as *vulture*. *Vellere*. "To pluck." "To tear." "To wound." Earlier that week we had hosted a two-day visit by an external evaluation team at the Family Medicine Residency where we were employed as medical educators. This was a series of meetings for which we held all the knowledge, possessed all the expertise, had all the answers. It had been intense. Meanwhile, I had been planning for a two-day faculty retreat scheduled for the following Monday and Tuesday. I would be the facilitator. Facilitate—*facile*—"to make easy." More than five years later, I am uncertain why either of us felt compelled to attend that retreat. We had suffered a significant loss—perhaps the most significant loss of our lives.

Vulnerable. Elissa had left a meeting early on that Friday for her 12:40 appointment with Holly, her primary care physician and our colleague on the faculty in the Department of Family Medicine. Sometime after 2:00, while I was conducting an interview with a job applicant in the School of Nursing lobby, Holly and Elissa came briskly through the lobby, right past me, another colleague, and the applicant, and through the double doors toward the faculty offices. A minute later, Holly appeared back at the double doors, signaling me to come with her. "Didn't you get my page?" She seemed irritated.

"No," I replied. Guilty. I wasn't wearing my pager that day. I excused myself from the interview and joined Holly. When we reached Holly's office there was my life partner, so obviously distraught. Tears streaming, her cheeks brindled, quite fixed in emotional agony. I knew immediately, of course, that something bad had happened but in the microsecond before we moved simultaneously toward each other, I still held out hope that the "bad thing" was something other than the loss of our child.

In my analysis of infertility in the popular press the word *devastate* surfaces constantly. Etymologically, to devastate is "to lay waste completely." From the Latin *vastus*—"empty, *desolate*." And desolare—desolate: "to make lonely completely." In the late fourteenth century—"without companions." By the fifteenth century—"joyless."

Later, Elissa asked me whether I had thought anything might be wrong when she and Holly had come back through the lobby, past the candidate's interview. No. It had not occurred to me that something was wrong. My only thoughts were that they were headed to Holly's office to look something up, some form of helpful information, something to explain, to interpret. I hadn't paid enough attention to the time to realize that there had been an exam in Holly's office and then a visit to the diagnostic lab where it had been determined that our baby was "no longer viable."

"Silence." I said this out loud as Elissa described the absence of movement she had somatically experienced and that the diagnostician had confirmed. "Silence," I remarked. Silent but sincere empathy was the tender expression signaled by her physician. Our friend. Holly.

Holly drove Elissa home that day and waited with her until I got home after canceling my remaining appointments for the day as well as the dinner plans we had with friends. It had been a rainy, cool day—autumn was upon us early in eastern Pennsylvania while the news reported that a hurricane was battering Galveston, Texas. The Major League Baseball pennant race was heating up.

Telling. We had been deliberate about telling some people the news of our pregnancy. We will tell family first, we decided, and then some close friends. Besides Holly and Brian (my physician), Brenna and Heidi were coworkers who also knew. Brenna, being the sly detective that she is, noticed that Elissa was not imbibing one night at the Allentown Brewworks. Brenna, the nurse, knew we'd been trying.

Not many knew how long we had waited to get pregnant and how many disappointments there had been. And yet, with our good news we were surrounded by support. But even among these friends and relations, few knew the whole story, the context that framed the significance of events. Just the night before, I had opened the front door to find a package from Josephine Wise—Elissa's best Australian mate. A necklace of bright green beads. Christine Kiesinger had also sent a necklace—a tiny figurine. Madonna and Child. We received a bonsai from my brother Alan and his wife, Jen. All symbols and sentiments of life and vitality, optimism and good fortune. Grins, hugs, and handshakes from those who we were able to tell in person. Hope springs eternal.

Over the phone, I told my old friends from Tampa—Bill (who has a child): "Yeah!" and Joe (who does not): "Cool." We did not buy into the superstition of waiting for the mark of three months before sharing the news. Now, after our miscarriage, we had to make phone calls of a different nature. Sad news. News for which the only response is—"I'm so very sorry." Or from Joe: "That sucks."

You can get anything you want …. It was sometime back in 2004. I don't remember what I said to Nina the time we went to Alice's Restaurant, in Niederwald, Texas. Alice's was our favorite restaurant near Maxwell, Texas, where we had our first home together. Following our commitment ceremony in 2003, our paradise was a cottage in the middle of a pecan orchard, fifteen minutes from San Marcos, and about forty minutes from Austin. We liked Alice's because Nina, who waited on us (and who also just sort of stood in for the *idea* of Alice), and Walter, the chef (and Nina's partner) always made a big fuss over us. Alice's—where there was always somebody playing guitar really well and where Walter created amazing Texas-themed fare. We were comfortable at Alice's. The last time we'd been in there, Nina was visibly pregnant. And this time it may have been three or four months later—I really don't remember. But Nina wasn't pregnant anymore—or at least she didn't look pregnant. And I just flat out asked her about the baby. "Oh," said Nina quietly, "We lost the baby. I miscarried." I hope I said, "I'm so sorry," but the truth is I don't remember what I said. I remember what I thought. And I know I didn't say anything to Walter.

Melancholy. The sadness one feels for something that cannot quite be named. Mourning is a different experience entirely: I know why I cry for my dead father. Melancholy. Melancholia or, from the Greek, *melankholia*. Sadness. In my Health Communication class I am discussing the roots of modern Western medicine. I explain "balance," the harmony perspective, and the four bodily humours of ancient Greece: sanguine choler, phlegm. And melancholy. Melancholy. An excess of black bile. Just as in Joseph Campbell's (2008) interpretation of the Frog Prince fairy tale, our child, our golden ball, was out of our hands and had disappeared into the black bile swamp of reproductive technology, statistics (not favorable ones), and *New York Times Magazine* stories about dual-career couples and postponed pregnancy. We don't know why we miscarried. And we don't know who this child was. Or would become. What I do know is that I want my love for this child to remain, even if that means that my sadness is perpetual. When a miscarriage occurs, what dies is an unknown future. Melancholy is that sadness for a loss unknown. In the Frog Prince fairy tale, the melancholy experienced by the princess when her golden ball falls into the well represents the loss of her childhood and the inevitability of adolescence that she refuses.

In her essay "Melancholy Gender/Refused Identification," Judith Butler (1995) writes of the bodily ego as gendered ego. We have obligations as gendered bodies. And our bodies, Elissa's and mine, it seems, are in a race against time. Butler writes, "When certain kinds of losses are compelled by a set of culturally prevalent prohibitions, we might expect a prevalent form of melancholy" (p. 27). As a culture we simply don't talk about miscarriage. The social (as well as the academic) prohibition of discussing pregnancy loss is what Rambo Ronai (1997) refers to as discursive "constraint." As a process it is foreclosed. For Butler, "foreclosure" is different from repression. In our culture, this absence of miscarriage in conversation suggests that, as in Butler's use of the term "foreclosure," talk is rigorously barred.

Miscarriage. We miscarried. Whoops! Fumble. "Miscarriage" is a terrible term. Pun intended. We did so love the little life that inhabited Elissa's body. Several weeks earlier, we had been blown away during the visit to the Maternal & Fetal Health Center when we "saw" this little being. Watched and heard its heart beating through the strangeness of the ultrasound. We had imagined the winter months ahead of us as Elissa's tummy would grow and I would spread on the "tummy butter." With the baby due in April, I had worried in advance of Elissa walking through the hospital parking lot and over the prevalent Pennsylvania ice. You will please be careful, I thought to myself. I loved spooning her and holding her stomach, believing that my hands on our baby were delivering the message, "Here is Daddy."

We received an email from Elissa's sister, Jo (so many Joes!). My father was Joe. Good Old Joe. Joey. A baby kangaroo. Jo would be visiting the United States in November from Canberra and was "looking forward to being with you and baby bump." We played "bad news/good news" with our San José friends, Anne Marie and Brian. Bad news: We would not be able to make the trip to Italy in March after all. Good news: Elissa would be delivering in early April. One night I had imagined the sound of our creaking hardwood floors being activated by footsteps other than Elissa's and mine. Obviously I had been able to project this child well into the future.

We had also received a marvelous pregnancy diary in which we were recording the changes to Elissa's body. We read each day's entries to each other including the descriptions of the baby's growth, recommendations about diet, and other useful facts for first-time parents. All these gifts. All these artifacts so lovingly selected. With the miscarriage we wouldn't throw them away but, for now at least—they must be set aside until ... when? We know not for whom we grieve or where we'll go, only that we want to keep on going. How to go on? We sought a grief counselor who would help us create a story of what happened and why. Kiesinger (2002) describes how this kind of reframing is an active reinvention of our life experiences and "permit[s] us to live more fulfilling lives" (p. 107).

So who was that little human? Perhaps letting go of that projection would be a good first step to forging ahead. But we didn't want to forget our first little heartbeat. We had named this growing presence in Elissa's womb "Cheerio" after being told in the pregnancy diary that this was the baby's size at such-and-such a date. And we wanted to remember our Cheerio. And we would keep trying to have a baby. And we wouldn't forget. In what some might depict as yet another kind of well-intentioned but poorly timed platitude, Dr. Holly reminded us at our dining room table a few weeks after the miscarriage that "at least you know you can get pregnant." Some of our other physician colleagues made similarly reductive remarks. "It's common in 25% of all first pregnancies." How is a statistic like that helpful? Knowing that we were able to get pregnant did nothing to minimize the loss of our child. It could be argued that a pregnancy following a miscarriage is widely applauded in our culture because it can mean (for some) the end of grief. Grief, it would seem, is something to be feared. But feared by whom? The grief-stricken or those who must bear witness to the grief? For Judith Butler (2004), fear gives "rise to the impulse to resolve it quickly, to banish it in the name of an action invested with the power to restore the loss or return the world to a former order, or to reinvigorate a fantasy that the world formerly was orderly" (pp. 29–30).

Spring, 2009: Interpreter of Maladies

I become the reader of the tests—the keeper of the keys—the messenger. Both ovulation and pregnancy test readings have fallen to me. In May 2009, eight months after the miscarriage, we are heading to Australia to visit Elissa's family. I am flying to San Francisco from Allentown a day before Elissa, who is coming from a conference in Illinois. We will be staying at my cousin Claudia's house in San Carlos before flying to Brisbane. Elissa calls me from the conference. "I think I might be pregnant," she divulges. "When can we test?" I inquire. "We'll test when I get to San Francisco." I tell Claudia, "She thinks she might be pregnant." Claudia grins her huge grin. Elissa isn't in the door fifteen minutes before she goes into the bathroom to, as she puts it, "pee on a stick." We sequester ourselves in a guest room. Elissa hands me the stick. I move toward a window to read it, holding it up to the late afternoon California sunlight.

NOT PREGNANT

I reveal this result to Elissa. Her face falls. "I really thought I was." I am wordless. I wanted so much to be able to deliver good news.

Late Summer, 2009

We still haven't gotten pregnant. Yet. And, in all seriousness, it's not "fun try-ing" as so many people like to suggest. At our monthly meeting with Virginia, our grief counselor, I declare, confidently, "We *will* parent." We are now in the realm of the IUI procedure. To maximize our chances we wait for ovu-lation; when that occurs, we make a same-day appointment and sit in the waiting room while the "active ingredient" is defrosted. We are then ushered into the procedure room while a nurse—some with skill and some without—employs the speculum, locates the cervix, and injects the sperm. It is an op-portunity for closeness; I position myself at the other end of the action and stroke Elissa's face as we begin the process of waiting and hoping. I would be hard pressed to call this "fun."

Liminal space has become important for us. For every ovulation there is a procedure. And for every procedure there is possibility. The two weeks of lim-inal space that exists between the ovulation, the IUI, and a pregnancy test is loaded with optimism. Both Dr. Holly and the reproductive endocrinologist are hopeful. And so are we. I remember delivering an earlier version of this miscarriage narrative at a conference and concluding my presentation with the admission: "We are in liminal space right now."

Saturday, September 13, 2008

I don't think either one of us could have predicted the pain that Elissa experi-enced the next day during the "expulsion." This is the word used to describe what happens when the baby's tissue is expelled from the body. I wasn't there when this happened. I wasn't there. When I woke that Saturday morning I went immediately to the gym and then, later, to the record store. I was gone for almost four hours. I almost never check my cell phone for messages. At an independent record store in Bethlehem, I purchased Eddie Vedder's (2007) soundtrack for *Into the Wild*.

> *Such is the passage of time/Too fast to fold*
> *Suddenly swallowed by signs/Lo and behold*

Mandolin in a minor key. Haunting. Melancholy. And so I wasn't there for her when the pain came, and the fear, and the blood, and the expulsion. I told an aunt about this. My no-nonsense aunt who then told me about her miscarriage. New York City in the 1960s. How my uncle wasn't there. And how she never forgave him. But Brenna was there—lovely Brenna. A home-care nurse, Elissa called Brenna when I couldn't be found and she came. Straightaway. I am so grateful to Brenna. My physical absence resulted from another absence: the absence of knowledge about what would happen. I blame myself for not knowing I should have known to ask but I also blame the institution of health and medicine for not knowing to tell me, to tell us, what we might expect.

September 2008: Ritual

We needed a ritual. So with a beautifully landscaped garden as a feature of our home, we took the bonsai plant and its arboreal symbolic smallness and with some quiet words and physical closeness, buried the plant along with the tissue from Elissa's body—the products of conception—in a corner by the garden gate. The ground is already dry and cold this time of year in eastern Pennsylvania. Dried leaves. Earth. Autumn. Melancholy. Greek mythology. Demeter searching for her daughter, Persephone. You remember the myth: One moment Persephone was there. And then she wasn't. Nobody can tell Demeter why.

It isn't fair, we sobbed to each other that first night in our tight embrace after we finally made our way to bed. Our bed. In our stylish 1930s home in Allentown's west end that everyone says is so cool. When we found out we were pregnant, Elissa had managed to convince me that I should give up a vice and I agreed to give up alcohol. On that night of our miscarriage, I consumed my first glass of red wine in almost three months. And then we both fell asleep on the couch. Despite being annoyed by the staleness of the television sounds, we had just not yet been willing to call it a night. Did we think by staying up late we could change the results? No. But I do think we wondered whether there were answers to be found by waiting out the day.

I am jealous of all the pregnancies around us. Only one friend who, along with her husband, suffered five years of miscarriages *deserves* her pregnancy.

That's a sentiment you might find shocking. I am shocked by it myself. I'm ashamed of this and yet I did feel it even though I know it's wrong.

And I'm angry at my family, our families. For calling us within days of the anniversary of our miscarriage to tell us that one of my brothers and his partner were four months pregnant. Whoopee. I'm ashamed of this and yet I do feel it even though I know it's wrong. And still later in that same month, my brother-in-law and his wife called to tell us they are pregnant with their fourth. We don't care.

A lesson for the culture wars. Eleven weeks. This was a baby because we loved it and because we were ready for it. We grieve the loss of this child because we planned for this child. Feeling this profound agony with the loss of our eleven-week-old embryo is not fuel for the Anti-Choice crowd, or an admission that "life begins at conception." This was a "baby" because we named her … him … so. "We are having a baby" is a much different condition from "I am pregnant." I have been asked more than once whether experiencing a miscarriage resulted in a change in my Pro-Choice stance. I find this to be a rather peculiar question. And the answer is "No."

February 7, 2010 (Super Bowl Sunday)

Liminal Space … filled. So we did get pregnant … again. And we are four months pregnant. It took us fourteen months to get pregnant again. I type "fourteen months later" and I'm struck by how effortlessly fourteen months seems to fly by in narrative time. But nothing flew by. Time dragged before—finally—success. And yet here's how precarious it can be. Friday night and most of Saturday it had snowed. So much, in fact, that I went skiing at nearby Blue Mountain. An excellent day of physical activity followed by a night out at the movies. After pizza at a local favorite of ours, we saw Colin Firth in *A Single Man* at the 19th Street Theatre. Sunday morning we made love and, while Elissa dozed for another hour, I practiced for my guitar lesson and soon it was time to go to church. At church we disclosed the news of our pregnancy to Anne (the volunteer coordinator) and the pastor, Reverend Kidd.

Back at home we sent out our Valentine's Day Party invitations via email. Elissa was tired and went upstairs to take a nap. I talked to my brother Alan on the phone and he shared the news with me that he and Jen were five weeks pregnant. Elissa suddenly appeared before me. She was clearly upset.

I hurried Alan off the phone. "I'm spotting," she confessed. We called Holly. After about ten minutes, she called us back. We explained the circumstances. She asked us to give her about thirty minutes and we could meet her at the Family Health Center (FHC). In the meantime, she asked Elissa to drink something sweet and cold in order to stir the baby. We were quite nervous. Elissa asked me whether I was scared. Not scared, I said, but worried. At the FHC, we waited in the car for Holly who soon appeared. We went into the FHC and within minutes Elissa was on her back with Holly spreading ultrasound lubricant on her eighteen-week pregnant belly. After a few short seconds of uncertainty, Holly found the heartbeat. And we cried with joy.

In March, we went on a "babymoon" to Key West. Everybody smiled as I strolled the sidewalks with my visibly pregnant partner. On a three-hour boat ride out to the Dry Tortugas, Elissa lost an enormous breakfast of fruit to seasickness. Earlier in this pregnancy both Holly and Brian had unapologetically displayed relief (even smiles and high fives) as Elissa experienced month after month of morning sickness. Evidently, morning sickness can be a sign of a healthy pregnancy.

Today

Aria Joy Foster Baglia was born on July 7, 2010, after a thirty-hour labor. In October 2010 Aria attended her first academic conference in St. Petersburg, Florida, where this chapter opens and the same conference at which I had presented a version of this miscarriage narrative a year earlier in Los Angeles. In August 2012 we moved from Allentown to Chicago with our two-year-old. By then, we had been trying to get pregnant again for almost a year via the IUI procedure with no success. This means we are categorized as having "secondary infertility." We had decided that IVF was not something we were willing to undergo. At a fertility clinic in a Chicago suburb I can feel pressure from the endocrinologist as she begins to pitch IVF to us. "I'm worried about the stress to Elissa's body from IVF," I begin, "along with the side effects." From behind her large oak desk and with a half dozen degrees framed behind her, the endocrinologist, Dr. Davi, wears a funny smile. "What side effects?" she inquires. "You tell me," I reply. We had been here before with medical professionals who seemed to embrace the procedure rather than the people.[2] Dr. Davi didn't answer my question. Instead, she says, "I love IVF!" Who *loves* IVF?

Months later, after the decision was made to abandon medically assisted reproductive efforts (and yet it sounds so sexy!), Elissa had her initial appointment with a new primary care physician who informed her that she should begin screening for breast cancer as a result of taking Clomid and other hormone therapies. I would call that a side effect.

In July 2013, Elissa and I celebrated the tenth anniversary of our commitment ceremony and the advances made by the Marriage Equality movement by getting married. Of course, having our three-year-old daughter in attendance was poignant and significant. At three and a half years old, our daughter began asking us regularly for a little brother or a little sister. And sometimes for a big sister. We tell her that "anything can happen" but we have—I think—come to terms (!) with the fact that our child will likely be an only child. Something else happened as a result of our having experienced both a miscarriage and infertility: I am always on the lookout for the vulnerability of others. I am aware that when we are in the public sphere (whether at the airport or the beach, a restaurant, or on Facebook) there are would-be parents who are looking on at our happiness (I have posted hundreds of pictures of our daughter on the social network site), having suffered a miscarriage or, perhaps, experiencing their own frustrations with fertility.

We are so proud of our daughter who runs and yells and sings and talks a blue streak. We feel so lucky. And we do miss our Cheerio.

* * *

"The world unfolded by every narrative work," writes Paul Ricoeur (1984), "is always a temporal world (p. 3). Ricoeur (1980) suggests that narratives can present this temporality in two dimensions. There is the episodic dimension, which depicts the story as composed of pieces, of events; and there is the configurational dimension, which superimposes—from these episodic moments—"a sense of an ending" (p. 179). But to return briefly to Judith Butler and her explanation for how melancholy occurs as a result of foreclosure, the pregnancy loss narrative has no ending.

When I recount the episodes of our miscarriage and infertility, I intend to make sense both of the liminal space between events as well as those events that have not yet revealed themselves. As phenomena, miscarriage and infertility contain both episodic (micro) and configurational (macro) forms of temporality. Returning to the threefold aspect of mimesis, with emplotment (as mimesis$_2$) serving as the transitional space between practical experience and conclusion, the micro moment of miscarriage (when a woman is "having" a miscarriage) is always experienced through a macro lens of a life story. In our case, our life story—our relationship story—includes our choice to live as an unmarried, heterosexual couple, our struggle to get pregnant, as well as our ages as first-time, would-be parents (and particularly, from the perspective of reproductive endocrinology, Elissa's "advanced maternal age"). If we look at infertility (which becomes the diagnosis when a miscarriage occurs for a woman older than age thirty-five) and our particularized IUI remedy, then the micro moments multiply. There is the micro moment of the ovulation test, followed by the micro moment of attempted insemination through the

IUI procedure, followed by the pregnancy test. Each of these micro, episodic moments contains all three of Ricoeur's distinctions of mimesis. The decision to try the IUI procedure follows the positive ovulation test. When compared with the minutes of liminal space that exist between the decision to undertake an ovulation test and discovering its result, the liminal space that the IUI procedure generates is substantial. Nevertheless, each micro moment offered us possibility; each and every ovulation and pregnancy test offered us a glimpse at what we perceived to be our future as parents. And, just as frequently, each time those tests indicated a negative result, I would wonder (present) about why we hadn't started trying to get pregnant sooner (past) and what we would have to do next (future).

Ricoeur's (1984) use of emplotment, however, is more concerned with the macro level. How a story is temporally ordered is what both defines emplotment and, arguably, produces the effect in/for the audience as they consider the story as a whole. For the storyteller of a pregnancy loss narrative, the loss is a disruption. The life story is disrupted. Etymologically, *disrupt* means "to break into pieces, to shatter." And so the meaning of disruption here (as well as in many examples of what Arthur Frank terms quest narratives) is two-fold. For Frank (1995/2013), "the present is not what the past is supposed to lead to, and whatever future will follow this present is contingent" (p. 60). Both this contingency and the episodes that reveal what the past was supposed to lead to (but doesn't) are broken into pieces, each piece a possibility drawn from myriad choices. For the teller, any chronologically imposed order for storytelling (and the one that is generally represented by the patient's medical chart) is usually rejected in favor of a series of episodes that makes sense, even if this sense-making stops short of providing for the audience the sense of an ending.

Notes

1. See Fairchild and Arrington (2012), Murphy (1998), and Puddifoot and Johnson (1997) for excellent qualitative analyses of men who have experienced miscarriage.
2. See Foster (2010), "My Eyes Cry Without Me."

15. Dying Inside of Me: Unexplained Recurrent Early Pregnancy Loss

Jennifer Morey Hawkins

> People who have had losses may find comfort or validation from hearing how
> another person has reacted to and dealt with a similar loss.
>
> (Baddeley & Singer, 2009, p. 206)

Telling one's personal narrative allows an individual to make "sense of embodied
disruptions" and create "new normals" (Harter, Patterson, & Gerbensky-Kerber,
2010, p. 467). Personal narrative offers alternative insights into what occurs in
the world (Harter, 2009) and includes understanding the patient's perspective
beyond the confines of biomedicine (Harter & Bochner, 2009). Reading personal narrative provides a window through which to view another's experiences
(Riessman, 2002). According to Riessman, narrative exists as a unit of discourse
in which derivation of meaning occurs and subsequent experiences may continue
to shape the story's meaning. Individuals are drawn to "narrativize particular
experiences in their lives, often when there has been a breach between ideal and
real, self and society" (Riessman, 1993, p. 3). This chapter provides a window
into my personal narrative of unexplained recurrent early pregnancy loss, a story
that challenges societal ideals of what to expect when expecting. The telling and
retelling of my story shapes my understanding of my normal. Personal reactions
to ways the world addresses early pregnancy loss and insights regarding experiences of grief, uncertainty, and coping are presented. Theoretical constructs from
communication and uncertainty management (Brashers, 2001, 2007; Brashers,
Neidig, & Goldsmith, 2000) provide me a conceptual framework by which to
understand how my uncertainty is navigated, coped with, and understood.

Loss #1: On the Way to Fetus but Stopped at Embryo

I emerged from my pale pink bathroom filled with excitement over the early
pregnancy test results. Thoughts reeled through my mind as I was on the way

to tell my husband, Alex. Would the child look like Alex, tall and slender with brown hair and almond-colored eyes? Or would the child look like me, short, average build, blonde hair, and blue eyes? When I showed Alex the evidence on the plastic test stick, he stood rigid as if lightning had struck. "Wow," he responded as the surge of shock regarding the path to parenthood flashed through him. I needed us both on board for the baby and inquired, "You want this too, right?" "Of course!" he confirmed. His frame softened and intense kindness and understanding radiated from his big beautiful eyes. Full of joy and excited to tell others, I asked him, "Can I tell friends and family?" Smiling, Alex replied, "Certainly."

People reacted joyfully to the news heard via phone. Girlfriends with children: "How exciting!" "If you have questions, don't hesitate to ask." "When's the due date?" I calculated the time since my last period with my fingers. "Thanksgiving," I replied. My mind and mouth exploded with questions when speaking with my close friend, Rina. "What fish do I avoid eating? What about cheeses? I don't want to harm the baby." My best friend with no children, Lynne, shared my excitement. "I'll live vicariously through you. Share everything!" Our parents reacted positively too. With solid jobs, a beautiful rental home in Newberg, Oregon, and a little extension of us on the way, the world was operating in our favor.

A tiny voice in the back of my brain interrupted my "living the dream" attitude, whispering, "Be careful, many women miscarry during their first pregnancy." I heeded the warning and stopped spreading the news.

***

At the sixth week of pregnancy, I wiped myself after I urinated and a pale pink viscous substance appeared on the toilet paper. "Oh my God. I'm miscarrying," I thought. My body felt numb, numb like a pinched nerve. There would be no child. I knew. I just did. I called the nurse at my OB/GYN to report the pink substance I discovered. She attempted to reassure me, "This can happen during pregnancy. Don't worry. Often a little spotting or bleeding occurs during early pregnancy. Could be blood left over from implantation." I expected leftover blood to look dark brown. Yet, I thought if this were serious, I would have more blood. I rationalized the pale pink substance indicated a slow leak. No more healthy pregnancy. Over. Although supportive and hopeful words came from the nurse, pink indicated an end to my pregnancy. No explanation exists for how I knew. I just knew. Sporadic visits from the pale pink substance continued. When no pink existed I wanted to believe the nurse. "Blood left over from implantation." But the pink returned the morning of my eight-week ultrasound appointment.

Prior to my ultrasound with Dr. Giani, my OB/GYN, I attended a mandatory pregnancy information session designed for newly pregnant patients. I checked in for my appointment, and received a gigantic four-inch binder. The binder held information regarding pregnancy issues, choices, prenatal testing, what to eat, and what to avoid. The baby photo adorning the cover of the binder upset me. I doubted I'd have an adorable baby face smiling at me in less than nine months. Cynical, I did not want to attend the pregnancy information session. I knew I was miscarrying.

I endured listening to the information session while sitting in a small caramel- and tan-colored conference room with four other newly pregnant women. Only the nurse spoke. We sat quietly, listened, and referred to our information binders. Toward the end of the session, the nurse asked, "Are there any questions?" Silence. "Am I miscarrying?" I inquired. "I've been wiping and seeing pale pink off and on recently." No other woman spoke. I did not look at them. I concentrated on the nurse who provided a similar scripted response of hope heard previously, "Spotting in early pregnancy is often normal. Don't get upset. Today you'll know more when you see your doctor." I felt inappropriate for daring to ask the question in front of pregnant women. Yet, I needed confirmation of what I already knew. That need circumvented the need to demonstrate socially acceptable behavior. Me: the only one in the room experiencing a miscarriage. I did not want others experiencing issues. But, why me? Why … ?

"Are you sure of the conception date?" Dr. Giani inquired after viewing the ultrasound images. "Yes. I recorded it on my calendar." He looked at me sincerely, placed his hand on my arm, and confirmation of loss began. "Well, the heartbeat is eighty to eighty-five beats per minute, which may be fine if conception had occurred six weeks ago. Your conception date puts you at eight weeks today. I'm sorry to tell you, your pregnancy appears non-viable. The embryo didn't develop normally beyond six weeks." Is my baby the runt of the litter? Was something wrong? I wondered, but did not voice. Seconds later I understood and asked, "Am I losing this pregnancy?" "Yes," Dr. Giani confirmed. I listened as he provided choices. "You may experience the miscarriage naturally, within a week or two. Or I can prescribe Misoprostol. The medication taken vaginally induces miscarriage." To avoid surprise disruptions to my normal routine, I opted for Misoprostol.

The next day, Alex set up the blowup bed in front of the TV in our living room to allow me to attempt to relax while I experienced the inevitable. Together we placed clean white sheets adorned with pink roses on the bed and pillows, and topped the bed with a feather comforter housed in a red floral duvet. We closed the drapes and created a cave-like space. I had no idea what was to come. Alex went to work. I administered the pill vaginally and waited. I recalled Dr. Giani's instructions: "If you experience heavy bleeding beyond a thick pad per hour, contact me." Nothing happened.

Suddenly, a warming sensation in my lower abdomen urged me to get up. I walked into my tiny, pale pink bathroom, where the pregnancy test confirmed the pregnancy, and where I first saw the pale pink substance. When I sat down on the toilet a tide of blood came. Patiently I sat until the blood flow subsided. Knowing I protected my underwear with thick pads, I stood up after I wiped. Curious, I turned around and looked. Red blood surrounded the toilet bowl as if painted in swirls by the toilet bowl brush. Thankful for the containment of the massacre in that tiny toilet bowl, I bent over and looked more closely. No identifiable items existed in the bowl, just a few blood clots. Upon flushing I watched shades of red swirl and disappear into the pipes.

I returned to the blowup bed. An overwhelming sensation of my connection to women who had experienced pregnancy loss throughout history provided me comfort. I was not alone. After all, miscarriage is common. I could only imagine women living in times of less medication and less understanding of early pregnancy loss. When bleeding slowed to that of a regular period, the book *The Clan of the Cave Bear* came to mind. I had read it as a child and I recalled that people in it feared the powers believed to exist in menstrual blood and banished women from the clan during menstrual times. "I will be okay. This will be over soon," I said to myself. If prehistoric women handled being alone, I could get through April 20, 2006, alone. This shit happens. Thoughts of connecting to women throughout history provided me a sense of strength that helped me through that day. I cannot explain why thoughts of those women calmed me; it was as if those women were with me. I was not alone.

With my birthday two days away, I received a plush, pale pink robe in the mail. The note from my sister-in-law said, "I wish I were there to wrap my arms around you. I hope this provides comfort in my absence." The timing of the gift was impeccable.

***

I chose the option for assisting the loss, the medication, to control what I could amidst the uncertainty of the experience. I held no interest in the "wait and see" option. After that loss, I never thought I might experience another early pregnancy loss.

A second miscarriage occurred later that fall, followed by a chemical pregnancy a few months later. I call chemical pregnancies "near misses." One day the home test showed positive, the next day or so later menstruation began. Our silence intensified with each loss. Although unwelcomed, the third loss provided the argument for insurance to cover genetic testing, which Dr. Giani recommended. The test results provided no explanation for our losses. Therefore, as we continued forward into the unknown, we cautiously hoped for the best.

***

The uncertainty felt like riding a seesaw up and down. Uncertainty compounded the grief of early pregnancy loss. Lack of explanation for the losses and lack of knowledge regarding the potential of future pregnancies added an element of anxiety to thoughts of conceiving again. Sometimes the uncertainty swung up to continued thoughts of positivity and optimism (Brashers, 2001). Then the seesaw of uncertainty swung back down again. In a society with such great medical knowledge, the lack of explanation for early pregnancy loss frustrated us. When family, friends, or medical personnel told me I was not to blame, understanding the reasoning behind my losses proved difficult (Frost, Bradley, Garcia, Levitas, & Smith, 2007). Some couples remain silent about loss, protecting their intentions of bringing a child into the world from becoming public knowledge (Adolfsson, Bertero, Larsson, & Wijma, 2004). Silence was one way we coped with the situation. After undergoing multiple unexplained losses, avoidance of publicly talking about the topic of children made life simpler.

Loss #4: The One That Got Stuck

One cold January night in Wisconsin I awoke screaming because of a horrible piercing pain in my lower right abdomen. I sat straight up in bed and felt the pain radiating from a focal point on my right side. Was the pain radiating from an ovary or my appendix? A few weeks earlier a pregnancy test result showed a positive result, so I assumed the former. I told Alex, "I'm experiencing an ectopic pregnancy." I left a message on my OB/GYN's emergency line, and Dr. Frederickson promptly called me back and advised it was too early to confirm an ectopic pregnancy. "We will not know until you're eight or nine weeks pregnant. Take Tylenol and use a heating pad for the pain."

At work the next day I confided in my colleague, Sandy, who looked out for me as if she were my mother. She would be helpful should an issue occur while at work. Two days later I felt sharp pains in my abdomen as I sat at my desk in my office next to Sandy's. I took two Tylenol and focused on my work. More pain. Pain worse than cramps. I ingested two more Tylenol.

Pain. Pain. Pain. "Have you taken Tylenol?" the doctor asked when I called. "Yes, and it doesn't touch the pain!" I exclaimed. "Get to the ER," he ordered. Doubled over I walked into Sandy's office, "Sandy, the doctor said 'get to the ER.' I don't want anyone to know I'm pregnant. I'll tell Collin I think it's my appendix." Collin, the assistant dean, drove Sandy and me to the nearest ER under the guise of my story. "Shit! This hurts!" I exclaimed. Cognizant of my volume and language I apologized to my colleagues. "No need to apologize," Collin replied. Clenching my teeth in response to pain, a muffled "Shit, shit, shit, shit, shit" escaped. When I checked in at the ER, Sandy remained at my side while Collin waited at a distance per my request. As I headed in to see the doctor, I told Collin and Sandy to return to work. I would contact Alex.

Unbearable pain replaced patience. Unable to stick a vein to determine my blood type prior to giving me pain medication, I snapped, "O negative, my blood type is O negative! I need a painkiller, please! I'm in PAIN!" My nurse—who looked like the stereotypical beautiful young, thin, blonde, sweet nurse—appeared apathetic. Left alone without any medication for pain, a calm came over my body, almost a tingling. Overwhelmed by pain, the receptors in my brain shut down to protect me. I called Alex. He could not leave the first day of his spring semester in graduate school. I called Ann, a friend who experienced loss, and asked her to talk with me while I waited for a doctor. She lovingly obliged.

Pain pills were administered, then I was whisked off through the ER halls to ultrasound. Disallowed to say anything, the grim look on the sonographer's face said enough. Brought back to my original ER room, I waited alone for the doctor to deliver my results. He said, "You're having a miscarriage. I saw the bleeding. Go home. It'll be over soon." This was NOT a miscarriage, I thought as I watched the doctor leave. Why would no one listen? I told the ER staff, doctors, and nurses I previously experienced symptoms similar to ectopic pregnancy but my OB/GYN told me he could not confirm whether it was an ectopic until later. I was frustrated.

The next day I went for a blood draw to determine my human chorionic gonadotropin (HCG) levels. The amount of hormone, produced after conception, indicates successful progression of early pregnancy by doubling every other day. Results from blood draws taken every other day indicated increasing, although not doubling, HCG levels. Dr. Fredrickson's nurse reported, "Well today they're 800." I'd respond, "Well that's not good! It should be 875." She'd reply, "We cannot confirm an unhealthy pregnancy." Each time I called for results her positivity annoyed me more. Things were not okay. Why wouldn't she say, "Yeah, this sucks. You're probably experiencing an ectopic pregnancy"? The fact that my HCG numbers increased just short of a healthy pregnancy, coupled with sharp pains on my lower right side led Dr. Frederickson to believe the pregnancy was ectopic. However, ectopic pregnancy would not appear on an ultrasound until week eight or nine. All I could do was wait and take Tylenol for pain relief.

At week eight, the HCG numbers appeared less than expected for a healthy pregnancy. The nurse confirmed the ectopic pregnancy. "You may elect to have surgery or take Methotrexate to end the pregnancy." "What does Methotrexate do? What is it?" I inquired. The nurse explained, "Methotrexate is a drug often used for cancer. It kills living cells. Methotrexate may work and it may not. If not, we would do surgery. We'd know within a week whether the medication had worked. The surgery is laparoscopic. The surgeon creates a small incision in your belly button and on your right side." I attempted to determine the best option for rapid recovery. "I have a conference next week. If I have emergency surgery tomorrow, will I recover by next week?" "It depends on how your body heals. I'll leave you two alone to discuss this, " she replied. A tear escaped my eye. Alex embraced me while we discussed our options in private. "Alex, I don't think I want a drug meant to fight cancer in me. I'd rather have the surgery and be sure it's over." Alex agreed. "I don't want you to take chemicals either." We heard a knock on the door and Dr. Nirav, a colleague of Dr. Frederickson's, entered. Dr. Nirav said gently, "Dr. Frederickson's out of the country, knows your situation, and asked me to perform the surgery." Dr. Nirav provided us our options and asked whether we had questions. "Will the fallopian tube be removed?" I asked. Dr. Nirav replied, "No. We try to keep your fallopian tube intact." I responded, "I don't want the tube." My history of multiple miscarriages already placed me at high risk for future miscarriages. I did not want to worry about a heightened chance of ectopic pregnancy due to a potential tubal defect. "I want one less thing to worry about if I get pregnant again," I told the doctor. The doctor replied, "We do everything we can to keep the fallopian tube. We cannot be sure this was caused by a defect located in the tube." We scheduled the emergency surgery for the next morning.

Once home, I called my parents and told them of my impending surgery. "Why didn't you tell us you were pregnant again?" Mom asked. "I had enough stress. I didn't want to cause anyone stress. We had no idea what was happening. We just found out today about tomorrow's emergency surgery," I reported in a calm matter-of-fact manner. I wanted her to know I'd be okay. "Can we come to the hospital tomorrow?" She asked. "Of course. It'd be good for Alex to have company." That night I was very worried the ectopic might rupture prior to surgery and kill me but I did not want to alarm my mother, so I said nothing. Dr. Frederickson had told me all along that ectopic pregnancies could become very dangerous if not properly monitored and treated. The rapidly scheduled surgery indicated a serious situation.

The next morning in a pre-surgery holding area with a curtain drawn around my hospital bed for privacy, I was thankful that I had made it to the hospital without an ectopic explosion. The serious threat to my own health made me less concerned for the life that might have been. I was more concerned with eliminating anything that could threaten my life. Although Dr. Nirav was not Dr. Frederickson, I trusted any member of that team with my life. I was in good hands. I would be okay.

***

Post-surgery, Dr. Nirav provided a detailed report. Standing close to my bed he asked, "How are you?" "Doing okay," I responded. He handed me a thick, shiny piece of paper with pictures of the surgery. Dr. Nirav continued, "We successfully found and removed the ectopic pregnancy. However, cauterization was performed and did not stop the bleeding so the right fallopian tube had to be removed." Relieved I responded, "Thank you Doctor, I understand." While I looked at the pictures I noticed red dots resembling bloodstains spattered over the page. The ink on the printer must have been on the fritz? Some photos included the surgery utensils used to complete the task. I focused on the photo of the ectopic. A thin line of reddish fleshy tube displayed a bubble suspended in the middle stretching the limits of the tube's walls so far the tiny capillaries covering the bubble looked ready to burst. These pictures provided the reason for my current and past physical pain. Imagine a peanut trying to squeeze through a shaft of hair. Alex and I call it "the one that got stuck."

Hopped up on painkillers the day after surgery, I looked down and observed that my pale white belly appeared black, blue, and purple. Home alone and horrified something went wrong I called the nurse's line and she explained, "Bruising is normal due to the surgery." I was probably told this would happen but was so drugged up at the time I did not remember. Although relieved that the culprit that caught this pregnancy, my right fallopian tube, was removed … I felt invaded. Instruments went into my body to extract an item that could have killed me. My right fallopian tube and pregnancy were taken from my core. Viewing my bruised belly somehow made what modern surgery accomplished with virtually no scarring very real. Although not physically scarred, I was emotionally scarred, but I had yet to discover that. It all had happened so fast. I don't know how anyone could tell another what to expect in the aftermath of this type of experience.

***

During my week of recovery, supportive acts of kindness surrounded me and brought warmth to the cold February of 2007. Alex cut up fresh vegetables and left other foods on the top shelf inside the fridge before going to work so that I would need to exert only minimal movement in my midsection to reach the food. One day a gorgeous arrangement of white and yellow flowers placed in a white, woven wooden basket arrived, sent from my colleagues. Cards and additional gift baskets arrived from my parents and in-laws. Another day, my best friend, Lynne, visited and brought me a delicious Italian sandwich and food for Alex. She sat with me on our purple couch in our front room while I went in and out of consciousness as we watched the movie *Ratatouille*. Her visit provided the break Alex needed from the stress of the situation and taking care of me. I welcomed the care of a supportive female friend. The responses from my family, friends, and colleagues that week made life after ectopic surgery more bearable and reaffirmed my decision to confide in a select few about the pregnancy.

***

Frustration regarding the lack of explanation or understanding behind why loss occurs increases among women who experience multiple miscarriages and/or ectopic pregnancies. The idea of loss being a random chance begins to wane when the experience continually occurs (Maker & Ogden, 2003).

Loss #7: Another "Near Miss"

The summer of 2010 I was enrolled in a Woman's Developmental Health course offered through Nursing. My professor approved my final paper topic: early pregnancy loss. A few weeks later I tested positive for pregnancy. "Really? You've got to be kidding me!" I said to myself. No, I wasn't using birth control. I welcomed pregnancy. But with only one tube, and my increasing age, I had doubted I'd get pregnant. I was dumbfounded, excited, and freaked out all at once. Sheer joy of pregnancy was a thing of the past. After all the unexplained losses, I felt more like an experimental test kitchen than a woman who would hold a baby in her arms in nine months. Ugh! How was I supposed to write a paper on loss now that I was pregnant? I called Lynne and told her I was pregnant again. "I know you're going to be there for me no matter what. You may as well know now," I said. She was a confidante I could call at any time whether the news was good, bad, or indifferent. She never passed judgment and always listened.

***

My HCG levels doubled every other day. That was good. Was this my seventh pregnancy? After a few chemical pregnancies I preferred to forget. It didn't help to focus on all the losses. Each new pregnancy offered a new possibility. After so many losses, I really saw pregnancy less and less as a possibility of anything but yet another loss. History kept repeating itself. Prior to writing the paper for my nursing course, I had intentionally forgotten how many losses I had had to avoid the "distressing certainty" (Brashers, 2001) that the large number of losses provided. I chose to remain uncertain. I was reminded.

***

According to Brashers's discussion of uncertainty management theory, individuals "learn to live with chronic uncertainty" (2007, p. 232) by accepting and adapting to the situation. In my case of unexplained recurrent early pregnancy loss, no answer existed. No evidence to explain why. No prediction regarding future ability or inability to give birth to a child. With each new pregnancy all we could do was hope. People would ask, "How did you two get through it?" Our only option was to manage uncertainty by accepting our situation as *our* normal and then adapting. Help from supportive others assisted.

***

The day after receiving a positive pregnancy test result, the articles I read for my final paper provided me information that assisted me in understanding that I had trivialized my early losses. One article by Lasker and Toedter (2003), "The Impact of Ectopic Pregnancy: A 16-Year Follow-Up Study," brought a flood of tears. Pain released when I read that grief levels for women experiencing ectopic pregnancy were similar to grief levels of women who had later miscarriages and/or stillbirths. This information gave me permission to mourn. Pain locked up within the depths of me suddenly was freed. And I cried and I cried ... and I cried. I understood and felt the significance of all my losses. My sadness surrounding "the one that got stuck" overwhelmed me. I cried for that ectopic loss. Why did it get stuck? What if that had been *the one* that would have been okay? We would never know. We had to live our lives never knowing whether the "one that got stuck" would have been okay. My heart was heavy.

From that point forward I knew I would be open to tears that might appear for no reason. I was not going to be ashamed or afraid of grief sneaking up on me.

***

Pregnancy loss is complicated because of the wide range of meanings people attribute to the pregnancy itself (Corbet-Owen, 2003). These meanings may be socially and/or individually constructed (Corbet-Owen & Kruger, 2001). Often, at the societal level "miscarriage is seen as a private, minor event in a woman's life, which entails a short visit to a hospital, full recovery and the expectation of a successful pregnancy afterwards" (Conway & Russell, 2000, p. 531). Practical, tangible, symbolic representations of the loss of an unborn child remain uncommon in our society. To many, miscarriage is a representation of the loss of a potential person: the loss of memories to be created versus memories that exist (Layne, 1997). Therefore, some reason the grief and loss that exists is in response to potential hopes for the future that have been halted. Yet, just as grief may be experienced differently in times of other significant loss, there exists an array of grief experiences that may occur after experiencing miscarriage (Brier, 2008; Lasker & Lin, 1996). Descriptions of grief in early pregnancy loss resemble descriptions of other significant losses and include "yearning, sadness, crying, fatigue, appetite and sleep changes, preoccupation with the loss, and guilt" (Brier, 2008, p. 454).

The meanings people attribute to the pregnancy may greatly impact coping, as can the number of prior losses (Black, 1991). The trivialization of losses because of the early nature of my losses allowed me to buy into the societal belief of miscarriage as "not that big a deal," especially with the chemical pregnancies. Reading the Lasker and Toedter (2003) article allowed for validation. My deep understanding of the emotional impact of the ectopic loss happened as a result of reading that article. In the privacy of my own home, alone with my journal articles obtained for my research paper, the possibility of recognizing and validating my losses opened up for me.

***

At exactly week five, I wiped and a pink viscous substance appeared. I felt cramping mostly on my left side and feared another ectopic pregnancy. I tried not to dwell on my current situation. I struggled to keep my intrapersonal communication positive. Thoughts darted. The little one may some day come into existence. I just need to make it past week eight, to week twelve to week twenty, and then to the end. I'll believe I am having a baby when one is in my arms. Okay, enough of that, time to remain positive for those cells that are doing whatever they are doing inside of me.

At five weeks and one day the color on the toilet paper continued. Not every time, so I remained hopeful. Similar to past situations, staying positive proved increasingly difficult. Alex maintained a positive outlook and worked to keep me positive, too. More than he ever had before. Tears flowed. Not only did I want the baby for me, but also for us.

The next day, cramping that felt like period cramps set in. Alex held me tight as I bawled on his chest. I was upset and sad for both of us. I knew the pregnancy was ending. I shared my anger with Alex: "Why the hell does this keep happening? Why is there no explanation? Why is there no way to stop a loss? I can't keep going through this. I want control of my body again! I'm willing to hand over full control to a pregnancy, but when indicators point to loss, I just want it over with!" The anger subsided as I attempted to calm down, exhausted from years of experiencing the ups and downs of recurrent early pregnancy losses. Tears remained as I continued, "I'm sick of being told by doctors and nurses that 'It's too early to know,' Alex. I know. I know what is happening. I just want it over." Alex listened quietly. He reached out his hand gently and wiped the tears that streamed down my face, and placed the tears on his cheek.

Good news! I did not spot for two days! The pregnancy might make it.

I spoke too soon. After dinner with a colleague, cramping came on hard. I went to the bathroom and confirmed I was bleeding. The loss presented as a late period, similar to prior "near misses."

***

At my appointment after my last loss Dr. Frederickson offered, "You know I have a patient who lost thirteen times and then had a perfectly normal baby." That idea was not enticing. I was tired. Tired of the ups and downs associated with getting pregnant and then losing the pregnancy. Tired of halting any other life plans because of a potential pregnancy. Tired of the emotions that accompanied loss. Tired of sex as a means to an end. I was done. No more experiments. I wanted my life back. I was no longer concerned with giving birth to a child. Done.

***

Maker and Ogden (2003) report that a woman alters the picture of her future expectations according to experiences. Previously unfamiliar with the concept of recurrent early pregnancy loss, I became increasingly aware that my situation was far from normal. I might never experience a pregnancy that would result in a child. Each loss brought me closer to that reality. Of the three early loss stories highlighted in this chapter, two clearly provided evidence of pregnancies that were dying inside of me, the nature and impact of which were not fully realized until I read the Lasker and Toedter (2003) article for class. The last loss was pivotal in our choice to stop trying. We chose to live life to the fullest and not regret circumstances we could not control.

"Adapting to chronic uncertainty also includes redefining tasks. If people cannot achieve predictability in their lives, they can change the way they plan or make decisions" (Brashers, 2001, p. 484). Returning to one's normal routine provides a mechanism for coping with loss (Abboud & Liamputtong, 2005). When it appeared clear to me that successful pregnancy was not part of my future because of what kept occurring, I resigned. Anxiety caused by the uncertainty was replaced with resignation (Brashers, 2001).

***

Women cope with early pregnancy loss differently. Some women construct stories reducing the importance of the pregnancy loss, some focus on returning to a normal routine. Some women prefer silence, while other women prefer reaching out and sharing the loss with hopes of receiving social support (Corbet-Owen & Kruger, 2001). Arguments exist in support of keeping silent about loss, as do arguments regarding sharing the information to receive support. Baddeley and Singer (2009) report, "Individuals who have experienced what are known as disenfranchised losses, that is, losses whose significance is not socially recognized or validated" such as miscarriage "may have similar trouble getting appropriate social support for the telling of their story" (p. 214). Brier (2008) notes the importance of social support as a moderating variable in coping with grief, pointing to the need for further study in the area of supportive communication after miscarriage.

In my situation I found utilization of a network of trusted individuals that I confided in instrumental to my overall well-being throughout each loss. According to Brashers (2001), "Supportive others affect the experience of uncertainty by providing a stable relationship through validation, opportunities for ventilation, or instrumental support and by minimizing social uncertainties through acts that project availability of support and lack of stigmatization or rejection" (p. 485). This was true in my case exactly. In most cases in which I reached out for support, or support was offered freely, I was completely validated. I was rarely made to feel like a freak for having such an anomaly. From colleagues, to friends, to parents, to my brother, to my spouse, I was never made to feel as though anything happening within my body were my fault. Nor was I badgered with ways to fix the situation. No one pushed for answers or an account of causality. I was upheld with love and support. And for that I am forever grateful.

My story and storying of unexplained recurrent early pregnancy loss provides some insight into how social support from friends and family impacted my ability to adjust to the uncertainty of my situations with pregnancy, and then loss, time and again. Although no absolute sense can be made of my unexplained events, I found that most often sharing my story proved beneficial. Each time my story was met with gentle, loving support and acknowledgment of the difficulty caused by struggling with uncertainty, I felt validated. These reactions from others greatly impacted my ability to cope. With the acceptance of the uncertainty came the acceptance of *my* normal.

In addition to owing my ability to cope with the uncertainty of the situation to those who sat by my side and helped me through what most would consider the most unbearable pain, I am thankful for the conviction I held within that kept me strong. I advocated for myself. I chose the key individuals who served as my support. I chose to accept when others could not provide support. And I chose to keep certain topics of conversation at bay when I needed to (Brashers, Neidig, & Goldsmith, 2000).

I share my story of loss in hopes that if you or anyone you know has experienced pregnancy loss, my story might bring comfort or validation. You are not alone. You do not have to be silent.

16. *Moving Through Miscarriage: A Personal Narrative*

RENATA FERDINAND

> Getting pregnant seems as natural as exhaling, especially for Black women. Infertility isn't our problem; it's White women's mess. At least that was the myth.
>
> (Villarosa, 2004, p. 174)

Nothing but empty space showed on the ultrasound screen. No heartbeat. No tiny limbs steadily moving within me. I looked. I searched. I found nothing. *Nothing.*

This wasn't supposed to be my reality. I had done everything right: completed an undergraduate and graduate degree in English before returning to graduate school to explore Communication Studies. Like many other African American women, I was the first in my family to attend and graduate from college. I married a loving man and gave birth to a beautiful baby girl. I started a tenure-track career as an Assistant Professor at my alma mater. At twenty-seven, I thought I had it all. With my personal life intact, I dedicated myself to establishing a career as an academic scholar. It was only when my husband and I sought to give our daughter a sibling that we tried for a second child. We got pregnant on the first try. We were ecstatic. I had already begun to think about how I was going to complete all of my scholarly duties while being pregnant. Then, suddenly and unexpectedly, I had a miscarriage at ten weeks.

I can remember the last time I wrote about loss. The writings were based on my summer abroad trips to West Africa, where I completed research for my dissertation. This afforded me the opportunity to travel extensively throughout West Africa, conducting research on slavery and its effect on African American culture and identity. I wrote about the things the Africans lost: their memories, their identities, their loved ones, their homes, their way of life, and most important, their names.

But I had never considered the things I could lose, especially a baby. Why hadn't I thought about this before? According to most studies, Black women are prone to having more miscarriages than are other women. RESOLVE: The National Infertility Association (2011) suggests that African American women could be at greater risk of infertility compared with women of other races. Callister (2006) finds that "the rate of perinatal and infant loss for African American women is twice the rate of perinatal and infant loss of Caucasian women" (p. 229). Further, Price (2008) writes, "African American women are at elevated risk of both singular and multiple pregnancy loss" (p. 110). Apparently, the odds were against me and I didn't even know it. I was caught up in the myth aptly described by Villarosa (2004): "Infertility isn't our problem; it's White women's mess" (p. 174).

Yet, apparently, it was our problem. According to most studies, many African American women have fibroid tumors, which may affect their ability to become pregnant or even carry a child to full term. Some may suffer from sexually transmitted infections (STIs), or even stress, which may affect ovulation. Brenda Wade, Ph.D., an author and clinical psychologist, discusses stress and its effect on Black women's fertility, stating, "The enormous amount of stress that we face as Black women is directly related to the hormone imbalances implicated in infertility and miscarriage. We Black women don't take care of ourselves. We overwork until we get to the point of exhaustion. We don't stop to say it's time to rest" (as cited in Villarosa, 2004, p. 175). And like many other women, African American women are waiting longer to conceive for various reasons, including the desire to pursue a career and find a suitable mate, which ultimately affects the quality of eggs needed for successful reproduction.

Considering that African American women are disproportionally affected by infertility and miscarriage, I wonder why it is not well discussed among African Americans. Dr. Meyer (2007) believes that African American women are reluctant to discuss health-related issues because we are "afraid to be labeled because society labels us" (p. 74). Other scholars point to the myth of the "strong Black woman," a controlling and dominant image that has been used as an alternative symbol of Black womanhood, hoping to offer a better portrayal of Black women than the sexless mammy, the lustful Jezebel, and the welfare queen. Yet, feminist scholars harshly criticize this image because it attempts to construct Black womanhood in contrast to normative, largely White, middle-class womanhood. Beauboeuf-Lafontant (2007) writes, "The strength discourse focuses on a Black woman's outward behavior, ignoring her actual emotional or physical condition. Being strong is essentially about appearing so, affecting a persona and performance of managing a difficult life with dignity, grace, and composure" (pp. 38–39). Therefore, African American women may sometimes hide or remain silent in the face of adverse issues so as not to be perceived as weak or feeble. This myth may contribute to the lack of discussion regarding the prevalence of miscarriage and infertility, as some African American women may see it as a challenge to Black womanhood.

But, oh, how I wish I had known. Then maybe, just maybe, I could have been prepared for this miscarriage. But how does one prepare for a life-altering event? And there was no comfort to be found. No comfort in reading studies exploring miscarriage. No ease in learning about the number of women who experience pregnancy loss, or the frequency of miscarriages. No hope gained from the books that explore depression, grief, or the need for a support system. Instead, it is Price's (2008) words that offer encouragement: "A woman's personal experience cannot be known without her willingness to disclose and discuss her loss. An important caveat to any research surrounding reproductive loss is that not all individuals have the opportunity, the ability, or the willingness to divulge the details of their experience" (p. 116). I take Price's words seriously, and therefore have decided to share my story of loss.

This is a personal narrative, which, according to Goodall (2004), is "about communication as it is experienced in everyday life, which is always first person, deeply felt, rooted in our past, not always rational, and often messy" (p. 188). As an African American woman, personal narratives give me an opportunity not only to be a voice for those who are otherwise marginalized, subjugated, and silenced, but also to reflect on my own experiences as a Black woman. Langellier (1999) writes, "Theories of the flesh are indigenous performance traditions in which black women theorize themselves. Personal narrative is a way of knowing carved out of experience, experience as it is inflected by particular cultural, geopolitical, and material circumstances" (p. 137). Therefore, this story is not framed around statistical analysis or discussions; it will not highlight the number of pregnancy losses documented throughout the United States, nor will it offer a comparison of the various experiences of different women. Rather, it is the narrative itself wherein merit lies. I hope to think that my narrative adds to the work of Van (2001), whose work on pregnancy loss and African American women became the first research study published that focuses exclusively on the experiences of Black women. She encourages us to begin "breaking the silence" regarding African American women and pregnancy loss (p. 229). I hope to contribute to the tradition established by Patricia Hill Collins's *Black Feminist Theory* (1991), adamantly described by Denzin (1997) as producing cultural texts that are "evocative, poetic, direct, personal, and biographical" (p. 69).

This personal narrative is enhanced by performative writing. Pelias (2005) describes performative writing as beckoning "empathy, allowing others to not only see what the writer might see but also feel what the writer might feel. It is an invitation to take another's perspective. ... They [readers] come to feel that they and others are written, given voice, a voice that they did not have prior to the reading" (p. 419). Performative writing allows me not only to capture the human experience of miscarriage, but also to connect it to readers in the hopes that they will understand and emotionally feel the nuances of this particular experience. Pollock (1998) writes, "Performative writing evokes worlds that are otherwise intangible, unlocatable [*sic*]: worlds of memory, pleasure, sensation, imagination, affect, and in-sight" (p. 80). This type of writing falls in line with Collins's (1991) recommendation that we try to learn from others' experiences because no one group has ownership of a particular type of knowledge, and that "groups can come to better understand other groups' standpoint, without relinquishing the uniqueness of its own standpoint or suppressing other groups' partial perspectives" (p. 236). Collins's work echoes that of other feminist scholars and is an epistemological tradition of standpoint theory.

Standpoint theory guides this research. Denzin (1997) describes standpoint theories as moving "in two directions at the same time. The first direction is toward the discovery of knowledge about the social world as that world works its way into the lives of oppressed people. Second, there is an attempt to recover and bring value to knowledge that has been suppressed by the existing epistemologies in the social sciences" (p. 58). Standpoint theory allows me to speak for myself within the clearly communicated context of, and the tensions created by, the myth within the African American community that infertility and miscarriage are "White women's mess" (Villarosa, 2004, p. 174) and the research that says that African American women have a greater risk of infertility and miscarriage without the onus and impossibility of speaking for all Black women. T. M-ha Trinh (1991) and Gloria Anzaldúa (1981) help me further understand the significance of standpoint theory as it relates to my research. Trinh helps me in understanding the representations of experience, and how writing from a culturally specific space makes this all possible, while Anzaldúa cherishes lived experience, and sees the multidimensionality of experience as liberatory. Denzin (1997) writes of the path of these two authors: "[F]or these writers, the science questions no longer operate. Nor is there any break between empirical activity (gathering empirical materials or reading social texts), theorizing, and social criticism" (p. 86). This is the path I hope to continue. Therefore, this writing also stands as a form of feminist cultural criticism.

This is a story about the loss of a pregnancy at ten weeks. This narrative will explain the impact of this sudden loss, and the clear signs of depression that I dealt with: avoidance masked by a strong desire to be invisible by hiding in plain sight; the constant tears that seemed to flow without regard; and my battle with guilt, embarrassment, and shame. And yet, there was another loss here: the loss of my perceived world. Until this experience, I understood the world to function in a certain way. I had accepted things in my life as is, no questions asked. But now this occurred, and it rocked my solid foundation, a loss of innocence, per se. My world had changed, and nothing, truly, would ever be the same again. This is *my* story.

Sitting Up

The doctor never told me that I was losing the baby. Actually, it was what the doctor didn't say. She didn't say to look here at the screen. She didn't tell me to notice the fetal sac on the monitor. She didn't rush to let me hear a heart-beat. She didn't use some creative tool to measure the length of my unborn child. Instead, while I lay on the table looking at the monitor, she gently tapped my leg and told me to sit up. Those two words, *sit up*, had sealed my fate. I knew it was over.

Everything became a blur after this, so much so that I couldn't remember the ride home. All I remember doing is retrieving my five-year-old daughter from school. But the doctor must have told me that I was miscarrying. She must have informed me that I was about ten weeks and that the baby had actually stopped growing about two weeks earlier. Maybe she was speaking too low. Was she whispering? Or maybe I must have simply ignored her when she said that I probably noticed that some of the pregnancy symptoms had vanished. Why was she speaking so softly? Speak louder! Yell the words to me so that I understand. Scream that I must have a D&C! She didn't shout it, so I guess I didn't hear it.

I only heard my heartbeat. Faster and faster and then faster. At times, it seemed to skip a beat. At others times, it totally stopped. I heard the voice in my head that told me she was wrong. I heard my body slump over like a sack of wet laundry. I heard horns honking, phones ringing, the clicking sound of a woman's heels, the slight cry of a newborn baby, the murmur of voices, a curious cricket stuck in the doorway. I heard all of this, but *her* voice created noise. Her voice loomed over me, attempting to make way through all the other sights and sounds. She competed for my attention, trying desperately to relay this important information. Yet, she spoke the words I could not hear. And as long as I could not hear her, she was not speaking.

Maybe it was the walk home with my daughter that made me finally listen to the doctor's words. But how could I process these words with a five-year-old accompanying me? I couldn't, and even more, I didn't want to. I walked with my daughter, still in a daze. Just as the rain unexpectedly began to pour, tears burst from my eyes. My daughter's soft voice attempted to wake me from my reality as she asked me why I cried. "Tears of joy, baby, tears of joy," I replied. But there was no joy, only sadness. The bag on my shoulder became heavy from the emotional baggage I was carrying, and I struggled to make it home. I pulled the weight of them both. My daughter saw my struggle and insisted on helping me, her little body tugging at my satchel in the pouring rain. I only remember her saying, "It's okay, Mommy. I got you!" She repeated this mantra the entire way home. She watched the rain, attempting to hold the umbrella we shared. She watched the cars, making sure we didn't cross against the lights. She watched me. We made it home unscathed because of her. But she couldn't save me from the depression that I would soon seep into.

Crawling

I wish I were a superhero for purely selfish reasons. Not to save the world or eradicate poverty. Not to stop criminals from robbing old ladies or from stealing property. I merely wish to be a superhero so I can be invisible, and then I wouldn't have to bother with the lies. To mask my miscarriage, I lied and told people that I had the flu. I called into work sick with the flu. I told friends and family who called that I had the flu. In fact, flu became my synonym for miscarriage. And so I wished for invisibility. I did not want to be seen or heard. I only wanted to crawl into bed and keep the covers over my head.

I felt a bit of shame, both for the miscarriage and when considering what others would think of me. To me, a miscarriage made me an anomaly with all its inherent connotations: abnormal, odd, peculiar, strange. I mean, a miscarriage is "White women's mess" (Villarosa, 2004, p. 174), and not the experience of a young, healthy, African American woman, especially one who had already given birth. I felt as though I had dishonored and disgraced myself. I had done something improper by miscarrying, and I felt ridiculous. Kundera (1991) nicely sums up my position: "The basis of shame is not some personal mistake of ours, but the ignominy, the humiliation we feel that we must be what we are without any choice in the matter, and that this humiliation is seen by everyone" (p. 254). I didn't want people looking at me and seeing my imperfection, seeing that my body was unable to bring forth a new life, seeing that my emotional state was momentarily ruptured, seeing me and the imperfection, the scarlet letter burning on my chest. I thought if they saw me, they would judge me.

I could almost hear my family, as they would continually question the reasons for the miscarriage. They would talk of how this isn't common in our family, of how the women in our family had lots of healthy babies, and how this must be a result of something I had done wrong. Or that God made this decision, so live with it. My friends would offer some comfort, yet stop short of saying that something must be wrong with me to have this happen, or that I could just try again, simple and easy. They would stress to me not to let this get me down, that struggling is a part of a Black woman's life, that trials and tribulations will help me be a better person, and that I should continue to show strength and strive to be a good wife and mother, despite the miscarriage. This is what I suspected they would say. I kept silent to avoid this conversation. The bigger implication of this dialogue hints at the definition of being a woman. To my friends and family, being a woman means the ability to give birth. Hence, a woman's fertility is directly tied to her existence as a woman. And I guess I support this rhetoric, for I too saw this miscarriage as a stunning departure from the narrative of a woman. If I couldn't produce a child, I wasn't really fulfilling my life's purpose. In actuality, I had succumbed to society's expectations of a woman, including the need to fulfill gender roles to be socially accepted. It is this realization that furthered the shame.

And so I crawled under a sheet of avoidance. Although I informed my husband and mother of the miscarriage, I didn't discuss it with them because of sheer embarrassment. Like many of the participants in Van's (2012/2013) study, I too embraced avoidance, "where participants either did not tell others (e.g., beyond partner and mother) or avoided others, especially those with babies" (p. 76). By avoiding, I wouldn't have to explain anything. I wouldn't have to explain that we really wanted this baby, and that we had already selected baby names based on the anticipated gender. I wouldn't have to talk about my feelings. I wouldn't have to keep up appearances as if everything were okay. Being invisible afforded me a type of silence. There is comfort in avoidance.

And so, I lay there in my bed of shame, mentally destroying myself by accepting the blame for the miscarriage. I mean, a miscarriage means I'm a terrible person, right? I must be defective and deficient, inadequate and inaccurate. I wasn't deserving of grace, or pity, or sorrow. Instead, I deserved everything that I was getting, to be punished. A bad person, morally reprehensible. Truly an enemy to myself who deserved to suffer. These thoughts became my cushion. I wrapped myself within this fantasy. But I was jolted into reality when the hospital phoned to inform me of my scheduled D&C.

The simplicity of these letters, D and C, had become massive in my life. Two letters, whose pairing would otherwise mean nothing to me, held my future. Even as the nurse uttered these words, I thought about how harsh they sounded coming from her mouth, how abrupt and obtrusive they seemed, how offensive and cold they sounded to the ears. I hated these letters! Or maybe I just hated what they stood for, not the dilation and curettage procedure itself but what it represented: loss, infertility, spontaneous abortion, and the list goes on. How did I end up in this reality?

Falling Down

I envy Alice from *Alice's Adventures in Wonderland*. She fell down a rabbit hole and found fanciful and magical creatures that introduced her to a world of imagination: a talking rabbit, a smoking caterpillar, a grinning Cheshire Cat, unruly playing cards. Her adventurous journey, however, was actually a dream. My rabbit hole looked a lot different from hers.

I tried and tried not to fall into this hole, but this depression was so powerful. I tried to keep to my regular routine, but sleep overcame me. Apparently, I even cried in my sleep, evidenced by my tear-soaked pillowcases. But I tried to stay out of the hole. I actually teetered on the edge of it. I continued to walk my daughter to school; I would just cry on the way back home. I finished dinner most nights, although it would be my first meal of the day. By the time the day of my scheduled D&C arrived, I was numb, not the kind of numbness felt in cold winter months, or the numbness felt from touching ice, or sometimes the numbness brought on by a throbbing pain. Instead, this numbness produced no emotional sensation. I felt no feelings of grief or sadness, no feelings of apprehension or nervousness, no feelings of remorse or regret. No feelings, period. I had come to the conclusion that it was easier not to feel. I wouldn't have to feel unhappiness, or be mournful or drab. No "what if" thoughts to cloud my judgment. If I remained nonchalant and mentally absent, I could at least keep my composure. And so I was dead on the inside. But at least I was still physically breathing. I sat in the area designated for outpatient operations, and I can remember telling myself to breathe. Breathe. Breathe. Breathe. It's funny how breath becomes precious in an instant. The same breath that I thought I would use to deliver my baby was the same breath I was using to keep myself alive.

A few people filled the room, my obstetrician, a medical student, the anesthesiologist, and a nurse. Isn't it ironic that these same people would have been in the room had I given birth? Nevertheless, surrounded by these faceless people wearing white robes, I thought about my baby that would remain faceless, never having the opportunity to grow into a full person, stripped of any ability to form a nose, or lips, or cheeks, or eyes, or small dimples, or a crooked chin, or freckles, for that matter. Never knowing what he or she could have looked like. Like the others, the baby remains faceless, yet significant, the presence of absence.

I can remember my doctor holding my hand until I was finally unconscious. When I awoke, it was over. I remember a harshness in my throat, as if I had been screaming. I felt sluggish, but extremely well rested. When I was finally taken to outpatient recovery, I overwhelmingly thanked the anesthesiologist. Why would I thank the anesthesiologist? Because she gave me the best sleep I had had in weeks.

I returned home, and there was that hole, staring at me. It was massive, having grown since the last time I had seen it. I tried and tried not to go near it, to keep some semblance of normalcy in my life, to try and maintain an ounce of courage. In zombie-like fashion, I tried and tried to keep sane. I knew what was waiting for me in the hole, and I feared it. So for days I managed to stay out of the hole, but I flirted at the edge of it, feet barely touching the rim, just enough to keep from falling completely in.

And it didn't help that there were no answers. No reasons I had a miscarriage, no discovery of some chromosomal abnormality that my doctor had promised would be a result of the D&C, no explanations of why my body failed me. I had to deal with not knowing why this happened to me. And this definitely exasperated my depressive symptoms. In fact, it is this "unknown" element that became the cornerstone of my depression, this unidentifiable, nameless, invisible, uncertain thing became the weight of the world. For the first time, I wished for a name for this unspeakable tragedy that had befallen me. Giving it a name, just one little title, would have given it meaning in my mind, or at least an explanation of why it occurred. Questions began to fill my mind: Will I have another miscarriage? Does this mean I am infertile? What did I do to make this happen? The questions go on and on, but the answers were none. Without one, I was left emotionally and mentally tattered.

Standing Still

Depression is exhausting. It takes a lot of effort to be depressed. Television commercials make it seem as though it is easy to slip into depression, as though all one has to do is think sad thoughts. But I find it hard. Hard because it takes energy to do that. The mere thought of how much energy I put into being depressed almost drained me. In fact, it was the depression itself that was debilitating. I understand why Van (2012/2013) encourages health care professionals to consider PTSD (post-traumatic stress disorder) as a by-product of miscarriage for many women. She writes, "A final and critical suggestion is for healthcare providers to assess bereaved women for PTSD symptoms if avoidance and escape coping styles prolong grief resolution after IPL [involuntary pregnancy loss]" (p. 83). I thought about why I grieved.

I grieved the loss of this baby. Yet I also grieved the loss of being able to experience pregnancy, of being able to see my body changing and growing with new life inside of me, of seeing the smiling faces that would ultimately inquire about how far along I was, or whether I knew the gender. I grieved the loss of knowing those who wanted to touch my belly and feel the quick movement of limbs. Simple grief over not being able to buy the cute flowery dresses for newborns, or those tiny baseball shoes, or to experience those moments of anticipation during which I would sneak off to be by myself and pretend to change diapers, or imagine life in the new nursery. Oh, how I longed for those moments when my colleagues would ask me about my well-being, and I would coyly talk of the terrors of pregnancy but secretly enjoy every minute of it. I grieved for the possibilities.

And yet I also grieved the loss of being able to do something that I thought was natural. I had a child previously without any complications. I was still young and healthy. As my daughter aged, people would always ask me whether I would have another child, and I always said, "Maybe later." Even when my daughter began asking for a sibling, I would say, "Maybe later," assuming I could magically grant this wish at my convenience. I think now about how loaded those words are: "Maybe later." The connotations of these words imply that it is solely my decision and discretion to have a child, that there is an easiness to getting pregnant, and that I determine the outcome of expanding my family, a kind of certainty in these words.

But, apparently, I didn't have this right. In fact, I felt as though my reproductive rights were being challenged. No verdict had been handed down in an effort to halt my fertility. No unanimous ruling had been determined to intervene in my childbearing capabilities. I am not Elaine Riddick, one of many African American women who were forcibly sterilized as a result of North Carolina's eugenics program that spanned 1929 to 1974. The state has mandated payment of $10 million in compensation to the victims of this horrible and atrocious movement, although Riddick believes, "There is no amount of money that can take away the humiliation of someone stealing your ability to reproduce and castrating you" (as cited in Crossman, 2013, paragraph 3). But someone surely had stolen mine. And there was no finger to point, no expectation of compensation, no vindication from a victory. All I had were questions with no answers.

So "maybe later" turned into "not able." And it is this loss, especially, that caused me to grieve the loss of my perceived world. My fertility was never an issue to me before this miscarriage. But now that my fertility was being questioned, it challenged the solid foundation upon which I built my life, my understanding of the world, my perception of being a woman, and my view of death. Nothing could be taken for granted anymore. No guarantees, no promises, and no predictions of the future.

I've since healed physically from the D&C, but my emotional scars are still in the process of being remedied. I've learned that grieving from a miscarriage is similar to other forms of grief due to loss. Some days are good; some are bad. Sometimes I can look back on the experience with stoic countenance, other times I can watch a program featuring a pregnant woman and burst into tears. It is the ebb and flow of recovery. Yet, I expect that I may always carry a sort of war wound from this experience, one that is not easily noticeable to the human eye, but is imprinted on my imagination, and probably my soul.

First Steps

I am not a number. I am not a part of some data algorithm or a multivariate analysis. I don't belong to a longitudinal study or fit neatly within a mathematical equation that can be defined or confined by a demographic category. I am not a figure to be placed within a generic model.

I am not a theory. No need to cram books on theory to find me, no searching in Freud, or Foucault for some understanding of my life. No urgency to take a theory course to see whether my experience fits neatly into your paradigm. I am "theorizing myself," as Langellier (1999) noted as a quintessential device for Black women. I don't need to understand Goffman's (1986) theory of stigma to know that my experience is wrapped in it. In fact, there is no theory that could adequately capture the "messiness" of my life. This narrative is of my experience, and it reflects all the things that Goodall (2004) describes as "first person, deeply felt, rooted in our past, not always rational, and often messy" (p. 188). This is exhibited throughout my text. I hope you can see it when you read the words of my personal narrative, my personal story, my personal life, my personal standpoint. I hope you can feel the ways my legs twitched while in the stirrups when I was *sitting up.* If you can refrain from judging me for seeing the miscarriage as shameful when I was *crawling* in avoidance. I mean, as Goodall (2004) writes, narratives are "not always rational" (p. 188). If you can only read this while looking in a child's face, then you can understand the longing I had to see mine when I was *falling down.* Maybe what I offer here is too "deeply felt" (Goodall, 2004,

p. 188), so much so that you may not understand numbness from a lack of emotion. Maybe "theorizing myself" comes at the expense of you not fully grasping how this experience "is inflected by particular cultural, geopolitical, and material circumstances" (Langellier, 1999, p. 137), for suddenly my reproductive rights were being destroyed while *standing still* and there was no culprit to blame. Vengeance is not mine! The "messiness" of this situation is precisely the reason I decided to offer you a fleeting glance at a moment in my life. It is often stated that a picture is worth a thousand words. Can you picture the words I offer here?

Can you appreciate the fact that I openly disclosed something so taboo in my own culture, the idea of depression? I mean, this is not something often discussed in the African American community. Many African American women believe that "only 'white women' got depression" (Amankwaa, 2003, p. 311). Danquah (1998) describes her depression to members of the African American community, and their impending response: "'Girl, you've been hanging out with too many white folk'; 'What do you have to be depressed about? If our people could make it through slavery, we can make it through anything'; 'Take your troubles to Jesus, not no damn psychiatrist'" (p. 21). Clearly, depression in Black women is seen as a sign of weakness. And this makes diagnosing depression in Black women very difficult. Jones and Shorter-Gooden (2003) describe it as the "Sisterella Complex": Black women's ability to masquerade their own needs by asserting a veil of strength. They write, "Sisterella suffers quietly. ... If you're trying to identify depression in Black women, one of the first things to look for is a woman who is working very hard and seems disconnected from her own needs" (pp. 124–125). This ultimately influences how African American women experience depression and their discussion of it, even shown in Beauboeuf-Lafontant's (2007) study in which participants revealed that they were only familiar with Black women who "entailed a stoicism, a quiet acceptance of what they could not change. A repeated refrain in the data was that the women rarely saw the strong Black women in their families cry or fall apart" (p. 39). The myth of strength is not only confined to African Americans, as Van (2001) even cautions clinicians from subscribing to the myth of the strong Black woman, writing, "Clinicians may consider questioning the myth that African American women are strong and can handle anything" (p. 239). Well, I've chosen to cross this wall of denial and begin a path that will I hope encourage other women of color to openly and truthfully share their stories, not as a sign of weakness but as a symbol of empowerment, a true edict of standpoint theory, which recognizes the importance of experience as the "starting point for social change—the site for a politics of empowerment" (Denzin, 1997, p. 59).

There is strength in saying this: I experienced the loss of a pregnancy, and I accept that. What I do not accept is literature that continues to downplay the significance of miscarriages. What I do not accept are studies that continue to limit our understanding of the process of grieving a loss due to miscarriage. I won't get into the debate about when life actually begins, or when a fetus is considered a child, or the appropriateness of the various nomenclatures used to describe miscarriages. But what I will acknowledge is the lack of studies that focus on miscarriages and women of color, especially the lack of research that explores African American women from various socio-economic backgrounds. Van (2001) writes, "Existing literature reflects profiles of African American women who have experienced pregnancy or infant loss as being unemployed and unmarried, and as low educational achievers who often succumbed to the use of illicit substances and other unhealthy behaviors that contributed to the demise of their pregnancies and infants" (p. 239). I hope that my voice contributes to the experiences of all women, but especially women of color who have experienced loss, and find their lives in unexpected turmoil and chaos. I hope this text follows Collins's (1991) examples of powerful cultural texts infused with lived experience that speak directly to the "lived experiences of African American women" (p. 210).

There is no absolute resolve to overcoming pregnancy loss, and this writing certainly does not endorse a specific strategy; rather, it hopes to expose the journey taken, with the underlying hope that voicing the issues may be as important as healing from them. I think about a quote from Anzaldúa (1981): "Writing is dangerous because we are afraid of what the writing reveals: the fears, the angers, the strengths of a woman under a triple or quadruple oppression. Yet … a woman who writes has power. And a woman with power is feared" (p. 171). This is my attempt to regain some semblance of power in the midst of a trauma that rendered me helpless. As a piece of narrative and performative writing—it is cathartic, highly therapeutic, and allows for an emotional and mental escape when none may be provided, or sought. It is the process of writing that has aided me, and continues to encourage me along this journey.

17. *Barren and Abandoned: Our Representations Left Unshared and Uncharted*[1]

JULIE NOVAK AND EDUARDO GARGUREVICH

I didn't get pregnant and my husband left me. I am bereft of family.[2]

Health and Fertility/Infertility

The World Health Organization (1946) defines health as "the total state of physical, mental, and social well-being, not merely the absence of disease" (p. 694). Our journey through infertility and health care intersects with dedicated professionals and eight years of treatments that narrowly target my physical well-being; nothing explains our *problem* (thus, there is an absence of disease), yet failed treatment after failed treatment is recorded in the medical chart. Without the dreamed of pregnancy, I am physically unwell. Even more, I am mentally and socially unwell. I am in a total state of *un*well-being. Our doctors leave me physically unwell and are guilty bystanders as my mental and social well-being—and to some degree Eduardo's—disintegrate. I am unable to fathom how deeply bereft I am. It is/was unimaginable, yet we lived this experience.

Beginning Context

It is 1995 and I am a woman of thirty-two with health insurance coverage who regularly schedules checkups and complies with preventive health measures. During my annual physical, I inform my primary doctor, Dr. Gaffney,[3] that I am stopping birth control since we are ready for a pregnancy. I explain, "We do not plan on 'trying' to get pregnant; rather, if it 'happens,' great." She encourages me to begin taking prenatal vitamins.

At the end of the same visit, she suggests that I schedule a follow-up appointment if I am not pregnant within the year. This mention of a possible, future appointment precipitously medicalizes the experience of pregnancy and plants the fear of difficulty in becoming pregnant. Whereas I expected best wishes—as we purposefully discontinue contraceptives and anticipate the interactions of lovemaking and conception—Dr. Gaffney posits pregnancy as a medical phenomenon rather than a natural one and even hints at trouble.

* * * *[4]

One year later, Dr. Gaffney says, "I am going to refer you to Dr. Elliot, a fertility specialist." After the consult, I imagine the medical chart entry in SOAP[5] note format, which I learned while studying and interning in hospitals.

S: Couple expressing desire to have child. Married 1993. Referral from primary Dr. 1 yr. post birth control pills and no pregnancy. Female menarche at 14 yr. Reports hx[6] of irregular periods, but no other complaints or related hx. No known pregnancy. Male has daughter with first wife, 1987. Couple would like to meet with therapist.

O: 32 yr. old White female and 36 yr. old white Hispanic male.

A: No identified fertility issues. Maternal age may be factor. Appropriate for r/o[7] labs/tests and first-line fertility treatments.

P: 1. Order labs for hormone levels, sperm count/activity.
   2. Begin Clomid and respective protocol.
   3. Schedule f/u[8] appt.

Understanding Our Infertility Journey

In Rita Charon's (2006) elaboration of narrative medicine, she claims as foundational the biopsychosocial medical model and the premise that a human being is by nature a narrative being and, therefore, understands one's self through narrative (see also Fisher, 1987). She writes, "When we human beings want to understand or describe singular people in particular situations that unfold over time, we reach naturally for narrative, or storytelling, to do so" (p. vii). Narrative medicine, as she defines it, is "medicine practiced with the narrative competence to recognize, absorb, interpret, and be moved by the stories of illness" (p. vii). Such competency she contends is essential for "effective doctor–patient relationships" (p. vii) and for doctors "to bear witness to suffering and, by that act, to ease it" (p. xi). Narrative medicine at its best enacts three movements: attention, representation, and affiliation.

In order to listen to patients—the movement of attention—Charon (2006) suggests that health divides, which separate providers from patients, must be bridged. These divides—differing perspectives on health and illness—center on relationships with mortality; contexts of illness; beliefs about disease causality; and emotions of shame, blame, and fear. When providers reflectively acknowledge the divides and competently employ skills of close reading, engaged and active listening becomes possible.

Inextricably linked with attention is representation of the narratives. To date, doctors employ as written representation the SOAP note, a standardized structure and method of documentation, complete with medical jargon. As such, the representations of the patient and doctor–patient interactions are redacted to the subjective, objective, assessment, and plan components in keeping with the biomedical medical model, medical education, and medical practice (Charon, 2006; Weed, 1964).

Medical practice seldom allows the charting of narratives that reflect the type of representation that narrative attentiveness might engender. Charon suggests "parallel charts" as an opportunity for medical students to "write about their patients in ordinary words" rather than the medical language recorded in charts (p. 155). The goals of such practice "are to enable them to recognize more fully what their patients endure and to examine explicitly their own journeys through medicine" (p. 156). Only by simultaneously engaging in the work of narrative attention and close readings do doctors gain an understanding of "how patients tell of themselves and their bodies" and demonstrate "a pivotal and enduring effort in their willingness and ability to care for the sick" (p. xi). Although writing parallel charts may encourage medical students to examine their interior lives and the narratives of patients, these parallel charts are separate from and not a part of the official medical chart. Moreover, the parallel chart persists as a physician-controlled representation. It is the physician who listens, reflects, and constructs the narrative/s in written form.

Eduardo and I react against this softer yet still persistent presence of physician control over the communication, its process, and written representations. The medical chart does not include patients' representations—those representations voiced, understood, and written by the patients. Neither is the medical chart written collaboratively. Charon's (2006) elaboration of narrative health as a symphony with movements of attention, representation, and affiliation posits the physician as the conductor, who improves her performance through narrative and the writing of parallel charts. While this permits the patients to have voice in the movement of attention, the patients have significantly less, notably unequal, and definitely not collaborative involvement in the representations. Such exclusion, Eduardo and I contend, still skews "what constitutes health and what signifies an effective response to it" toward a physician-constructed perspective, albeit one that embraces the biopsychosocial model (Charon, 2006, p. 26). Since representations prompt affiliation and response (the third movement discussed later in the chapter), we assert our need to retrieve, share, and write our representations as we too bear witness to our suffering and act to care for ourselves.

In this chapter, Eduardo and I engage in narrative work and document our representations of our journey through infertility. We offer them in the form of a patient parallel chart. These representations were mostly unshared with each other prior to writing this chapter and definitely cannot be gleaned from the medical chart, official or parallel. In the next section, we interlace experiences of infertility spanning eight years, culminating in zero pregnancies and two frozen embryos. Relational (marital) dissolution immediately followed the second and last course of IVF as well as my downward spiral into complete unwell-being. We invite you, the reader, to engage in our experience, to imagine the medical chart and the care of health providers without the following representations in oral or written form. We subsequently invite you to construct future representations of health (and health care) in meaningful collaboration.

* * * *

Julie's and Eduardo's Representations as (Patient) Parallel Charts

I open the box, the box in which I put all the notes, medical instructions, and leftovers of vials, ampules, needles, and records. My stomach is a knot, a pit of anxiety. My head starts to hurt. Can I remember the order of all the tasks, the purpose of each medication—birth control pills, Lupron injections, Folistrim stimulation injections, folic acid, doxycycline, human chorionic gonadotropin (HCG), progesterone in oil, tetracycline, and Medrol? What did I journal, document? How will I read and feel my notes from the past?

* * * *

Julie asks me to share my narratives from the process of infertility, and I will do it in spite of the pain these memories bring. My reasons to do it are threefold: helping Julie with this chapter, somehow helping others who might find themselves in this same process, and helping myself to see, years later, who I was at that time, who I am.

* * * *

Eduardo and I go to the visits together. Eduardo helps to mix and administer the stimulation injections. Eduardo and I anxiously await the follicles as they appear projected on the screen during the transvaginal ultrasounds.

* * * *

8/24   7 a.m. transvaginal ultrasound and lab draw. Will call with results ~ 3 p.m. re status of starting cycle.

p.m.   Labs: 53 Estradiol <50, 5 FSH (follicle-stimulating hormone)[9] <10, 6 LH <10 (luteinizing hormone).
Inject 2 ampules between 6 and 9 p.m. same time every p.m.

8/28   7 a.m. transvaginal ultrasound: endometrium double in thickness, follicles in R (right) & L (left) ovary.
Lab done—will call re number of ampules to inject.
Return date probably Tues. or Wed.

p.m.   Called at 12:30 p.m. Estradiol at 83; continue with 2 ampules and return Tues. a.m.

9/1   Transvaginal ultrasound
13 mm endometrium lining; R follicles at 16, 11, 10 … (number indicates size of follicle) L follicles at 18,11 …
Lab draw. Will call with results, likely to return on Thurs.

p.m.   Estradiol 128

9/3   Transvaginal ultrasound and lab draw R 21 … L 18 …
Administered HCG (to release follicles) at 7:25 a.m.

p.m.   Estradiol 334. Have intercourse at 24, 36, 48 hours.

9/?   I go to the bathroom and see blood on my underwear.
Results: Negative … Failed Attempt … No child.

* * * *

Why can't we say we want a child, make love … have sex … or fuck … and be pregnant? Instead, each and every month is filled with daily shots of hormones, multiple trips to view eggs by transvaginal ultrasounds, labs to measure estradiol and … there is no room for momentary doubt, deviation, forgotten steps or the entire cycle may be compromised and that would be irresponsible, that would be useless effort, that would be wasted money, that would be questionable commitment.

Really? Shit. Does anyone who lives an examined life desire a child every single second of every single day? This fertility process demands that I want a child more than anything else. And I do. But I don't.

I cannot imagine anyone or any couple ever feels completely ready to start a family and welcome a child. It's partly—*isn't it?*—a leap of faith and love. Yet ... the medical process squeezes out the faith and love.

* * * *

Not so many months before our wedding,[10] I ask Eduardo, "What would you think if I were to become unexpectedly pregnant?" He says, "I would want you to abort." I would, however, choose the child, whether or not the timing is "right." I want us to be in sync about this important issue. Since we are not, does this affect our wedding plans? (We individually decided it did not.)

We live together. We marry. We love each other. We experience good times, struggle in others. We move forward, at times gracefully and other times clumsily, learning how to embrace each other and create our being as family. I think we are committed to being our best, loving our best.

* * * *

In the spring of 1995, we decide to stop using birth control because we are ready for a possible child. We travel to Slovenia with side trips to Florence, Rome, and Venice. I fantasize about a conception in Italy. What I remember is an absence of sex. If he isn't in the mood, he isn't in the mood.

I imagine a family *with* Eduardo, Erin Amanda (my stepdaughter), and a second child. I do not want a child on my own. And, thanks to *Oprah* and *Dr. Phil*, I believe both Eduardo and I have to say "Yes" to the possibility of a second child before embarking upon fertility treatments. Do I imagine Eduardo's "Yes"? Are we both saying "Yes"?

* * * *

Prior to getting together with Julie, I was married and had one daughter, Erin Amanda. I fell deeply in love with Julie, although I was married. In order to be with her, I left my wife and my daughter. After the initial honeymoon period with Julie and once I resumed my relationship with Erin Amanda, I realized how painful it was for me to leave Erin Amanda, not to live physically with Erin Amanda and not to share a home with her. I still carry with me the image of me saying goodbye to her, an image that accompanies me forever.

I feel the need to share grief, guilt, remorse. Somehow to explain my initial refusal to have another child. If I had left Erin, someone whom I loved with all my heart, am I willing to go through an experience that might end in leaving another child? Of course. I believe history never repeats itself, not exactly. However, the past haunts the present. It haunts me, yet I keep quiet.

* * * *

Another cycle ... Results: Negative ... FAILURE.

* * * *

I peruse the stacks of music CDs, find and place Sweet Honey in the Rock's *Sacred Ground* (1995) in the machine. Over and over and over I select track six, and the strains of "Sing Oh Barren One" play:

> *Empty and lonely I was/Wordless and useless I felt*
> *Bounded and closed I wandered/Empty and useless I was*
> *Then I heard the Voice*
>
> *Sing oh barren one/Sing out and cry aloud*

Sweet Honey in the Rock, 1995

Despite all the tests with results that appear within normal limits, I experience cycle after cycle, fertility treatment after fertility treatment, and still no pregnancy. There is nothing to explain why I am not getting pregnant. At what point will we stop and yell in unison, "I AM BARREN"?

* * * *

Another cycle.

9/21   Transvaginal ultrasound and lab. Endometrium ~ 4
           Met with Dr. to start 2 ampules in a.m. and 2 ampules in p.m.
           Would like to see estradiol ~ 800–1000: may start inseminations after
           a couple of cycles.
           Will call in p.m. with results.

9/30   Office visit. Too many follicles ~ 12. Not safe.

p.m.   Estradiol 1722. Too many mature follicles, cancel cycle.
           Do NOT have intercourse.
           Results: FAILURE.

* * * *

In all of the notes and records in the box, I find only one written sentence of mine that contrasts the objective data. One line in eight years of remnants. The sentence is "I got emotional." Right in the middle of notations about a cycle is "9/27: I got emotional." I couldn't describe or write more than "I got emotional" because that would put into words all the fear of not getting pregnant, the doubts about medicalizing fertility, the worry that Eduardo or I—we—would say it's time to quit. It would mean the loss of a child.

I am so tired. My neck aches with tension; my eyes get heavy, feeling deeply tired.

* * * *

We tell Dr. Elliot we want a consult with a therapist. He replies, "That's fine. We'll schedule an appointment." We meet with Jane. "We want to try and have a child," we say. "We don't want to obsess. Although we could be happy without another child, we want to try. We know it will be stressful, which is why we wanted to meet with you as part of the process." I have my summary of the appointment. Yes, Eduardo and I are thinking clearly and ready to manage fertility treatments. Our desire and action to meet with the therapist indicate a commitment to supporting our relationship during a process known to be stressful on relationships. In conclusion, we are both saying "Yes."

A "Yes" to me means that I buckle down and try not to listen to any doubts during a treatment cycle. Why does it seem that Eduardo switches back and forth from "Yes" to "No"? I can't acknowledge this sensed vacillation, not *during* a treatment cycle. Just one day's deviation from the treatment protocol can sabotage the cycle.

No. Now is not the time to reconsider. We have to do every task. Give the hormone shots. Go to the doctor for a transvaginal ultrasound. Wait for the news about the follicles. Wait for the lab results about hormone levels. When do we have sex? When don't we have sex? Is this the time we do an insemination? Is this a time we do an egg aspiration? Is this the time we administer an intramuscular shot? If Eduardo can't be here to administer the shot, do I ask the neighbor who is a nurse?

I cannot expand the scope of my perspective. I cannot ask whether I am saying "Yes," not now, not at this time. I can't. I CAN'T.

* * * *

We have many treatments, including one IVF, to get pregnant. It is true that at first I hesitated. However, once we begin I share the whole experience with Julie. I go with her to all the doctor appointments, follow all the protocols, administer the shots (I still feel nervous at the memory of the big needle and the possibility of missing the right spot to bury it), go to the ultrasound sessions, and look with Julie at the embryos. I remember the frustration that follows the failures.

We don't talk much. It is something we are doing, that we decided to do. In the midst of my fears, I am happy.

I fear what Julie might feel. For her it is more difficult. I very well know that she feels responsible, and I try to make her feel that it is not her responsibility. I am very much aware that no matter what I do, she is going to feel responsible, but I still try to assuage her feelings.

Am I the perfect partner? I don't know. I get overwhelmed. I am doing and doing and doing. But doing is what I have to do at the moment. I have fears and doubts ... the same fears and doubts I had at the beginning ... fears about abandonment, about abandoning. It becomes obvious to me now that these fears have to do with something much more primordial than my having abandoned Erin. It has to with my own fears of having been abandoned as a child. It becomes obvious that this whole process of fertilization moves in me some primordial fears that I am willing to combat silently rather than to confront in an open way.

* * * *

Eduardo gradually stops helping with the injections. Instead, he reminds me by calling up from the downstairs living room when the hour arrives for me to inject. I sense his distancing (or is it his form of coping?). Rather than ask him questions (and open the door to doubt and his possible demand to STOP), I buckle down (choosing to think that I may be expecting too much from him) and focus on following the directions, complying exactly.

* * * *

Another cycle, and ...

I get a phone call from the doctor's office while driving home from work. She says, "Wait for forty-eight hours without having sex; then, have sex as many times as possible in the following thirty-six hours." I hang up and immediately call Eduardo; he doesn't answer. I feel the weight of all the steps taken in the past month. We MUST follow the protocol. Where is Eduardo? Why isn't he answering? The time for doubt is not now. I hope Eduardo will be home when I get there. I need us to follow the schedule and its rigid timeline.

Results: FAILURE.

* * * *

For me the story of our attempts to get pregnant has two phases: (1) prior to our year in Peru during my first sabbatical and (2) after our return to the United States until the end of my relationship with Julie as my wife. The turning point that starts phase two is my reencounter with Melinda, a girlfriend during my graduate studies and who, by the time we are in Peru, lives in France. The relationship had been very important. It ended absurdly, a story of missed encounters with the lingering question, "What would have happened if things had happened right?"

Simply put, going to Peru was getting out of the environment where I felt overwhelmed, full of fears and doubts. It is a parenthesis, a breath of fresh air … or so I think. Being in Lima makes me aware of how tired I am and how I am in need of something different. I go out with friends, while Julie stays with my parents. I seek other female company as a way to get some escape from what I experience as endless worry.

And then it happens. I get an email from Melinda and things take a turn that I never imagined. While Julie is downstairs with my parents, I begin communicating with Melinda. I guess the question is, "Why?" And the answer is that a relationship with Melinda will free me from the doubts and fears I am going through with Julie.

The emails go back and forth. When Julie and I return to the United States, the email correspondence continues and phone calls begin… .

* * * *

The plans once again slip into place and start to unfold as we leave Lima to go back to Fargo for the final IVF attempt. We agree that this second IVF will be the final treatment we undergo in trying to conceive. I think, I hope, I will get pregnant. After all, nothing was wrong with the implanted embryos in the first IVF. They were, in fact, of highest quality according to Dr. Eliot.

* * * *

We shortened our stay in Peru because it is time to continue the fertilization process. Do I feel that I am without say? In the moment I don't think so, but maybe I do. We are back in the United States and resuming the process. At the same time I am interacting with Melinda.

I am very confused. I tell myself that if the fertilization process is successful I am going to end the relationship with Melinda and devote myself to my family. I am afraid. Am I going to be able to do it? I begin sabotaging the IVF process. I am tired of trying, of feeling spent from so many emotions and having no results. I am torn between my commitment to getting pregnant and my wanting to continue my extramarital relationship. It is something new, fresh, with no expectations … or rather, with the expectation that in this new moment Melinda and I are going to be happy together.

And Melinda knows this. She knows that my wife and I are trying to get pregnant, and if it happens, our relationship is going to end. Melinda accepts this.

* * * *

I stop accompanying Julie to the doctor's appointments. I am tired of helping Julie with her shots. I distance myself from the medical procedures. I leave Julie alone. When Julie asks me to go to therapy, I refuse. When the time comes to have sex, I do it without being into it. As if thinking: If we get pregnant it will be because it has to be, and if it has to be, if it is, I will assume my responsibility. But at the time, it becomes—I put it in these terms—Julie's responsibility. If this time it doesn't happen, we are going to stop trying.

* * * *

On the IVF Information Session sheet from the fertility clinic is the heading "The Bottom Line." What follows are the beginning bulleted points:

- Not all eggs fertilize; not all fertilized eggs become embryos and not all embryos continue their development to the point of transfer.
- The more embryos transferred, the higher the pregnancy rate, but also, the higher the multiple rate.
- Not all transfers cause a pregnancy. There are many unknown parameters.

* * * *

We cry and hold each other intertwined on the bed upon receiving the phone call of the last, bad, baby news. "The results are negative," reports a voice from the fertility clinic. The words mark the beginning of the end of a vision of the future.

I think back. Was this the last time we talked with anyone from the fertility clinic?

I think back. Was Eduardo crying about us too?

* * * *

I am with Julie after receiving the phone call from the doctor's office. For the second time, it has not happened. We embrace each other and cry together. My tears are tears of pain, of frustration, of farewell. Farewell to the idea of having a child with Julie, but maybe also farewell to Julie. We have been through so much together. Not a perfect couple, but we love each other deeply. This second failed attempt opens the doors for me to pursue my relationship with Melinda. Not getting pregnant gives me the green light to leave.

* * * *

I walk along the banks of the Red River in Fargo, North Dakota. Every day I walk. My grief becomes my walk and my walk, my grief. All that will never be is a void that is bigger than all that is and will be. I breathe. The river flows on relentlessly.

Eduardo is spending more time in his office. He is gone *so* many hours. I walk alongside the river. I breathe. I follow the river. At times the river leads me. The sun warms. I release my body and mind to the rhythms of the walking and the river, this river that flows north instead of the usual southerly direction. Obviously Eduardo and I are not going to grieve together. I need to give him his space to grieve and me, mine. It is okay, I think, that we have different ways of grieving.

* * * *

Eduardo disconnects then reconnects to a time of the past. He conjures up a love from the past as he types, in his few-fingered tapping, Internet messages of disrupted love and re-ignited passion. He attempts to leap to a future by returning to a lover of the past. Will he tell me about the furtive emails? I choose to focus on what he is doing and not how I put the pieces together. Will he leave his office and return home?

* * * *

Fall arrives. The university term is soon to begin. Eduardo will start teaching again; I am going to be a graduate student again. All the plans become reality except for the pregnancy, yet only the pregnancy mattered, the rest was/is inconsequential. What cruel twist of fate has the world emerging just as I imagined except for the only part that mattered—the child, the changed family?

This barren fall brings a burning, crawling, stinging, sweaty sensation that grips my embodied me. I am all consumed and all defeated. I am overtaken by this sensation. The sweet, sweet escape to sleep is a distant memory, an ephemeral wish, and eludes me, hour after hour, day after day. I cannot get up; I cannot leave the bed.

Eduardo commands me to get up and come to the table set with the dinner he has prepared. The food tastes like sawdust, dry and inedible. I can't swallow; I gag. I can't eat. Not even one bite. Eduardo argues that I must get out. A trip to the grocery store with him ends with a tidal wave of panic as I survey too many brands and bottles of shampoo. I can't decide; I have to leave. I have to leave NOW.

How many seconds before I can go back to bed? Bed is no refuge. Bed is torture; yet, nothing is less torturous than bed.

* * * *

"I think you need to see Jane," Eduardo states. "Will you go with me?" I ask. "No, YOU need to see her," he clarifies. "Will you go with me?" I plead. "I need us to go together," I weakly assert. "Okay," he assents.

* * * *

Jane suggests and I agree on partial hospitalization. It gets me out of bed. I go every weekday for eight hours during a period of two to three weeks. I start taking sleeping medications and anti-anxiety/depression pills. Every morning after arrival, there is a round-robin check-in with the psychiatrist. I report how many hours I sleep, how many times I wake up, and my general levels of anxiety/depression. I learn to do thought records. I learn to pass time with distractions. I have short-talk therapy sessions. The psychiatrist makes me bristle. He has it *so together*. He even ends every session exactly on time, to the minute.

I talk only about the loss of becoming pregnant. They ask only about this loss. Family members (in my case, Eduardo) may be invited for a summary-type session at the end of each week and/or partial hospitalization, but Eduardo isn't interested and the staff doesn't encourage or discourage such a meeting. They are not *asking* about Eduardo or us.

* * * *

While I want to talk with Eduardo and together envision plans about the future, Eduardo says, "Julie needs to focus on herself and her next goals." Jane replies, "It is perfectly fine that Julie focuses on you as her family, especially now." I want Eduardo to stop corresponding with his ex-girlfriend and I make this request after voicing that Eduardo corresponds with Melinda yet denies doing so. Jane looks at Eduardo and says, "It is completely appropriate that you stop emailing with a past lover. Do you agree to stop?" "Yes," he replies. I want his word to transfer into action. I fear it won't. He doesn't stop.

Months later, I realize that I was grieving our marriage before he stopped denying his drifting ... before he tells me (immediately after I finish partial hospitalization) that he needs a vacation (to Paris where Melinda lives) ... before he tells me he doesn't want to be married to me any longer.

I walk out of the house hopeful and happy to see him when he returns from Paris. As I reach for his luggage, he fiercely pulls it backwards, distaste and dismissal on his face.

* * * *

While Julie spirals down into depression, I am blinded by the promise of something new. While Julie has to go daily to a medical facility to get better, I make plans to go to Paris on vacation. And I do. Then comes the breakup of the marriage; my leaving Julie. I dream of a new life with a "new" person, without pressures, demands, visits to the doctors, or failed IVF attempts.

* * * *

"Did my wanting a child and all the infertility treatments lead to you walking away from our marriage?" I ask. "No," he replies.

I am left alone and bereft. I mourn my child. I mourn my husband. I mourn my family. I mourn my stepdaughter. I mourn my Peruvian family.

I spend much of my days on the sofa. Suzy and Jonette, two of my sisters, call me most days and hear me say the same words over and over. I listen to the same words over and over.

> *Sing oh barren one/Sing out and cry aloud*
> *Sing oh barren one/Sing out and cry aloud*
>
> *Thou that didst not bear/Thou that didst not traverse with child*
> *Break forth into singing and cry aloud*
>> Sweet Honey in the Rock, 1995

* * * *

I have two Polaroid pictures of our embryos. They document our children, those that didn't continue to live and those that are suspended in a frozen state. At times I think about framing those pictures and hanging them on my walls.

I avoid opening the mail from the embryo storage company. Their letter arrives every year. Then a statement from my insurance company eventually follows the letter, and finally a bill arrives. I keep paying the annual $400 to cover storage costs.

I want to call the company and ask whether I can retrieve the frozen embryos. I would like our embryos to thaw and naturally continue to divide until they stop; then, I will bury our children.

I buried blood from the periods that occurred after the two IVFs. Eduardo stops the conversation almost before I mention my desire to enact such a symbolic action. I bury the blood (our lost child) on my own. The blood mingles with flowers from bulbs belonging first to my grandmother and then my mother. The ongoing generations of mother and daughter will stop with my mother and me. Eduardo and I as family will soon die too.

* * * *

Now when I have health care appointments, the health history form prompts me to check single, married, divorced, or widowed. The form asks how many times I have been pregnant. It asks how many children I have. Do

I get to count my stepdaughter? The form only asks about my birth family in regard to their medical history. Why does the doctor ask whether I have guns in the house, but not about my relationships?

* * * *

We—two sisters (Jonette and Lisa), my parents, and I—sit around the dining room table, while eating dinner and enjoying each other in conversation. After a lament about the general decline of common courtesies, I tell about having called one of our nieces (a brother's daughter who had recently celebrated her eighteenth birthday) by phone and suggesting to her that she write thank you notes after receiving a gift. "What right do you have?" my sister Lisa asks assertively. I stammer in my response. "Well, she's my niece—it takes a village—because I am an adult and she's still a child?" My sister replies, "Let's not talk about this or we will get upset and feelings will be hurt."

Two days later, Jonette, also childless, brings us back to the previous conversation by saying to me, "You should have answered 'because we're family.'"

I am haunted by the question, "What right do you have?" I hear a subtext, a statement often voiced by others too: You are not her mother. You are not *a* mother.

Unshared, Uncharted Representations and Fragmented, Woeful Affiliation

One dream became THE goal written in the medical chart and the health care providers continued with ongoing assessments and plans in SOAP format toward meeting that goal. Dr. Elliot saw "no reason to explain why you are not getting pregnant" and he continued to have treatment options. In turn, we adopted the medical approach to becoming pregnant, and we followed the seductive pull into more and more medical procedures and the medicalization of pregnancy.

* * * *

Eduardo and I didn't share many of our parallel chart entries. We didn't talk about other dreams, other futures. I don't think we knew how. We were overwhelmed. Dr. Elliot, our fertility specialist, did not ask about our mental or social well-being. He did not ask for our parallel chart entries. He did not guide us toward health. The SOAP notes—in keeping with the biomedical medical model, medical education, and medical practice—let him down, let us down.

* * * *

I plead for a more couple-centered perspective during infertility from the health care providers. "The patient" is the couple. While I understand that it is the female[11] who carries the weight of the procedure, it is equally important that the partner be considered. It is my recollection that during the entire fertility process, Julie took center stage. I do not say she did not have the right to be at center stage; however, I think not enough attention was paid to what I was feeling, what I was going through, what my needs were. ... I wouldn't want this to sound like a man once again crying for attention, but I also have needs, fears, doubts ... even in those therapy sessions, the emphasis was almost always placed on Julie.

* * * *

I realize that the physical, mental, and social facets of well-being are coupled, at times loosely and at times tightly, but always interdependently. Drs. Gaffney and Elliot singled out the physical, mostly mine, and unfortunately controlled the movements of attention and representation.

I know deep inside that health is a dynamic of physical, mental, social, *and spiritual* well-being. Health is neither the absence of disease nor is it the sum of the individual facets within the WHO definition of health. Best said, health is a spiritual dance of physical, mental, and social well-being. Is that why the song calls me?

* * * *

Affiliation (the third movement of narrative medicine) emerges from spirals of collaborative attention and representations and culminates in *contact* and *action* (Charon, 2006). "Contact, taken to its limit, is ... the sense that no matter what is about to be said, access to the object will not be lost. Without the belief in the safety of such contact, we are burdened with the threat that sectors of the mind, if spoken, will lead to abandonment" (according to psychoanalyst Donald Moss, as cited in Charon, p. 150). In complement, action becomes manifest through being moved by our narratives, bearing witness to and easing our suffering, and actively loving and caring for each other. Without collaborative attentiveness and co-constructed representations, affiliation seems unlikely or more accurately will be fragmented and woefully under-enacted. Rather than concordance, the symphony of health from inadequately enacted movements—attention, representation, and affiliation—is marked by discordance. We are marked by a state of unwell-being.

I perceive the providers as talented and well-intentioned, yet they paradoxically demonstrate little understanding of their power in the face of patient vulnerability, they rely on under-interrogated methods, and they enact a willingness to depart without completing care. If only they had prompted our voices a bit more. If only their actions had not emerged from their attentiveness to the physical SOAP representations. If only they had invited our representations.

I didn't get pregnant. I felt/feel/live loss. My husband left. I felt/live loss. I did not create family, one of choosing and co-creating. I am without physical, mental, or social well-being.

Notes

1. In this chapter we share many representations and create the chapter representation about our infertility journey. During the lived experience, we woefully undershared our individual representations with each other and also did not share (to any appreciable degree) these representations with our health care providers. Moreover, our health care providers did not ask questions to prompt the surfacing of these representations. Thus, we are quite certain that the essence of these representations was largely left unshared and cannot be found written in our medical chart. Our written representations exist now, here in this chapter.

2. This chapter was co-written by me, Julie, and Eduardo. I drafted the chapter proposal—narrative approach, dialogic voice and authorship, theoretical framework and critique—and sent it to Eduardo as part of my invitation/suggestion to consider. He accepted, and we began. I wrote the starting draft, which included the theoretical framework and some of my representations, and sent it to Eduardo. He responded by mailing his representations. After integrating his representations, we sent the draft back and forth between us. We engaged in an iterative and reflective writing process. We each made additions and changes only to our individual sections, yet we did so with an awareness of the other's sections and an appreciation of the developing co-written chapter and its co-created context. In latter iterations, I included and refined the theoretical critique. Upon receiving edited versions, Eduardo and I discussed (by phone and in person) the comments and made appropriate revisions.

   We differentiate Julie's representations from Eduardo's by use of font. Julie's writing is in roman font, while Eduardo's is in italics. The differing fonts distinguish the writers' identities. We do not ascribe other meanings to the differing fonts or the respective writer. Together, we lived the experience and together we share our representations.

3. We use pseudonyms for the two health providers named in the chapter.

4. * * * * is a subheading used to note a break in temporality, either in chronological time or, as often employed in the section of our representations, in patient parallel chart entries.

5. Introduced by Dr. Lawrence Weed (1964), the SOAP note is a standardized method of documentation employed by health care providers in a patient's medical chart. The SOAP note provides structure and process for communication among health care providers regarding a patient's health problems and care. SOAP is an acronym for subjective, objective, assessment, and plan. The subjective component of the note consists of information provided by the patient and without external measurement. The objective component consists of measurements and findings from physical examinations as well as results from any labs/tests. The assessment component consists of the provider's diagnosis/es and the basis for said diagnosis/es. Finally, the plan

component consists of what the provider and patient will do, including action steps such as additional labs, procedures, medications, referrals, education, and follow-up.

6. Abbreviation for history.

7. r/o is an abbreviation for rule-out. Providers order tests and procedures to rule out possible causes. This is standard protocol in the search for an identified etiology (cause).

8. Abbreviation for follow-up.

9. I have added parenthetical specifics for you, the reader. The nature and purpose of the hormones, physiological measurements, labs, and medications during the treatment cycles were often understudied by me. Such a response was part of how I coped with this often-overwhelming experience. I leave this to you as I was left to seek additional, perhaps clarifying and useful, information.

10. I remind the reader that this is a break in chronological temporality. Eduardo and I lived together and married before we began our infertility journal.

11. I use couple-centered because potential parents can be any combination of individuals. Nevertheless, I am grounded in our experience as a married, heterosexual couple. Therefore, I write about the female and the male. I do so not to exclude other couples, only to honor this narrative as part of my narrative.

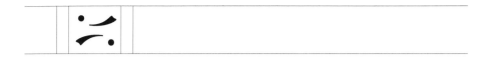

Section 5: Reframing Loss

18. *Cruel Optimism and the Problem With Positivity: Miscarriage as a Model for Living*

Desiree Rowe

After the first miscarriage, I went back to the gynecologist. During what I always think of as the preamble to the visit, the nurse sat me down in a tiny, hot room, just off to the side of where I had waited, to check my vitals and ask preliminary questions. The nurse had a cough. We were sitting close enough that I could feel a surge of warm air every time her chest heaved. The heat of her breath mixed with the dry, stale heat of the furnace made the room feel as if it were closing in on me. I watched her type my information into the laptop. Click. Click. Cough. Click. Click. Cough.[1]

Everything was a blur until the nurse asked:

"How many pregnancies have you had?"

"One," I replied.

"How old is your child?"

"I had a miscarriage."

"Oh," the nurse responded, "I meant real pregnancies."

Everything then remained blurry and out of focus. I was too proud to cry in that tiny, hot room with the throngs of patients waiting just outside the glass door. I felt all the need, the longing, and the want rise in my empty belly to my throat. It was hot, hotter than fire and moving fast like sewage rushing out of dirty pipes. I quickly apologized and changed my answer.

"None. I've had no real pregnancies. I'm sorry. I was confused. It is so hot."

She finishes with my blood pressure and the questions: "When was your last period?" "Do you have a history of diabetes in your family?" The questions rushed past me. We stood and moved. I waited in another space—just as hot—until I was called into the gynecologist's office.

He told me there was nothing he could do until I had at least three *confirmed* miscarriages. I wanted more. At least an exam. Is that weird to say? Peek around there, I thought to myself. Get a flashlight. Something. All I heard was that I needed to come back, bloody and bruised, and then, maybe, I will get treatment. Walking out, it was now my cheeks that burned with heat. The nurse with the cough said, "Goodbye." I never went back there again.

Recounting the stories of my miscarriages is not something that drips easily from memory to keyboard. The narrative takes on meanings that seem important only to me. I am always thinking of that nurse. She didn't seem to be aware of the rising heat or the tears that would come when I was safely in the car. The semantic power of her words slapped me hard in the face and still lurks within me today: "*I* meant *real* pregnancies."

The complexity of narratives about miscarriage is very difficult to engage in, in any kind of critical way. We listen. We listen closely to each other's stories but we do not question the larger normative subjectivity behind the need, behind the suffering. Tell the woman suffering through her second miscarriage that her desire for a child is irrational. That children are too expensive. That it is a marker of heteronormative, patriarchal dominance. Do it. Go up to her, and critically engage that need. That burning in the belly. It's not a need for a child, it's not a need to be pregnant. It's something else. A pull, a longing. What makes us need so much? What made my pain so real? What made my suffering and longing so great? The Need. The Want.

To write about these stories, to live with those experiences, I need to hold on to something deeper. Something that will allow me to finish this without you seeing me cry. I turn to narrative to work through my experiences. The pain becomes more manageable if I can talk through the experience in a critically reflexive space. As Pelias (1999, 2002), Spry (2001), Fox (2010), and others have said, the lure of narrative autoethnography is its messy implications and critical power. Narrative has the ability to alienate the object of miscarriage by taking apart the context and examining the twists and turns of affect. Miscarriage becomes the word that you closely examine. The curves and indentations of miscarriage-as-object deserve a closer look. Why did the gynecologist tell me that I had to have three *confirmed* miscarriages? Why did the first one not count because I never told them I was pregnant? In this narrative I am working to understand how the traces of miscarriage, expressed through stories, stick on to our bodies in complex ways. To unearth that complexity, I work to isolate the word—

MISCARRIAGE

—in order to examine a deeper understanding of the scene. This isn't just about my story, or your story; this is a collective understanding about what it means to be women with the shared experience of miscarriage. To be clear, my approach—the isolation and examination of a word—does not advocate a moving on from the traumatic experience of miscarriage. Rather, I am turning to Lauren Berlant's (2007, 2011) work around the understanding of depressive realism as a perspective to understand my own experiences and as a method of writing. Berlant (2007) tells us that depressive realism is a position "in which the world's hard scenes ride the wave of optimism inscribed in ambivalence, but without taking on optimism's conventional tones" (p. 434). I see depressive realism as a way to engage miscarriage as object through narrative, to take a detached approach to an event that, in a neoliberal climate, is read as an attainment of the good life. The good life, then, is the gold ring of attainment that is held out to us, over and over again. And, in this good life, having a child is one of the most vibrant objects of desire. I am using narrative to write beyond the enigmatic fantasy of attaining a child, to ride the wave and experience the object. As Berlant (2007) explains, "I do not want to move beyond a thing, as I am always still approaching it from within a scene of contact" (p. 434). I want to move through and around this "thing"—miscarriage—to revisit the point of contact and avoid narrative simplicity.[2]

On (Not) Writing Experience

Avoiding narrative simplicity is the reason, at times, I leave out the details that allow my narrative to spin out details that the listener craves. The details that allow the listener to round out the narrative with her own judgments and preconceived (!) notions. If you have ever had a miscarriage or have spoken to someone about her miscarriage, the first question is almost always, "How far along were you?" For many, this is a question that validates the pain and justifies the mourning. And for others, the answer is embarrassing. What if the miscarriage had been at twelve weeks? Is the mother only allowed a certain amount of grief in comparison with the loss at five months? Through the quantification of time, the trauma of miscarriage is judged.

Following Berlant, the anguish and pain of miscarriage are carried with us always and already, and not reducible to days and types of clots. You absorb everything about that pregnancy into who you are and who you become. In this narrative, to engage in simplicity, and move away from judgment, I mark my own two experiences as May/November miscarriages.[3] Each miscarriage was different. Each was marked with physical and emotional pain that I had never experienced before but many others have. My life had been complicated in a way that I never thought was possible.

Though the emotions were raw and powerful, isolating the object of miscarriage allows me to think differently. Pushing aside judgments, and dates, and blood, I realize that I had these intense experiences in relation to really normative aspirations. Aspirations that were centered and grounded in a very white, heteronormative, ideal life. I expected that getting pregnant would be easy. I mean, shit, I had been preventing it every time I had sex with a man. The experiences of miscarriage allowed me to complicate my normative expectations of an object. Which is, in this case, a baby. Thinking of a child as an object may be a bit depressing, but how else shall I think of the thing I do not have? It is a marker, an object that is waiting to be touched. A signifier without a signified. I was projecting a fantasy of a life I didn't yet have, complete with a happy, healthy pregnancy and baby. Before the miscarriages I could sit still enough to imagine entirely the life that I was projecting. I had/have a wonderful partner. I had/have a rewarding job. Isn't a healthy pregnancy supposed to come next?

During one of the miscarriages, my partner and I were living in a rented Craftsman-style home. The house was more than a hundred years old and spoke its age through creaky floors that made quiet nighttime bathroom visits impossible and drafty windows that made the Southern weather feel more extreme than it was. There is a lot of my blood in that house. Rather than have a D&C, I miscarried at home.

Pause. Note: This was a choice I made because of my experiences with medical treatment. I didn't want any more questions, needles, or sorrowful looks. I wanted my home, my bed, and my control.

The blood lasted for days. A river with rocks. The old house had only one windowless bathroom and I took it over. For days I would not allow my partner to go into the bathroom and turn on the light. A washcloth-covered flashlight or a candle was the only source of light permitted. You see, if you've experienced that much blood you know how hard it is to clean up. I was showering three times a day in candlelight. I didn't want to see the blood until it was over. I wanted to clean it up only once. "The days of the dark, bloody bathroom" is how we refer to that time in our life. We moved quietly through our lives until the rushing river stopped.

When he was out of the house I turned on the light. It was one of those big, overhead florescent lights. The kind that gives me a headache. The old light flickered on and shined on the river and the rocks. Blood. Everywhere. Everywhere. Everywhere.

I took a few steps out of that tiny bathroom and sat in the hallway staring inside. There was so much blood. But it was me. I gathered up cleaning supplies and cried through the smell of bleach and rubber gloves and scrubbed that bathroom until it was a dry canyon. I even changed the shower curtain. I bought a new floor mat. The bathroom was back to normal.

Thinking and writing through that experience I realize that my sadness and grief were rooted in deep misrecognition of the object. As the subject, I was unable to achieve that object and because of that failure I lost my sense of self. I lost my sense of continuity of life. I was mourning a fantasy. A fantasy of an ideal life that I did not have.

It is/was easy to talk about wanting a baby without getting into the hidden, gory details of miscarriage, to talk about the life we want rather than the present we are experiencing. "Yes," I would say to friends, "we are trying, but, you know, it takes time." Hidden behind platitudes are the rushing rocky rivers and hot, tiny rooms. We articulate so rationally (to doctors, friends, others) the normalized ideal life, yet fail to acknowledge the perversions and idealizations of what we are attempting to achieve behind closed doors. So, to offer a counter-understanding of these aspirations I turn to miscarriage as an object isolated within itself.

Miscarriage as a Model for Living

One of the worst things you can say to someone who is trying to get pregnant is the dreaded "If you stop trying so hard, it will just happen!" Fuck every single person who has ever said this. I'm sorry about the language, but really. Let's all be real with each other. That's just straight up 100% mean. Passive-aggressive mean. And we shouldn't be allowed to give them a free pass for being stupid. People should just know how stupid that kind of statement is. Through my experiences I learned that it was better for my own well-being to just be honest with everyone. Someone asks me whether I was thinking about having kids? I'm honest. I tell them I've miscarried twice and am working on it. Thank you very much. Lady at the grocery store? Honesty. Nosy aunt? Honesty. No one ever asked for more details.

My newfound blunt honesty had the unintended consequence of shifting the focus of my miscarriages from an inward sense of longing to an outward understanding of belonging. My straight-talking answer elicited unexpected responses from both women and men. I realized, quickly, that I was surrounded by people who had had the same experiences that I had. I spent hours talking to that nosy aunt about her miscarriages, and after more talk with the women in my family, I realized there was a family history. All of the women I talked with shared the same sense of desire for that object that was like no other. The Need. The Want. Again and again. Talking about miscarriage, or the failure to attain the object, creates a sense of *communitas* that is wrapped in blood and shame. The conversations slowly unwrap the trauma, and were easy once they started. Once the liminal space of the taboo was crossed these women and I fell into easy conversation about the hard work of getting (and staying) pregnant. Everyone had shared this trauma.

The pain and longing are what binds people to the social. Our common experiences bring us together, and once we begin talking and engaging about those experiences, the conversations begin to flow. Making this apparent between me and other women allowed for a deeper engagement with those messy moments in ways that are not always about despair, but rather more about engaging in what Berlant calls "footing in worlds that are not there" for you (McCabe, 2011, para. 6). This is miscarriage as a model for living; this is depressive realism. As articulated by Berlant (2007), depressive realism is where "the world's hard scenes ride the wave of the optimism inscribed in ambivalence, but without taking on optimism's conventional tones" (p. 434). Depressive realism is an understanding that we will always be within the context of our trauma, that it is real, and it is not exceptional.

Miscarriage as an object illustrates the living of a depressive realism. The ups and downs of life that are pushed through, that are inscribed in blood, and lived by women. In this way depressive realism is as Berlant notes a "sense of realism that isn't dark or tragic, but less defended against taking in the awkwardness and difficulty of living in the world" (McCabe, 2011, para. 5). That is why the stories of miscarriage must be told. That is why voices must be heard. Because there should be no optimism in "trying to get pregnant." Our understanding of pregnancy and reproduction stems from a feeling of promise—that we are promised this type of life if we perform all the rituals of an American neoliberal life correctly. This promise is often broken. Rather, embracing depressive realism opens up the possibility of failure and does not consistently imagine an optimistic vision of fertility. Failure becomes another crest of the wave as we feel the pressure but see another wave on the horizon. All the while we remain in the water.

There is failure in the ordinary life. And miscarriage is, in fact, a failure. However, narrating life as if childbirth and child rearing are expected norms does nothing but exceptionalize a trauma that is widely experienced by women. Adopting the perspective of depressive realism would allow for a clearer vision of what failure means. Rather than allowing the failure of a pregnancy to be a private (dark, bloody bathroom) shame ("How many *real* pregnancies?"), women will be able to talk more openly with those who have shared the same experiences.

Notes

1. Watch for space. Watch for distance. You have felt that feeling haven't you? How words hang in the air. Waiting for the next sentence. Waiting for the heat to pass and waiting to move to the next (more important) room.

2. My phrasing becomes purposefully vague as I work to describe a picture of how I approach this narrative. Think of miscarriage—the word and the experience—floating in an empty space. My approach in this was and is physical, the way I walk up to and touch and feel that experience. The approach is also here, on the page, approaching the narrative of miscarriage straight ahead, working through potential reservations in detail with precision.

3. I am looking to be purposefully vague on the differences between the May/November miscarriages to move against the traditional judgment that comes with allocating a gestational age. Rather, I chose to mark them as different through the changes in seasons.

19. Turning Tragedy Into Triumph: A Hero's Journey From Bereaved Parent to International Advocate

SHEROKEE ILSE AND KARA L.C. JONES

Kara: In this chapter, I offer guidance to Sherokee through the Hero's Journey (Rebillot, 1993) as she explores her story of love and death. Together we explore Homeground, the Call to Adventure, the Guides, Hero's Initiation, Discovering Our Shield, Council of Heroes, Instruments of Power, Confronting and Summiting With the Shadow, Confronting Obstacles and Blocks, and Rewards and Re-Newed Homeground.

The Hero's Journey reveals itself like a spiral staircase. We come round and round to explore and re-explore, from a flight or two up or down, from a different perspective, always with new insights to our experiences. After a death, we can get caught up in the concepts of getting better, getting over it, "working" grief, or finding closure. But there is no cutoff. No end to the relationship with a child who died. No hard work to be done. Rather, there is a cycle, a way of walking through the post-death world through remembering and re-membering. Re-membering. As in repairing dismembered parts of expectations, dreams, heart, self, and identity that have shattered. A way of finding peace from the pieces. As well as remembering the child we love.

We all have the ability to re-make meaning and come into relationships with our loves and losses in ways that let our hearts be—not just broken—but rather broken *open* to making new meaning, to rediscovering or redefining our lives and identities. I hope Sherokee's story—as she revisits her Journey with miscarriage and stillbirth—serves as a guide for how we can help others explore their own narratives.

Sherokee: When beginning this chapter, I had envisioned a gentle, honest account of what it was like to have a baby *die*. I did not *lose* my babies; they died. I expected to share my story and hoped to teach others about how to survive and thrive after such a deeply painful loss. Simple. "I can do that," I thought. Looking back with Kara to review my experiences, resources, and coping techniques proved to be enlightening and surprising. When I came to this project, I did not understand the Hero's Journey and wrongly assumed that it might set me up to look like someone striving to *be* a Hero in the area of infant loss. Nothing could be further from my truth. Fame or being a role model was never a motivator for what I have done since my loss thirty-two years ago; nor is it today, despite the fact that I am one of the early pioneers who changed how we view miscarriage, stillbirth, and other infant deaths.

In November 1981, my husband David and I were shocked to learn our baby had died a few days prior to his due date. How can a baby die inside a healthy, well-prepared pregnant mother? The drama and trauma when learning of the death and the first days and weeks were overwhelming! I could hardly lift my head or get out of bed. We had left the hospital with no pictures, no mementos of any kind, no helpful literature. No one in our family saw him. The ten minutes we spent with Brennan after his birth, before we handed him back to the staff, was hardly enough time to meet him. No one offered us guidance or told us that we could have him with us longer; this has become a painful regret. I had few memories of his birth during the days that followed.

I felt scared, unworthy, and full of shame, feelings that resurfaced vividly when working with Kara on the Hero's Journey. I could not do what most mothers could—produce a healthy baby. This was our second failure (it felt like *mine*, solely mine). A miscarriage two years earlier had knocked me off my well-planned life. But then the miscarriage was stuffed away, inside a trunk in my mind's attic, put to rest, only to be painfully rediscovered after the second loss.

I sought ways to survive and ways to honor a son no one would ever know, a son who could not do anything to make the world a better place (one of my hopes for my children and me). A new mission to help others emerged.

Did I have the right to call myself a mother? I wondered. In our society, are dead children seen by others as members of a family? A common message is that there is no reason to dwell on them since they are gone. This led me to wonder what a *non-mother* should do. Remember the child or forget? Should I keep talking about my children or clam up? I did not know where to find others who could guide me or who had walked this path before me. I was at a crossroads. A decision needed to be made. There it was—laid at my feet in a very painful way. Following my own instincts, I felt compelled to include these children in my daily conversations and my *new* life going forward, despite pressure to bury them.

I realize now that I chose to take up the challenge and charge ahead, not knowing where I was going. The path I chose for my life's adventure would give my children a voice, make them real to others, and create meaning for me and for the thousands of others who were also left falling, not knowing where they might land. I was without a map, but willing to tackle the future no matter what it would bring.

Homeground

Kara: Homeground is a starting place for the Hero's Journey, where the Hero has lived, worked, made meaning prior to a major change, loss, or adventure. Homeground may have been a safe space before death invaded and gave the Hero the experience of grief. When death arrives, something shatters. Grief may bring groundlessness. It is disorienting to have death take us out of the everyday pace of our impatient world. Senses are slowed. Hearts and expectations have shattered. Everything in the physical body has geared up to feed and care for an infant and there is no one to feed. Ready to be stay-at-home moms or on maternity leave, mothers now find they are haunting an empty house. Home does not feel like home anymore. I asked Sherokee to explore her Homeground experience.

Sherokee: With my eyes closed, feet up, and a busy mind that I tried to quiet, I saw a green, open field, a calm place of beauty and serenity. As I tried to visualize it more deeply, I realized that I barely recalled that time of naïve happiness and hope. It was so long ago and I couldn't see the picture clearly anymore. I was a graduate student working as a business consultant teaching about communication, assertive interactions, and team-building in corporate America. I had a comfortable, rather ordinary, hope-filled life in which all was in order and the beauty of fields, streams, lakes, and running trails made up my life.

What happened next, I liken to crashing into the darkest, coldest, loneliest corner at the bottom of the Grand Canyon. Or I was in murky, muddy, smelly water that engulfed us all, taking our breath away. I was drowning. Was this more of Homeground? This felt like the starting point for my Hero's Journey, the place where the hero starts on a reluctant path.

Call to Adventure

Kara: While many heroes willingly set off to have an adventure, others find themselves reluctantly shoved out the door of Homeground, set on a path they never wanted to walk; they come to the Journey at the hand of trauma.

A reluctant Hero may try to reject the Journey. Reluctance can show up as attempts to return to some sort of pre-death normal in this world that gravitates toward resolutions, desires, and cruel curiosities. Are you better yet? Can you come back to work now? You have three days of funeral leave from work; why do you need more time? Why should the baby shower of a coworker bother you? You need to get over this so you can be healthy. Don't you want to be healthy? You are young and can try again. You have other living children.

With all that pressure and expectation (placed on us by ourselves or others), it is no wonder we don't realize we are allowed to take the time needed to create a new normal or to discover new meanings. A Hero can be reluctant because it feels like loss upon loss. Not only did the baby die, but now we must redefine what it means to be a mother, what it means to do meaningful work, what it means to still feel love even after the physical being of our love is gone. Not only did the baby die, now parents must decide what to do with the space created for the baby. It becomes a physical metaphor for the rearrangement of our hearts as we set out (or are pushed out) on to this reluctant path.

Sherokee: Kara's description of the reluctance to answer the Call fit perfectly with my story. I did not want to face reality; I wanted my old me back.

I recalled visitors in my bedroom or my kitchen. Aghast and disbelieving, I kept asking them and myself: Did this really happen? Is this a nightmare? Will I wake up to find I actually have a living, cooing, sweet baby in my arms? Do babies really die? Why did I never hear about this? Did I cause it? My thoughts, my sins, my worries abounded. Why didn't I go in earlier to be checked? How could a healthy, positive-thinking, blissful, naïve mother let her baby die?

I have memories of feeling raw with overwhelming fear; it was nothing like the safety and calm of Homeground. Feelings of guilt and shame and anger were pushed deep inside. Unable to feel them at the time, I spoke and wrote of their reality and explained why they were a normal response for most mothers at times such as this. But that does not mean I could deal with mine. While exploring this Journey, some notes I took revealed that I had feelings of being unworthy of love during those dark days. I was surprised by this revelation. I don't remember being aware that I felt unworthy of love and I can't explain that. I suppose, since I felt responsible for both babies' deaths, I did not *deserve* to be forgiven and loved. It was not a place in which I was comfortable or prepared to go.

Soon after the death, my mom helped me take down Brennan's nursery— it was so soon and so hard! The sobs came from somewhere so deep that I did not even recognize myself. The unfairness and bitter grief engulfed me and my mother, too. I could not imagine her feelings, only mine. Self-focused, selfish, I was in my own world of pain and anguish, not sure whether I could endure any of it.

Instead, I asked more questions of myself and out loud: Why did we do it that way? Why did we say "no" to photographs, to more time with him? Why did we neglect to invite our family—many of whom lived within thirty miles of the hospital—to meet him? Why did the staff not prepare us or teach us how to meet our baby? Why were there no mementos of any kind? Why did we tell everyone *not* to join us as we scattered his ashes? Thankfully, a few of my husband's relatives didn't listen and showed up anyway. The regrets rose up quickly and none could be undone. It was too late. There are no do-overs!

My friend Sharon, who knew my philosophy of not complaining, asked, "Well, Sherokee, what are you going to do about it?" The challenge was laid out. The answer came quickly, with little contemplation. "You are right!" I said, "I need to do what I can to change how families experience their baby in the hospital after a miscarriage, stillbirth, and other early infant deaths."

My Call to the Adventure turned into a goal to write a pamphlet for every hospital labor and delivery unit. Such a practical, self-help piece would also share a little of our story and our regrets in an empowering and enlightened way. I began to write, night and day, for months. It turned into an eighty-page book, with a question and answer format, for all those who would come after us. I hoped it would be a beacon to light their way through the darkness at such a shocking and overwhelming time. Enthusiastically and optimistically, I was on an unplanned, new adventure.

The Guides

Kara: Guides come to the Hero in many shapes and forms, some internal and some external. For some, the memory or spirit of their child may become a Guide. For others, just the building of a legacy to that child will guide Heroes in new directions. External Guides may come in the form of other bereaved parents, nurses or caregivers, a support group leader, a friend, or relative who has had a similar experience. For others, Guides may come with more intensive work, like delving into grief support via creative coaching, talk therapy, or art therapy. Guides may come in the form of archetypal characters, spirit guides, pop-culture icons, or what is known in Sanskrit as *dharma*.

In whatever shapes or forms they come, Guides host a safe and encouraging reception for our new path, for our re-exploration of the interior and exterior world, for our re-creation of new meaning in our lives. Guides see past the shattering of our hearts. They see us as already reintegrated, foundational, whole beings. They see that it was our experiences that shattered, not our selves. They see that our whole-hearted selves simply need help to make sense of our experiences.

Sherokee: I realize I was not alone, though I felt alone. I was drowning in an immense, stormy ocean. The waves were tsunamis most days; calm waters were rare. As I tasted my tears, I often felt pulled down where it was dark and surreal. Dangers awaited. Sharks and unknown creatures could end it all with a bite or a sting. The maelstrom metaphor only came to me as I reflected and Kara listened.

When he could, David, my Guide, held me up. He must have been treading water, paddling his feet, yet looking calm above water—how could he be so calm? So *there* for me? I now understand he was drowning, too. I knew he hurt deeply. Yet he held me, gave me strength, and floated beside me, keeping me from drowning on the days I wanted to.

In the early days and months, he did not rush me or challenge my intense feelings. When I began writing the book, I no longer went to bed when he did. Or if I did, I couldn't sleep, thinking about what needed to be written. I stayed up writing and rewriting. I organized and reorganized the structure and agonized over each word and thought, cutting and pasting paragraphs on the page, tossing pages into the trash. It had to be just right; vulnerable parents would need to be inspired and taught in a compassionate, thoughtful way. I felt pressure as I envisioned the outcome. I hoped parents would be able to say, "I made the most of a terrible and devastating event. I have no (or few) regrets. Meeting my baby was beautiful and we did it just the right way for us."

David was patient and supportive. He encouraged me and he saw that I was moving along in my grief as I worked on the project. If I needed advice or perspective, he always had something to share. When the book was finally finished, he threw a party inviting all our family and friends. We paid for three thousand copies to be printed with the memorial money we received in the mail from friends and work colleagues after Brennan's death. The book felt like another baby, birthed a mere nine months afterward. Months later, on our way home from the hospital with our newborn, Kellan David, we found hundreds of letters and orders for the book, *Empty Arms* (Ilse, 1982/2013), as a result of the first of many newspaper articles about my story in the *Detroit Free Press* newspaper.

The most important Guide was an unseen force who quietly guided, shielded, and taught me what I was to do and when. God carried me during that time. In looking back, I could feel the love and wisdom that could only come from one who knew what it felt like to have a child die. The letters I received described it as their bible and would say they felt that I was their best friend because I knew exactly how they felt. Such responses were humbling and seemed beyond my own personal capabilities. I was just a grieving mom trying to parent two children—Brennan and Marama (the name I gave to the miscarried baby). Though I had never written a book, God's love and guidance took away most of my doubts and brought me along each day of those many months of writing.

There were times when I felt deep, abiding love. For my babies. For my dear husband and family. For my editor, therapist, and caring friends. As my comfort grew in prayer (I was not a daily praying woman at the time), I felt God's love cradle me through the process of healing and growing after Brennan's death. I didn't have fear or worry and besides being feverishly driven to complete the book, I felt calm and peaceful during the writing process.

While working with Kara on the Guide concept, she asked me to think of what was special about people I admire. I wrote of two people who are accepting, thoughtful, funny, courageous, loving, caring, strong, truthful, and inspirational. In this self-exploration exercise, I came to see that I seek those traits and feel good when others see them in me.

Hero's Initiation

Kara: Up to the point of seeing themselves as initiated Heroes, many parents characterize their experience with grief as hardship, shadow, and other characteristically negative experiences. Struggle. Failing to get back to normal. Through many actions, we have the opportunity and possibility to become initiated as the Hero of our own story. This may happen once we begin to brave a reconnection with the world at large. We may find voice in a support group whereby another human can mirror for us that we are acting heroically. We may receive affirmation from others when they say, "I can see how much creativity it took to get yourself to support group today. Thank you for sharing your story." We may find it as we share our new story with others whereby they reflect for us the ways they see us now. We may hear that they are inspired to make changes in their own lives because they've seen the model of how we are moving in the world. It may be that we finally get a glimpse of what our Guides have been pointing to all along: that we are whole-hearted beings who have had a shattering experience, but our selves are not shattered. We are not broken, even when the experience felt broken.

As we begin to give ourselves permission to follow our hearts, to embody the new normal, to redefine a meaningful life, we are allowing ourselves to be initiated as the Hero of our story. We cannot change what death took. But we begin to be conscious that we can change the life we have left to live. We have agency. We are embracing the agency we have.

Sherokee: My initiation was intense and deeply challenging. I had the need to mother, but no baby. I was not the typical new mother—rocking baby, sleepless nights. Rather, I was a mother with a mission. This was not as satisfying and definitely not a part of my original dreams and plans. Yet it gave me purpose in my days and dreams for my future.

I cried for the first six months, *every day*. I know. I counted. Then when a day or two went by without tears, I was surprised and felt guilty. Could I forget him so easily? Did I deserve to have an ordinary day? Would I become hardened to the pain? Did Brennan and Marama think I loved them less? These questions felt like invaders jumping out at me as I journeyed down the path of my life after loss.

My writing was cathartic and all the people I met and interviewed allowed me to voice my feelings. Conducting workshops and in-service parenting events with nurses, doctors, clergy, funeral directors, and other care providers became weekly events. I was becoming comfortable in my Initiation into a meaningful life. I loved what I did because it mattered and it seemed to help, though it was also sad and hard.

People wondered whether I was stuck in my grief since I was not moving on. Others asked whether I was a nurse or perhaps a medical caregiver, since I spent so much time teaching in hospitals and clinics. The message I interpreted was, "There must be something wrong with her. She is a parent, stuck in her sadness and spending her days talking about death, grief, and other morbid things." My answer, boldly spoken, was, "I am moving on. This is how I *am* moving on. I have an important mission." *This* then became my profession, my business, and my calling. I was proud of this choice and happy with myself. The ultimate honor is having parents say they know I speak on their behalf. My new normal was evolving.

Discovering Our Shield

Kara: A Shield, like the shields used in battle, can be held out in front of the Hero for protection. A Shield might be created as an art project, such as the colored ribbons or rubber bracelets given to groups that promote awareness and say to others, "I am grieving." These symbols hark back to the black armbands or attire worn as Shields in the past. Parents experiencing loss may create language Shields when they are faced with platitudes. Someone may say to a parent, "You are young and you can try again." Instead of just accepting this, the parent can counter it with a language Shield: "Yes, I can try again, but that next child will be the *next* child, *another* child, and not a replacement for this child who has just died." By putting up these physical or linguistic Shields, parents have agency to prevent arrows from piercing them.

The mythical Hero's Shield—the armor used for protection—has two sides. There is that outer side that goes up, displayed to the world, raising awareness or visibility, communicating to the aggressor that arrows cannot reach the Hero. There is also a back side, the side with a handle that allows the Hero to wield the Shield skillfully. It is a physical contact, an extension of the Hero with an energy fueling stability and protection. Parents experiencing the death of a child may volunteer for a nonprofit that helps other bereaved parents. The outer part of the Shield is raising awareness and doing good for the nonprofit. The back side of the Shield is used to re-direct the love, time, money, and energy that would have gone to the physical child if s/he had survived.

Sherokee: When Kara asked me to consider my Shield and to draw it as a sort of warrior's Shield, it was a foreign idea to me. However, I immediately envisioned a cross with the words "Trust in Me" written on it. This surprised me a bit. I don't believe I had such a clear image at the time of my loss. I was on a mission that took courage and fortitude; such a Journey in the midst of early grief is not easy or even possible for many people. Yet I worked on it every day. People who met me at this time would probably say that I was serious, committed, persistent, and always giving of myself to others in need. But they didn't know the silly, fun, active, and lighthearted person I used to be.

After I wrote *Empty Arms* (Ilse, 1982/2013), I rather impulsively decided to start a nonprofit along with seven other hardworking, committed parents. It was the first national nonprofit organization in the United States created to shift the paradigm of care and understanding about early losses, a shift from what I call the "Dark Ages" to a more enlightened time. It was a very intense, overwhelming, and painful time. It was a time that required persistence and patience to make the changes we sought.

Our team gave it our all for ten years, leading the United States into a new day with newsletters, literature, direct care, and support to thousands of families. We even led the movement to make October National Pregnancy and Infant Loss Awareness month. I spoke at hundreds of in-services, workshops, meetings, conferences, and support groups inspiring change all over the United States and Canada and eventually the United Kingdom, Japan, New Zealand, and Australia. Over the years, I wrote and cowrote sixteen other books and booklets along with newsletters, articles, and whatever it took to improve the environment of care for bereaved families. Looking back

I remember how busy I was while also being an involved mother to my two living sons, Kellan and Trevor.

On the outside of my Shield I saw words such as "Don't give up. Don't give in," "Inspire," "Be persuasive and positive," "Act like it has already happened," and, of course, "Trust in Me." God had my back and although there were some very dark and difficult times, I persevered and did not give up. For thirty-two years I have lived and worked this mission.

Also, on the outside of my Shield were hearts—small baby hearts and larger parent hearts. I often drew hearts and incorporated them as logos. We used various forms of baby feet and hearts on sympathy cards and in awareness campaigns. Recently, I have begun using the heart as a logo for our new venture—I have started to help others become Guides to the newly bereaved.

The Shield I carried was heavy most of the time, much like the armored shield of the knights of old. Now I see that inside my Shield were messages of love and sharing, along with financial stress, insecurity, and worry. I wondered about whether we could really change the minds, hearts, and protocols in every hospital and community. The pressure I felt on behalf of all the people for whom I was doing this work was immense, bringing many sleepless nights.

Council of Heroes

Kara: We come to find that we are not solo Heroes out in the world. We are not the only ones to experience death and be faced with learning to live again. We come to find that there are actually Councils of Heroes everywhere, consisting of people who stand in support of us, love us, maybe have had similar experiences, maybe jump in and help with some aspect of our Journey. It may be in attending a support group or gathering our friends and family that we find our Council of Heroes. By gathering our Council of Heroes around us, we begin to gather a Council of others who really understand what it means to live whole-heartedly after the death of a child. So we continue reaching out—one person at a time—into the world.

Sherokee: A Council of Heroes. What a great concept! I always thought of my like-minded people as a team. And they were, indeed, Heroes for taking up our cause to help families and to improve care in clinics, hospitals, and throughout the community and country. These dedicated folks gave their hearts and souls. I wish I had called them Heroes more often.

After Kara introduced the concept of a Council of Heroes, one of the first people who came to mind was Susan Erling, our Executive Director at the Pregnancy and Infant Loss Center. She was a perfect partner to change the baby loss world. Our relationship brought our different skills together, which resulted in a successful organization and awareness-building campaign. We helped thousands of families each year, taught and empowered thousands of caregivers, and brought miscarriage, stillbirth, and other kinds of infant deaths out of the shadows. Our staff, board of directors, and many volunteers worked tirelessly to attain our goals. We worked as a team and had many successes, laying groundwork that helps us still today.

Friends from organizations such as SHARE, RTS Bereavement Services, HAND, NEOFIGHT, AMEND, and UNITE played important roles in shifting the paradigm from silence to acceptance. Many parents who have reached out to me with their own projects and books stand out in my mind as members of my Council of Heroes.

Instruments of Power

Kara: Feathers given to Native American warriors. The wand in *Harry Potter*. Even Popeye's can of spinach. Instruments of Power are often very common objects, but they are objects that become infused with numinosity. They become touchstones to newly recreated lives and meanings. Many parents will come up with physical Instruments of Power. They carry rubbing stones in their pockets, or wear pins displaying hummingbirds, dragonflies, or ladybugs. Some parents will create Instruments of Power that demonstratively show the world how meaningful the life and death of their baby has been. They will perform random acts of kindness in the name of the child. They will create or commission public art installations. Instruments of Power become signifiers of empowerment and agency. They say we are going in the right direction or calm and encourage us as we continue on a new path.

Sherokee: At first, I couldn't imagine what an Instrument of Power was and what mine might be. When my friend Polly's husband died, we walked the beach and I searched for heart-shaped rocks. When I sought a memento to give fathers (often forgotten in the labor and delivery room), I found some perfectly sized stone hearts. I believe that my broken heart needed healing and so finding heart pictures, stones, ribbons with hearts, and heart logos must be my Instrument of Power. My Babies Remembered heart symbol on the cover of *Empty Arms* (Ilse, 1982/2013) also serves as my web site logo. As I look at it now, it makes sense that hearts are my Instrument of Power. There is no doubt about what brings healing and meaning to me. The heart holds multiple meanings and soothes my own heart and, I hope, the hearts of others who are touched by my work.

Confronting and Summiting With the Shadow

Kara: Unfortunately, the concept of the Shadow is often discouraged. Family and friends want parents to be positive, to get better, and to get back to normal. Even in the new age, self-help, or other spiritual support systems, there can be a resistance toward anything deemed negative, and often the dark emotions are deemed bad, for fear that parents will get stuck in negativity. In the Law of Attraction and thought-change movements, it can be deemed that even thinking about something negative will only bring more bad experiences. Even in some mythology, the Shadow may show up as a Dragon to be slayed. For many parents, the implicit or explicit direction to "stay positive" can cut them off from the insights and love to be found when we accept the whole of our experience, the Light *and* the Shadow. For instance, if a mother of a dead child never admits or explores how jealous and envious she feels of other pregnant women, she may never get the opportunity to discover what is driving those Shadows of jealousy and envy.

When a mother is given safe space to explore and admit to these Shadows, she discovers that what she really fears is that her child and her motherhood will be silenced. She discovers that while other mothers have their children physically present to signify motherhood, her motherhood will become invisible because her child has died. Once she has this insight, she then has the option of becoming her own best advocate. She can begin sharing with others the fact that Mother's Day in the United States was founded by bereaved mothers during the Civil War, so Mother's Day is indeed a day for honoring all mothers, those with living children and those whose children have died.

There are many ways to facilitate people's experiences with the Shadow. Miriam Greenspan's *Healing Through the Dark Emotions* (2004) is an amazing guide for exploring the Shadow. We may counter violent reactions to the Shadow by countering what is normally considered proper in the confrontation of Shadow. For instance, rather than seeing grief as a dragon to be slayed, what if we were to dance with grief? What could we learn about our Shadow if we explored it without judgment, to learn more about what we are experiencing?

Sherokee: I hardly remember the Shadow much anymore, though it was always lurking and still visits on rare occasions. I can remember that darkness and accompanying fear; they were overpowering. I feared living, dying, and the emptiness of my arms and life. It was the darkest and most overwhelming for me at night. I worried I might never be *normal* again. I wallowed in pain, but also stood up with a sword in hand, giving me the energy to face CEOs of hospitals or intimidating interviewers—I was intimidated; they were kind and welcoming—such as Phil Donohue and Oprah. I was committed to making the changes needed in our institutions and in our culture.

I pray that the Shadow keeps its place in my life, since it is part of my story and my whole. I work against being frightened or controlled by its presence and power.

Confronting Obstacles and Blocks

Kara: You don't master the art of yoga after one class, and so you keep practicing. In this same way, parents on the Hero's Journey after the death of a child will find that every day is a continuation of the practice. Practicing skills of agency. Learning daily how to be creative in the face of grief. Finding continued fuel and inspiration from Guides, Shields, Instruments of Power. We continue to explore both the Light and Shadow with curiosity rather than judgment.

Some parents continue their practice by attending support groups, eventually learning how to facilitate a group. Others continue to practice awareness of unanswerable questions such as, "Why me?" They continue to ask questions such as, "What can I do today to help another person in the name of my child?" They continue to challenge themselves to understand what they are called to do in this post-death life.

Sherokee: At one point my husband asked me whether I wanted to go back to school and get an advanced degree in counseling or grief. After much thought, I decided against that idea. I wanted to become respected as a parent voice—a parent advocate. I suspected that the professional path, with all the theory and research, would alter my voice and my message. I share parents' stories. That voice is one I know and one that allows me to use the first person (I and we) in a powerful way. Many professional caregivers use the third person voice (they, she, he), even if they have had their own loss. They often depend upon research and theory when speaking, teaching, and even storytelling. There is a place for both voices and all experiences.

The choice I made to be the parent voice as I advocate for change and awareness represents one obstacle that continues today. Over the years, I have noticed that there are some who use their academic titles as a way to compete rather than collaborate. It can be difficult to stand strong as a parent advocate without academic credentials. I believe my contributions and those of parents are important and deserve to be valued. After thirty-two years of experience, I continue to be happy that I chose the parent voice, as it has served my community well and provides personal fulfillment.

Rewards and Renewed Homeground

Kara: The Hero's Journey is a practice that allows death and grief to transform our hearts into open vessels. As the Hero continues to be in the world, she discovers the rewards of re-creating that world, of finding new meaning, of re-defining self and Homeground. The Hero may not always be out on the path. She will often return home, changed, and with the discovery that she is also an agent of change. She has discovered how to give herself permission to live whole-heartedly again in this post-death life. She continues to practice finding peace within the pieces of shattered experience while allowing for the reality that she herself is not shattered. She has a whole-hearted approach to life now. And she is a powerful agent in the world, sharing the gift of her voice and story, as well as receiving the gifts and rewards of connecting to others in whole-hearted relationships.

For some bereaved parents, this means they've found new careers, co-created foundations, or had their priorities rearranged. For others, things may look much the same on the outside, but their interior landscape of Homeground is more heart-centered, with more compassion toward themselves and others.

The possibilities of where the Hero's Journey can take us are endless. We don't take this path just once and suddenly all is perfect. Rather, we are on the spiral staircase of this path, always moving up or down a level or two, getting different perspectives, living a life of practice and curiosity.

Sherokee: I often speak of the fragility of life and the miracles that are easily taken for granted. I make time to enjoy sunsets, flowers, amazing people, and life experiences. Experiences are transformative and offer personal rewards that define me as a different person. Mountaintops are higher because of the valleys I have survived.

Many of the rewards of this life work come from the feedback I receive from parents, family members, and caregivers. I have saved every letter and email sent to me. I reread them when I am sad or in need of guidance. They help me to remember that this mission is not about me or about my own babies. Rather, it is about those who suffer and what we can do for them and each for other. I reflect on what there is to learn and how grateful I am for my life just the way it is. Today I love to spend time on social media validating people's rights to their feelings and offering them understanding, compassion, resources, and, most important, hope. Mentoring and teaching, along with sharing my philosophies and helpful resources, give me satisfaction. The spiral that Kara speaks of and the repetition at different levels is a metaphor that I relate to as I live in my new Homeground.

Conclusion

Kara: There are so many ways that we can explore the Hero's Journey. We might come to explore it on our own as a bereaved person. We may come to facilitate the exploration for others in our capacity as caregivers. We might use conversational creativity or making art to explore the various areas of the Journey structure. We might look at Joseph Campbell's (2008) framework or Paul Rebillot's (1993) version of the Hero's Journey and use those as guides, but we can also break open the various steps to explore all the spaces off the path. Explorations of the Hero's Journey include both the practice and the process. There is no final destination. There is no closure. There are continually evolving meanings, experiences, relationships, co-creations.

Sherokee: Recovering from the loss of a baby or any death is hard work. How we grieve, what tools we use, and what path we take often happens with no framework. The Hero's Journey offers such a framework. As for me and my life lessons during this guided Journey—I was able to differentiate that being a Hero in the world, as seen by others, is not the point or purpose. Rather, I came to see my Hero's Journey as a fight for survival after suffering tragedy. Thankfully, I survived and changed in many positive ways. It has also been a call for greater purpose and meaning.

How will I use the Hero's Journey paradigm to understand my life as I go forward? With new awareness, I feel confident that when I need it, it is in my bag of tools. For that I am grateful to people such as Joseph Campbell, Sherene Zolno, and Paul Rebillot—pioneers in exploring the Hero's Journey. I am grateful to Kara for gently, wisely, and compassionately leading me through the Journey. Kara shared her wisdom and her gifts in a way that honored all of my life experiences without judgment. I was able to be authentic, vulnerable, open, and honest. What a gift that was to me!

Now I have a new Hero in her; I have added Kara to my Council of Heroes. I love that I have continued to change and grow every year since the events that permanently altered the direction of my life! Who knew that the chapter I envisioned would become so much richer and deeper than I could have imagined?

20. Breaking Through the Shame and Silence: A Media-Centered Approach to Consciousness-Raising

RACHEL E. SILVERMAN

In season seven (1997) of the epic television series *Beverly Hills, 90210*, lead character Kelly Taylor (Jenny Garth) suffers a miscarriage during her senior year at California State University. Although she fears that her condition, endometriosis (which led to the miscarriage), may cause future complications in getting pregnant, she is nonetheless relieved to avoid the difficult decision about whether to have an abortion. In an emotional scene, she and her boyfriend, Brandon (Jason Priestley), cry over the loss of their potential child and with relief because they were not ready to become parents. As a freshman in college, an avid fan of the show, and a recently sexually active (sexually experimenting) adult, I too was relieved for Kelly. The week before, when Kelly realized her period was late and learned she was pregnant (a secret she shares only with best friend Donna Martin [Tori Spelling]), friends and I debated whether *90210* would be daring enough to show an abortion on television. Conveniently, they did not have to. Little did I realize at the time, but Kelly's miscarriage was one of many "convenient miscarriages"[1] to appear in popular media. In fact, I probably equated miscarriage with being relieved of making a tough decision about an unwanted pregnancy until Charlotte York repeatedly miscarried and declared herself "reproductively challenged" four years later on *Sex and the City* (2001–2004). Admittedly, my initial viewing of Charlotte's infertility did not leave much impression on me. I was recently out of college and still far from the time when my peers would be trying to get pregnant and begin dealing with their own reproductive challenges.

When the time did come that the women I knew had switched from astutely taking their pills to actively pursuing what they had spent most of their lives avoiding, I also began to hear more and more about friends suffering from miscarriage and ectopic pregnancies, discussing in vitro, and considering freezing their eggs. In the midst of my doctoral program, I was busy teaching feminist theory and doing dissertation research. Charlotte York's conversion to Judaism on *Sex and the City* was the focus of one of my dissertation chapters and therefore her infertility added to the recurring discussion of pregnancy loss going on all around me.

Over the course of the next few years, the number of stories about pregnancy loss and infertility seemed to be growing within the media and the representations of pregnancy loss were becoming more poignant and thus more powerful. Rather than pregnancy loss happening off screen, the mediated narratives began showing the actual physiological aspect of loss. Meredith Grey (Ellen Pompeo) bled through her scrubs as she miscarried during a hostage takeover of Seattle Grace-Mercy West Hospital (*Grey's Anatomy*, 2010) and audiences saw a bathroom full of blood as Celia Foot (Jessica Chastain) miscarried multiple times in the film *The Help* (2011). Khloe Kardashian's ultrasounds and infertility are chronicled on a variety of E! network reality shows (2011–2013), and in the film *The Other Women* (2009), Natalie Portman's character Emilia Greenleaf relives the death of her child from SIDS over and over throughout the film. From the Dixie Chicks' song *So Hard* (2006) and Jay-Z's song *Glory* (2012), to the novel *Luscious Lemon* (2004) and the memoir *The Baby Chase* (2011), everywhere I turned, the popular media seemed to be offering yet another storyline of infertility or celebrity account of miscarriage—and not convenient ones.

When I sat down to lunch with an old friend who was dealing with infertility, she complained of having nothing to read that resonated with her experience. Too many books offered coping strategies that she found trite or overly religious; other books told stories far too different from her own and she was unable to relate. Throughout our conversation, I was impressed by the ease with which she was able to discuss what too often seemed a taboo subject. I thought that maybe I could help her by finding some scholarship on the subject—surely there were feminist writers tackling the issue of miscarriage who could offer her some grounded, practical ideas rather than emotional sentiments and guides to self-help. Hours of searching produced minimal results. What I discovered was that because the issue of pregnancy loss treads on the issue of "fetus versus baby," the feminist intelligentsia has largely avoided the topic.

* * *

Chira (1994) succinctly states, "The debate on abortion has contaminated our discussions and feelings about pregnancy and miscarriage" (para. 1). On one hand, she admits to difficulty in reconciling her grief from experiencing a pregnancy loss "with [her] belief in the right to abortion" (para. 5) because to claim a fetus is a (wanted) child is "inconsistent, hypocritical and politically maladroit" (para. 8) with abortion rights. On the other hand, Welch and Herrmann (1980) argue:

> It should be obvious, but it isn't: an abortion and a miscarriage are qualitatively different experiences. Where the woman who chooses abortion controls her body's use, the woman who miscarries has lost control through no fault of her own. And while the physiological outcome may be the same, the psychic effects are … a different story. (p. 14)

Layne (1997) suggests feminists fear the topic of pregnancy loss for two reasons: (1) because pregnancy loss takes the control of reproduction out of the control of the individual woman; and (2) because pregnancy loss straddles definitions of what is considered a baby and what is considered a fetus. In her 2003 article, which followed the publication of her book *Motherhood Lost*, Layne expounds on the reasons pregnancy loss is excluded from feminist texts. She offers three detailed reasons this is so: (1) Pregnancy loss overlaps with the politics of abortion, rights to individualism, and the meaning of loss; (2) pregnancy loss counters the feminist stance to depathologize pregnancy; and (3) pregnancy loss unduly emphasizes the patriarchal "seed."

According to Layne (2003a, 2003b), the primary reason for the silence among feminists concerning pregnancy loss is that feminists, like anti-abortionists, fight over individualism and essential rights to personhood, that is, whether the fetus is or isn't a baby. If the pregnancy is a person, if the fetus is a desired child, then arguably it deserves full civil rights and abortion is not an option. By acknowledging that the loss of a pregnancy/fetus is the loss of a desired person, then the rights of that fetus/baby as an individual put feminists in a bind over abortion politics. If the desire for a pregnancy to grow into a person is the determining factor between a fetus and a baby, and therefore between choice and no-choice, then acknowledging the desired human being is tricky. And because the right to choose is so fundamentally a right all women deserve, any discussion that might suggest the opposite is one that feminists have been unwilling to have.

The second reason for silence comes from the longstanding feminist tradition to depathologize pregnancy, which is countered when pregnancy loss occurs. Pregnancy loss evokes feelings of weakness, incompleteness, and failure; pregnancy loss implies that a woman's body has failed her and as a result she has failed as a woman. As a pathology, pregnancy loss is antithetical to feminism—again a bind and again silence, although the shame of failure is now added to the equation.

Layne's third explanation for silence comes from the fetus's growth process. The linearity of growth harks back to the patriarchal rendering of a male seed planted within a woman's womb. Because feminists have long fought against this heterosexist, patriarchal notion of pregnancy, discussing pregnancy loss as a loss along the growth process places feminists in a bind, and again there is more silence—although now a hierarchy of experience occurs because as the "seed" grows, the value of it changes and with it, the value of the experience. While Layne sympathizes with the reasoning behind the silence, she believes that ignoring the issue is "patronizing" to those who have experienced loss. Without an understanding of and discussions about pregnancy loss, people who suffer losses suffer alone, in silence, and without recourse.

***

In September 2012, a childhood friend and his girlfriend discovered they were pregnant. While not a planned pregnancy, it was a welcomed one. At five months, she was rushed to the hospital because of pains and bleeding. The heartbeat was gone. The doctor offered her two choices—a D&C, which could potentially harm her uterus and hinder future pregnancies, or a stillbirth delivery, which the doctor suggested as the option better for the health of her body. She chose the stillbirth delivery. Hours after the delivery a nurse came into the room carrying the stillborn. The nurse informed her that per New Jersey state law, what was in her arms was a baby and therefore needed to be seen by the parents and given a name; a birth and death certificate needed to be signed; and arrangements needed to be made for the body. Had she chosen the D&C, none of this would have happened. Because she made a choice for her body, a choice presented by her physician without repercussions, she was forced to contend with the realities of anti-abortion legislation.

***

Individual state laws about reproductive rights are not always made clear to patients when they are making the necessary choices that often come with pregnancy loss. Similarly, hospitals are often filled with literature about loss that does not suit the needs of the patient. Reagan's (2003) account of pregnancy loss describes being at the hospital surrounded by images and phrases pulled directly from anti-abortion literature. Tiny footprints, angels, and statements such as "All life is precious, even for just a moment" are as common in pregnancy loss literature as they are in anti-choice paraphernalia. Reagan suggests that the "use of the anti-abortion movement's language in *official* hospital material lends that movement medical legitimacy and political power" (p. 367 emphasis original). By making anti-abortion symbols ubiquitous with pregnancy loss, power is given to those symbols and an environment hostile to women's reproductive rights ensues.

When we don't discuss pregnancy loss from a feminist perspective and when we don't acknowledge the reality and diversity of women's experiences, the taboo nature of the topic grows and power is given to those who will discuss the topic. At a time when so many politicians are attempting to minimize reproductive rights, it is crucial that we learn to talk about loss in a way that breaks the silence and maintains choice. Likewise, as reproductive technologies become increasingly available and the system of baby-making changes, pregnancy loss becomes an even more varied issue. Pregnancy loss is an issue of women's health, just as much as abortion, birth control, and breast cancer, and the silence that continues to surround pregnancy loss is unacceptable.

Silence exists because of the fear that by acknowledging the loss of life, the fetus will become a baby and anti-abortionists will have a stronger platform. Silence creates shame when women feel inadequate because their bodies are pathologized as a result of their inability to live up to pronatalist social expectations. Silence and shame create a culture wherein the amount of time a woman is pregnant impacts the level she is supposedly allowed to mourn the loss.

This twofold framework of shame and of silence within which pregnancy loss exists is the reason for this book. But more so, this framework points to a larger social problem, one that needs increased awareness—an awareness that moves the discourse out of the clutches of those who work to limit reproductive freedom and an awareness that each story matters and no one loss is greater or worse than another.

***

In the spring of 2011, in my last semester in graduate school, amidst my family's and friends' experiences with pregnancy loss, during the school's annual Take Back the Night[2] (TBTN) event, I began to think about the social construction of pregnancy loss as a phenomenon comparable to rape. While the experiences are vastly different, to the point of being incomparably different, the social responses to each and the personal feelings that emerge as a result of both are similar. Both are topics shrouded in silence. Both create feelings of incomplete or inadequate womanhood. Both cause women to question themselves and their culpability. And both create feelings of guilt, shame, failure, and remorse. As the survivors of sexual assault took the stage and asserted their right to wear the clothing they wanted or to go running whenever they wanted, I thought about the women I knew who worried their years on birth control were at the root of their infertility or that training for a marathon had resulted in their miscarriage. I began to see the parallels between the feelings of failed womanhood, the secrecy, the endless comparisons about whose situation is worse than another's, and the needless but penetrating feelings of remorse and doubt.

Sometime not too long after that TBTN event, I sat with my sister, her friends, and their kids as the women discussed their bouts with infertility and experiences of miscarriage with the ease that comes from having healthy children. I wondered what it would have been like for these women to have had this conversation during their infertility or immediately after their miscarriage. This session among the women felt similar to the TBTN event on campus—I thought about the power of finally sharing your story, of release, and of the changes that happen when people realize they are not alone. I wondered, where is the TBTN for pregnancy loss? Why did these women remain silent and suffer alone rather than share their stories with each other when they needed support the most? How can we remove the guilt and shame that comes as a result of pregnancy loss? What does it take to begin a discussion about pregnancy loss, one that is grounded in the right to choose while also acknowledging the pain of losing a wanted pregnancy? In Audre Lorde's words, "when your silences will not protect you ... What are the words you do not yet have?" (Lorde, 2007, p. 41).

* * *

Years before pregnancy loss was a reality among my friends, my mother lost a baby who was less than two weeks old. Benjamin Harris Silverman was born September 1981. Ever since, at Yom Kippur, my mother cries. When Benjamin died, my mother was left alone in an empty nursery to grieve. My father went back to work and my sister and I continued on at nursery school with only a cursory understanding of what had happened. In fact, I can't distinguish the pregnancy of Benjamin with the following pregnancy that produced my brother Matt. I remember being angry at my mother for not bringing home the baby brother she had promised, but I can't remember a second pregnancy—just a baby brother arriving sometime later. A psychologist had told my parents it would be good for them, and for my sister and me, to have another baby, that another baby would help them heal from the wounds of loss and help my sister and me in our developmental stages of memory. In the years since, the tears that always come during the High Holidays are for Benjamin. But until recently, I never really understood what they meant.

Benjamin was born with Down syndrome and a number of other health issues. My parents made it clear from the moment of his birth that there were to be no extreme lifesaving measures. During the time he was alive, he had a *bris* at the hospital, per Jewish custom, in case he lived. When he died, he stayed at the hospital because it was less than thirty days and again, per Jewish custom, there was to be no funeral. When he was born, he was immediately taken from my mother in the delivery room and she was left in silence to wonder why. During the next few days my parents were in and out of the hospital and my mother began to realize that she had lost not just her son, but also the community of women with whom she was bringing up my sister and me. For these women, my mother had become their worst nightmare and no one wanted to be near her. While many sent letters and food, few came over to our house or over to the car when she dropped us off at nursery school. Looking back at the situation, she describes her experience as feeling like she had something the other women feared "catching"; no one wanted to get too close to her for fear they too might lose their babies.

My mom had nowhere to go and nothing to do. Without the baby to care for, her time at home was unfilled. There were no support groups, no books about loss, no one to talk to, and no way for her to talk about it. The empty room where Benjamin was supposed to sleep was on the second floor and so my mother retreated to the third floor of the house where she could sit in the silent darkness and cry. For years she was angry and for years the sight of children with Down syndrome made her cry. Now the crying mostly happens in the fall.

***

My mother's experience has informed my experience of loss, my sister's experience has informed my loss, my friends' experiences have informed my loss, and my own life has informed my loss. I am thirty-five, I am in the third year of my first job as an assistant professor, and I am in a committed lesbian partnership. I have always wanted to be pregnant, to have a baby, but never so much to bring up a child. Until recently, having kids was never my thing, but being pregnant and having a baby was. I joked with friends that I would carry their babies for them. I looked into being a surrogate, even offering my womb for free, but without already having given birth I am a non-viable candidate. I am too risky. My partner is twenty-nine, and in the past few months we have been discussing having a child. Neither of us is quite ready, and if or when we are, her body will be better suited because of her age. Her body is also better suited because my brother will donate the sperm—the child will be as close to biologically ours as possible and that is important to both of us. I know I will struggle watching her belly grow round. I also know that the cost and risk it would take to implant an embryo comprising her and my brother in me is beyond what we are willing to do. I long for the experience of being pregnant, and I mourn the loss of an experience I will never have.

In editing this collection, I realize that each new story of loss further informs my understanding of the experience of loss and my ability to speak about loss. The authors in this collection take an important step in creating a language of loss and recreating the discourse surrounding pregnancy loss. The authors provide a variety of experiences of loss, but by no means have the stories spanned the diversity of loss. Importantly, the collection does not have enough non-white voices nor enough diversity among the people of color included; the collection lacks gay and lesbian couples; it lacks single women attempting motherhood; it lacks class variety, religious variety, and variety of physical abilities. While we have all worked to bring awareness to an issue that for many feels like an isolated incident, we have only taken the first step. We have narrated the complexities of pregnancy loss as a means of negating a single story. We have worked to reconceptualize loss outside the discourses of medical pathology, self-help literature, and anti-abortion rhetoric. We need to do more. We need to hear more stories. The media provide places to find such stories.

Knowing that any understanding of pregnancy loss is socially constructed by our cultural and historical contingency, looking to media can provide another source from which to understand how pregnancy loss is and can be understood. As the author of the final chapter in this collection and, in many ways, ending up where we began, I offer the possibility of a media-centered approach to consciousness-raising (CR) as a method for working through the silence and shame that comes with pregnancy loss. CR is at the root of feminist thinking and events such as Take Back the Night; it is a strategy for change, a way of developing new perceptions, a technique for approaching difficult issues, and most important, a way to increase awareness about an idea.

During the second wave of feminism, women gathered in small groups to tell their individual experiences about oppression. These CR groups allowed women to analyze the conditions of their lives and discover that their experiences, which many had thought were isolated incidents, were actually cultural phenomena. According to Koedt, Levine, and Rapone (1973), the process of CR is "one in which personal experiences, when shared, are recognized as a result not of an individual's idiosyncratic history and behavior, but of the system of sex-role stereotyping. That is, they are political, not personal questions" (pp. 280–281). Stories about sexual assault, sexual harassment, health problems, and unsatisfactory family lives were revealed through CR, and these issues were discovered to be plaguing women everywhere. By raising people's consciousness about an idea (or a situation, event, etc.) the importance of that idea was elevated and previously ignored issues were brought to light. In other words, the personal became political.

In the introduction to this book, we offer narrative as a third-wave rhetorical methodology for CR. Here, I extend the narrative methodology and take cues from second-wave feminist literary scholars to argue for a media-centered approach to CR.

Feminist literary scholars such as Hogeland (1998), Frye (1986), and Register (1975) claim the act of reading feminist novels and sharing the novels with other women as a method of CR; I suggest the act of consuming mediated representations of pregnancy loss and discussing those representations as a method of CR. Important to note is that nowhere do these scholars define what a "feminist novel" is; rather, they assume that novels written by women about women's experiences are feminist. Likewise, I suggest that consuming media about pregnancy loss that move beyond the "convenient miscarriage" offers an opportunity to better understand the experience of loss. Hogeland (1998) cites literature such as Erica Jong's *Fear of Flying*, Marilyn French's *The Women's Room*, Margaret Atwood's *Lady Oracle*, and Joan Didion's *Play It as It Lays* as examples of CR books. In each of these novels, "the protagonist moves from feeling somehow at odds with others' expectations of her, into confrontations with others and with institutions, and into a new and newly politicized understanding of herself and her society" (Hogeland, 1998, p. 23). Frye (1986) adds to the description of literary CR by explaining how:

> feminist change derives from the reader, especially the woman reader, who might find through the reading of novels the growing edge of her own humanity, extending beyond available roles and categories and into a renewed future. As she learns from female characters new ways to interpret her own and other women's experiences, she helps to reshape the culture's understanding of women and participates in the feminist alteration of human experience. (p. 191)

Register (1975) suggests literature has the potential to "augment consciousness-raising" and help "reshape the culture's understanding of women and assist in humanizing and equilibrating the culture's value system" (p. 19). If literature has been a source for CR, then media can be a source for CR as well. As a conclusion to this book, I offer a media-centered approach to CR.

Media scholar Fiske (2011) argues that audiences are active interpreters of the media. As such, people "read television in order to produce from it meanings that connect with their social experience" (p. 84). In particular, Fiske cites Hobson's (1982) work, which focuses on the role of television in the home and the ways in which media can be used by women to "kick against patriarchal domination" and "become part of their (women's) resistance" (Fiske, p. 75). Radway's (1984) work also supports the idea that media can help women create "their own cultural space" and enable "a self-generated sense of feminine identity" (Fiske, p. 75). Following the work of these media scholars and literary critics, I suggest audiences and those who have experienced pregnancy loss take an active approach to reading today's media texts as a form of CR. By using the texts to create a cultural space wherein we reshape our understanding of the human experience, we can thus remove the silence and shame surrounding pregnancy loss. This political act will increase awareness of pregnancy loss and will work to prevent a hierarchy among narratives of pregnancy loss.

Each media text can be seen as an individual voice, as an individual story that, when combined, acts as a coming together to create a common experience. While the "convenient miscarriage" trope still exists on television and in film as a harmless alternative to abortion, and there is no doubt that the media continue to promote ideal versions of motherhood and failed versions of childless womanhood (Lauritzen, 1990), an increasing prevalence and diversity of pregnancy loss experiences are happening within popular culture. More and more television shows and films offer stories of pregnancy loss in which the miscarriage is not a problem solver but a plot driver; fetal death is a full storyline, not a secondary tale; and infertility is a problem without a solution. The shift from stories such as Kelly Taylor's, whose pregnancy and loss came and went in two easy episodes, to stories such as Charlotte York's, whose struggles span three television seasons (and two feature-length films), is increasingly common.

Meredith Grey's miscarriage did not solve her relationship problems; in fact, it complicated her relationship with her husband and her friends. Her miscarriage and infertility led to a tumultuous adoption struggle and hours of questioning the choices she made to become a surgeon. Khloe Kardashian remains childless and the pain in her eyes as she watched sister Kim grow large with baby North was apparent to her fans. On *The L Word*, when Tina (Laurel Holloman) miscarries, she and her partner Bette (Jennifer Beals) mourn their loss for months afterward. In Anita Diamant's *The Red Tent*, the biblical story of Jacob comes to life for readers as his four wives repeatedly struggle with miscarriage, infertility, and infant death. And while the adoption of a Chinese baby girl does offer a happy ending to Charlotte York's reproductive challenges, the story itself offered viewers a chance to understand the difficulties of pregnancy loss, social expectations, and adoption. (See the appendix, "Pregnancy Loss in the Media", for a complete list of media resources.)

The diversity of stories of pregnancy loss in the media is itself beginning to create a new sort of dialogue of loss. As stories of loss are told on television and in film, through lyrics of songs and a growing number of books, and in interviews with those who have lost, a new discourse emerges. This new discourse, while emerging from popular culture, must also be read actively in order to remain consistent with feminist values. We must be the active interpreters of media and we must use media to shape a contemporary discourse of pregnancy loss. There are two frames that shape how we must interpret the media discourse and how we create a media-centered form of CR for narratives of pregnancy loss; the first frame is in support of reproductive rights and the second frame deprioritizes different types of loss. Crucial to creating a feminist discourse of pregnancy loss is that we move away from any and all anti-choice rhetoric that limits women's reproductive freedom. In other words, we must read texts in ways that allow us to acknowledge the pain of pregnancy loss without fear of losing our reproductive rights. In addition, we must read texts with an understanding of the feminist belief that no oppression ranks higher or lower than another. In other words, there is no pregnancy loss that is better or worse than another pregnancy loss—each story matters equally. From these two frames, we can form a discourse of loss, one that will shape our current socio-cultural conceptions of pregnancy loss to be better and more inclusive.

Notes

1. Pollock (and many others; 1999) notes that "positioning miscarriage as plot relief, as a way of eliminating a pregnancy that had served its plot function by complicating a romance or forcing moral reflection and yet that would overdetermine subsequent events should it remain" (p. 253) is a common phenomenon and a regularly used media and literary trope.
2. Take Back the Night is an annual international speak-out, march, rally, and candlelight vigil held to protest against rape and sexual violence. The event began in 1975 in Philadelphia, Pennsylvania, after Susan Alexander Speeth was stabbed to death while walking home. Since then, college campuses and community centers around the globe have hosted the event as a way to increase awareness about and prevent sexual and relationship violence.

Afterword: How to Do Things With Stories[1]

JAY BAGLIA AND RACHEL E. SILVERMAN

The stories in this collection give voice to those who have lost a pregnancy. Nowhere does there exist such a collection, one that gives each contributor the space to tell her or his own story with this level of intensity and vibrancy. The women and men who suffer pregnancy loss are rarely given the opportunity to speak and to tell their stories. They are often silenced by the medical community, by their well-meaning peers and families, and even sometimes by books intending to help people cope with loss. Narratives of pregnancy loss (whether those found here or those shared among close friends) are easily read through the lens of the personal and yet feminists have good reasons to identify connections between contemporary political moments and the significance of sharing or silencing personal narratives of pregnancy loss. In today's political climate, those who have experienced losses may also be silenced by the elected officials meant to protect them.

Famous for giving voice to women, Gloria Steinem embarked on a speaking tour in advance of the November 2012 elections, and on October 19, 2012, she spoke at the University of Central Florida (UCF) in Orlando to a modest crowd of approximately one hundred people. During the next few days, she traveled throughout the state of Florida, speaking at a variety of venues and stressing the importance of each person's vote. While at UCF, she told the crowd that her reason for the Florida tour came from a certain guilt she had been carrying for twelve years. In November 2000, Steinem was speaking in Fort Lauderdale about the now infamous Bush versus Gore election, which had taken place the day before. At the end of her talk, a veteran asked whether she would stay and help him, and his daughter's future, by attending a protest with the goal of demanding a recount. Steinem told the vet that she was unable to stay because she had other speaking engagements, and she told us, twelve years later, that she had been feeling guilty about her decision ever since. In those twelve years, the world as we know it has changed dramatically. America was attacked, we have engaged in two lengthy wars, we elected our first black president, the Tea Party rose to power, and in 2011, for the first time ever, more non-white babies were born in the United States than white babies (Reuters, 2012). Steinem addressed each of these changes; she praised a few and offered some explanation for others.

"Many people are scared by the world, which no longer resembles the world they were born in," she told the small crowd at UCF. "Fear," she continued, "causes people to act in extreme ways." Beautifully and provocatively, Steinem then told the crowd that the United States is slowly coming to mirror the population of the world, that people's minds are changing and equal rights for all are not too far away. However, she warned, freedom always comes at a price. She then compared the United States to a battered woman. Most women are killed by their abusive partners just as they are about to leave, and if they are not killed they are often beaten more severely than they have ever been. "America is like that battered woman. We are about to be free and this backlash against women's rights, and humanity in general, is our last and worst beating because we will not die" (G. Steinem, personal communication, October 19, 2012).

Examples of the kind of backlash Steinem refers to include Congressman Todd Akin (R–MO), who claimed in August 2012 that women who are victims of "legitimate rapes" rarely get pregnant (Moore, 2012). This claim was followed, several months later, by another equally ludicrous one from Indiana Senate candidate Richard Mourdock, who stated, "I think, even when life begins in that horrible situation of rape, that it is something that God intended to happen" (Groer, 2012). This remark was intended as a defense of his effort to outlaw all abortion procedures in his state, even in cases of rape and incest. Akin's attempt to redefine rape by claiming some rapes as "legitimate" and others as warranted and Mourdock's claim that God intends for the babies of rape victims to live are among the most repugnant attacks witnessed on a woman's right to choose and control her body. Then, in February 2014, Congressman Steve Martin (R–VA, who voted for his state's mandatory ultrasound bill and advocated for a fetal personhood bill) posted to his Facebook wall the notion that a pregnant woman is merely a "host" and should not have a choice regarding her pregnancy (Chozick, 2014). Martin, Akin, and Mourdock are emblematic of those in power who would repeal *Roe v. Wade* and who regularly assault women's health, endeavoring to wholly limit access to family planning.

What these politicians—and others like them in today's news (Chozick, 2014)—have in common is the underlying desire to take reproduction out of the hands of those whom it affects most and put it into the hands of conservative ideologues. Additionally, these news stories demonstrate a climate that necessitates the careful use of language about women's bodies and their reproductive capabilities. As early as 1992, Gilbert and Smart acknowledged, "Today, there is heightened sensitivity to fetal and infant death, perhaps in part because of elective abortion issues" (1992, p. 1). A year later, Jones (1993) wrote in the preface to Allen and Marks:

> Although medical art and practice has become increasingly sophisticated in treating women whose full-term babies are stillborn, there has been little emphasis on dealing with the loss experienced by women who lose their babies early on. This is no doubt due, in part, by the controversy surrounding the definition of life—when the miraculous division of cells can be regarded as first embryo, then fetus, then unborn child. (p. xi)

For a topic such as pregnancy loss—which is already shrouded in silence—we cannot afford to add another layer that suppresses our voices. And at a time when reproductive technologies are ever increasing, we cannot allow politicians to further polarize the issue of reproductive rights. What do the silences and alienation indicate other than uncertainty, ambiguity, and hostility?

Amidst the political backlash, we—Jay and Rachel—came together and found we had a mutual interest in the topic of pregnancy loss. Each of us has been touched by miscarriage to the degree that a scholarly approach to the topic became a logical professional activity to pursue in tandem. Because we share the belief that reproductive rights are a fundamental human right, that stories of pregnancy loss cannot be shrouded in the silence of an anti-abortion backlash, and that narrative is an absent methodology in the vast literature on miscarriage and pregnancy loss, we agreed that a collection of narratives was the ideal approach to pursue this interest. We began to share our vision with friends and colleagues and found ourselves overwhelmed with supportive voices. Many of those supporting voices are included in this volume, their stories became the foundation for our collection, and this collection, we hope, will become a source for change.

As we stated in our introduction to this volume, and as Silverman reiterates in the chapter that precedes this afterword, feminist consciousness-raising (CR) can result in both heightened awareness and legislative agency. These twin forces—personal and political power—represent the symbiotic outcome of narrative methodologies. In this afterword to the collection, we'd like to guide our readers through an understanding of these pregnancy loss narratives as an act of CR, as personal, cultural, and political struggles (Bochner, 2001; Bochner, 2014; Frank, 2013; Harter & Bochner, 2009; Harter,

Japp, & Beck, 2005; Lindemann-Nelson, 1997; Sakalys, 2000). Furthermore, we'd like to draw from the collective wisdom articulated through these narratives a call for improved communication practices among health care providers, institutional policy changes, language changes within the biomedical discourse, as well as heightened introspection and understanding among friends, relatives, and coworkers of those who experience pregnancy loss.

What can stories do? Hilde Lindemann-Nelson (1997) suggests that well-crafted stories engage both the personal and the public. Stories are told (whether through the written word or through oral performance). Stories, then, are read or heard by an audience. This interdependent storytelling triangle—consisting of story, teller, and listener/reader (Lipman, 1999)—can then result in the comparison and analysis of stories as well as invoking more stories. When we invoke a personal narrative—one that may have been told initially (perhaps even tentatively) by one person to another—it is usually to connect it to a larger, cultural issue, according to Lindemann-Nelson, "to make or illustrate a moral point" (p. xii). Miller, Geist-Martin, and Cannon Beatty (2005) further elucidate this sentiment: "At their best, narratives can be open-ended resources, sources of healing and comfort, spiritual maturation, privileged moments of self-change, epiphanies, turning points, and lessons to live by" (p. 299).

These pregnancy loss narratives can and should be considered for the ways they provide counternarratives to personal, cultural, and political master narratives. In *Damaged Identities: Narrative Repair*, Lindemann-Nelson (2001) asserts that "master narratives exercise a certain authority over our moral imaginations and play a role in informing our moral institutions" (p. 6). When master narratives indicate a propensity for ethnocentrism, classism, and sexism they are certainly oppressive. And it must be stated that the institution of medicine has demonstrated the capacity to construct master narratives of "normal" responses to infertility and miscarriage that serve to oppress or silence dissenting responses. In these instances, counternarratives become highly useful tools that can reveal exactly what the master narrative suppresses. For Frank (1994), the illness narrative becomes "a self-conscious effort" for the author "to hold her own against forces that threaten to overpower her voice and her text" (pp. 4–5). In this section, we point to scenes from the chapters in this book that illustrate personal, cultural, and political counternarratives of pregnancy loss along with proposals for an ethics of empathic care.

Personal

Julie Novak and Elizabeth Root each identify the different ways inept interpersonal interaction further exacerbates the impact of the pregnancy loss experience, whether from friends, coworkers, family members, or the medical community. Jennifer Fairchild and Michael Arrington share their desire to be competent communicators as members of emotional support networks and how uncomplicated such support can be for the motivated friend, coworker, or family member. As Baglia suggests in his chapter, the only words required of a caregiver—whether personal or professional, in the midst of infertility or miscarriage—are "I'm sorry this is happening to you." Many of the authors in this collection address the way interpersonal communication with relatives and friends affected their experience of loss and how they sometimes longed for better understanding. Each of these authors also stresses the ways in which their experiences with loss have made them more competent communicators. However, without the right language with which to speak of loss, an author such as Lisa Weckerle uses fairy tales to understand her experience and Deleasa Randall-Griffiths returns to Greek mythology for support. Combined, these narratives about interpersonal communication stress that while there may not be any one recipe for communicating about loss or concern for loss, there are changes happening among individuals—always the first step toward changing the system as a whole—and that communicating support can be as simple as acknowledging loss.

Maria Brann and Jennifer Bute hold the medical community accountable, including midwives and ER doctors, for failing to follow through on informational support and for failing to identify the particular psychosocial context of unique patients and partners. In each instance, follow-up care—a standard practice with an inestimable number of medical conditions—is neglected and, perhaps just as disconcerting, not even considered necessary. From these chapters it is clear that there exists no consistent medical protocol at the interpersonal level—whether from doctor, nurse, or receptionist *to* patient—for communicating what women can expect when they are experiencing a miscarriage. Unfortunately, this is not news. Research has demonstrated that comprehensive care following a pregnancy loss is needed and that, generally, medical management of miscarriage is thought to be poor (Rowlands & Lee, 2010; Séjourné, Callahan, & Chabrol, 2010). The clinician's platitude that miscarriage or infertility is not uncommon or that a subsequent pregnancy will relieve, minimize, or otherwise diminish the grief a woman or couple experiences is not nearly as effective as the need for clinicians to acknowledge and address the immediate physical and emotional well-being of the patient. Kristann Heinz and Elissa Foster unveil the physician's desire to help fulfill a dream, the capacity for a physician to positively change the patient's story, and the questions that emerge when scripts are inadequate and patients become "lost to follow-up." Similarly, Lisa Schilling and Rachel Silverman address the ways in which working within the medical field while experiencing pregnancy loss force an individual to help others fulfill their dreams while one's own dreams are confronted daily. This sort of personal–professional difficulty is experienced by many of our authors—from Caryn Medved's work on family life balance, and Fairchild and Arrington's desire to focus their study of health communication within the field of pregnancy loss to Silverman's conflict between her study of women's health and her desire to carry a child and Sherokee Ilse and Kara Jones's experiences of loss as motivators for career paths.

This blurring of lines between personal and professional identities speaks to the reality of our individual lives, how we exist within our world, and, most important, how our stories become the foundation for the changes within our world.

Cultural

If scripts are absent from the medical side, they are also lacking on the cultural side. In their chapter, Julie and Ben Walker refer to the concept of maladaptivity as a consequence when scripts for behaviors don't exist. We know how to celebrate the news of a pregnancy (as men, as women, and as couples whether gay, straight, or queer) but there is no cultural script for pregnancy loss, no Hallmark card (Fairchild et al., 2008). In this pronatalist culture, Medved grows weary of the question, "Do you have kids?" insofar as the expected answer seems to be "yes" or "no" with little acknowledgment that for many women and couples the answer isn't so simple. As Renata Ferdinand asserts, "Being a woman means the ability to give birth" and "a woman's fertility is directly tied to her existence as a woman." Desiree Rowe's chapter explicitly calls on the need to reframe these kinds of scripts.

Schilling and Silverman expose another cultural component in the complexity of pregnancy loss—the undeniable fact that individuals who work in medicine are subject to the very same sets of probabilities regarding the capacity to have children as the rest of us. Schilling's chapter is representative of the reason that the relationship-centered care model (Beach & Inui, 2006; Limbo & Kobler, 2010; Safran, Miller, & Beckman, 2006) is so significant; the model presumes the uniqueness of all those involved in the creation of a health care culture insofar as emotion is an important aspect of health care and occurs in reciprocity. Schilling, like Foster, Heinz, and McGivern, highlights the continuing movement between work and life. Simply because one works within the field of medicine does not make his or her experiences with loss—of patients, of one's own, of family—any easier or more understood. When

Weckerle compromises her voice in the presence of health care professionals in the effort to maintain her carefully crafted, obedient patient persona, we can see that she is Foucault's docile body personified. Other authors, such as Desiree Rowe, Jennifer Hawkins, Brann, and Randall-Griffiths, all describe moments when they too were pathologized by the medical field and made to feel silenced. For those of us who are well-educated and have experienced a similar self-silencing, we can ascertain how these kinds of interactions play out for those members in our society who do not have this same privilege.

Medicine is its own culture (Lupton, 2003). And that culture has facets that are visible (language, logos, uniforms) and invisible (beliefs, values, attitudes, assumptions) and there are even cultures within cultures in medicine (DelVecchio Good, 1998). When Heinz describes her holistic practice as a "medical outpost" it becomes plain that there are hierarchies within the health care community. Medved alludes to "coercive hope" as the attitude many women and couples will encounter in the terrain of reproductive endocrinology—the ever-expansive (and expensive) series of options made available when a woman or couple desires a child (see also Novak, and Heinz & Foster, this volume). In the arena of language, it is clear that the archaic use of terms such as "spontaneous abortion" is far overdue for change. Root describes how having "nulligravida" applied by the medical establishment to her identity left her feeling diminished and shamed. Foster (2010) experiences a similar discursive violence when she encounters "elderly primigravida" on her patient information sheet, a term that means a woman older than thirty-five who is experiencing her first pregnancy. And Novak's distaste for the SOAP format forces her to create her own medical journal within which to track her experiences. To emphasize the extent to which these terms reflect an outdated medical philosophy, consider this passage from Fliehr (1956) in the article "Management of the Elderly Primigravida":

> The elderly primigravida has always evoked a feeling of dread and foreboding in the careful obstetrician; he is most conscious of the added problems she presents. He knows that the processes of aging *present him* with such complications as cardiac disease, arterial disease, and the like. (p. 494, emphasis ours)

Clearly, the continued and acritical use of phrases such as "incompetent cervix," "spontaneous abortion," "nulligravida," and "elderly primigravida" represent an era of physician-centered medicine. As we move to patient-centered and relationship-centered care models that integrate the subjective experiences of patients to advantage both their health and well-being and to the efficiency of the medical encounter, it is time to abandon the phrasings that indicate an antediluvian, objectivist lens. We're confident that patients,

communication scholars, and semioticians are eager to partner with concerned representatives in health care to work to correct these kinds of lapses.

Political

Other changes may require sustained persuasive campaigns. If the absence
of scripted responses to pregnancy loss is acknowledged, then the paucity
of rituals that could be employed to help with coping becomes even more
evident. Mansell (2006) reports that women and couples along with medical
personnel are often uncertain regarding what is to be done with postmortem
fetal remains, the "products of conception." Layne (1990) refers to these absences as responsible for "the angst of an incomplete rite of passage." Rebecca
Kennerly writes about her pregnancy loss as post-traumatic stress disorder
(PTSD), citing the work of Lapp, Agbokou, Peretti, and Ferreri (2010) and
Olde, van der Hart, Kleber, and van Son (2006). In her chapter, Hawkins
calls our attention to the trauma of successive miscarriages, as does Patricia
Geist-Martin in the foreword to this volume. Independent of quantity, another silenced aspect of pregnancy loss involves grief. With no small amount
of frustration, and discussed by Silverman, Rowe, Ferdinand, and Medved,
women are prone to opinions—through support web sites, media, and personal relationships—that suggest that some pregnancy losses are worth grieving more than others. Cosgrove (2004) writes, "The conflation of distress
with gestational stage not only lacks empirical verification but it also flies in
the face of technology; an intense early bonding experience is made possible
by the visual image (and ultrasonic picture) of one's fetus" (p. 110).

One clear indication that miscarriage and infertility are not recognized by
our dominant institutions involves organizational responses to these experiences. Miscarriage, for example, is rarely an occasion for bereavement leave
in the workplace. Instead, employees are instructed to use personal leave or
sick leave if they desire time away from work following a miscarriage or disappointing results after infertility treatment. Both miscarriages and discouraging
news following the use of reproductive technologies (such as IVF) occur all of
a sudden, so that there is no anticipatory grieving. Indeed, Renner, Verdekal,
Brier, and Falluca (2000) have determined that the meaning of miscarriage is
often misunderstood by friends and family.

Both the Society for Assisted Reproductive Technology web site and the
Centers for Disease Control and Prevention web site provide extensive tables
that account for success rates of IVF facilities nationwide. However, visits to
individual clinic web sites favor a far more optimistic story, fulfilling a version
of Arthur Frank's (2013) restitution narrative: (1) woman/couple has no

baby; (2) woman/couple receives state-of-the-art technological assistance; (3) woman/couple has baby. Medved, Novak, Hawkins, and Baglia all articulate how decisions to cease assisted reproductive interventions are fraught, in no small part because of relational, cultural, and even industry pressures, because there's always one more procedure to attempt. And when there isn't another attempt, other sorts of loss emerge. Lauritzen's (1990) discussion of reproductive technology as an additional pressure on women to reproduce asks the question, "What price parenthood?" He suggests that reproductive technologies have drastically changed the concept of pregnancy loss, for while many use the technology and are able to become and stay pregnant, many others do not. When the difficult decision to stop trying via reproductive technologies is made, a new loss emerges—one that bears an additional burden of guilt, a guilt that emerges from the choice to stop, a guilt that compounds the guilt many already feel as a result of the medical pathology of loss. So it becomes clear that in our scientific and capitalistic democracy, more care should be exercised by the reproductive technology industry. This can be accomplished by placing greater emphasis on the welfare of the client and less on profit.

This same obligation of the "person first" model should be embraced as well by mainstream medicine. Here we are speaking specifically to those employed in fetal ultrasound facilities at hospitals. It is time for the medical profession to loosen its grip on the right to diagnose and encourage a partnership among sonographers, nurses, and physicians. As Foster and McGivern elucidate in their chapter, the sonographer is often the point person during a fetal ultrasound and frequently has expertise that the physician does not when it comes to identifying both a healthy fetus and fetal demise. Why then must the patient wait for a physician to dispense the news when a sonographer trained in communication skills will save time and possibly spare unnecessary anguish?

We recognize that many of these recommendations and suggestions will fly in the face of deeply entrenched standards and traditions in personal, cultural, and political arenas of health care. Nevertheless, like most stories, this collection is a conversation starter and one that we hope this diverse array of experiences helps to continue. In *The Vulnerable, Empowered Woman*, Tasha Dubriwny (2013) articulates media's power to construct dominant narratives by perpetuating aspects of the postmodern feminist. Sueellen Miller (1997) suggests that a similar embrace of postmodern feminism in medicine serves as a normalizing discourse when it comes to women's health care. For Buzzanell and Ellingson (2005), "Stories must be told for awareness and retold in counternarratives until they impact cultural and organizational delusions of ideal bodies and perpetuation of the sick/well dichotomy" (p. 293). For Sakalys (2000), illness narratives can be emancipatory insofar as they challenge dominant narratives. Sharf (2005) calls this the "exponential power of narrative, that is, the resulting force of stories that build on one another to deepen and accentuate meaning" (p. 341). The authors in this collection demonstrate Anne Hunsaker Hawkins's (1999b) ideal of narrative as pointing to "deficiencies in various aspects of patient care" and "alerting all of us to important problems in medical practice" (p. 128).

To ignore the truths remembered and shared through stories is to deny our interlocking personal, cultural, and political worlds the possibility for improvement and the hope for more just and compassionate communities. In our postmodern society, personal narratives join literature, film, and news media as part and parcel of Kenneth Burke's "equipment for living" (1938, p. 10). We need all the stories we can summon.

Note

1. This title is a direct reference to Hilde Lindemann-Nelson's (1997) chapter in her edited collection *Stories and Their Limits: Narrative Approaches to Bioethics.* Her title, we presume, is a reference to J.L. Austin's *How to Do Things With Words* (1975).

Biographies

Editor Biographies:

Jay Baglia (Ph.D., University of South Florida) is Assistant Professor in the College of Communication at DePaul University. Dr. Baglia's research explores the intersection of health, gender, and performance studies. He has published in *Health Communication, Journal of Dramatic Theory & Criticism, Family Medicine*, and *Cultural Studies ↔ Critical Methodologies*. His 2005 book, *The Viagra Ad Venture: Masculinity, Media, and the Performance of Sexual Health*, received the Organization for the Study of Communication, Language, & Gender's 2006 Book of the Year as well as the National Communication Association's Health Communication Division 2012 Distinguished Book Award. Dr. Baglia is co-editor of this collection.

 Rachel E. Silverman (Ph.D., University of South Florida) is Assistant Professor of Communication in the Department of Humanities and Social Science at Embry Riddle Aeronautical University. Dr. Silverman's research focuses on the intersection of Jewish and LGBT identities in popular culture, women's health, and food studies. She has published in *Sexuality & Culture, Health Communication*, and *The Journal of Religion and Popular Culture*. Dr. Silverman is co-editor of this collection.

Contributor Biographies:

Michael Irvin Arrington (Ph.D., University of South Florida) is Associate Professor and Director of Graduate Studies in the Department of Communication at Indiana State University, where he also serves as an affiliate faculty member in ISU's Center for Genomic Advocacy. Dr. Arrington's research interests include health communication, narrative inquiry, interpersonal and family communication, and communicating social support. His most recent work includes articles in *Health Communication; Illness, Crisis, and Loss;* the *International Journal of Men's Health; Popular Communication;* the *Journal of Family Communication; Journal of Aging and Identity, Journal of Psychosocial Oncology;* and *Sexuality & Culture*.

Maria Brann (Ph.D., University of Kentucky) is Associate Professor in the Department of Communication Studies at Indiana University-Purdue University Indianapolis. Dr. Brann's research focuses on the integration of health, interpersonal, and organizational communication. Dr. Brann's primary research interests focus on ethical communication in health care contexts as well as the promotion of healthy and safe behaviors. She has published refereed journal articles and scholarly book chapters regarding health care providers' confidentiality disclosures; women's health issues; promotion of healthy lifestyles; and tensions, support, and maintenance of healthy relationships.

Jennifer J. Bute (Ph.D., University of Illinois at Urbana–Champaign) is Assistant Professor in the Department of Communication Studies at Indiana University-Purdue University Indianapolis. She studies communication about health in interpersonal relationships and public discourses about women's health. She is particularly interested in issues related to privacy, social support, and gender. She teaches graduate and undergraduate courses in health, interpersonal, and gender communication. Her work has appeared in numerous edited books and journals, including *Health Communication, Communication Monographs, Human Communication Research, Communication Studies, Review of Communication, Qualitative Health Research*, and *Social Science and Medicine*.

Jennifer L. Fairchild (Ph.D., University of Kentucky) is Assistant Professor of Communication at Eastern Kentucky University. Dr. Fairchild continues to extend her dissertation research involving women's narrative reconstruction post-miscarriage and the social support offered to women post-miscarriage in addition to teaching a wide variety of courses, including interpersonal communication, health communication, and gender. Her dissertation work has been presented at meetings of the National Communication Association and the Southern States Communication Association. Her research also has been featured in such journals as *PRISM: A Journal of Regional Engagement* and *Illness, Crisis, and Loss*.

Renata Ferdinand (Ph.D., Bowling Green State University) is Assistant Professor of English at New York City College of Technology in Brooklyn, NY. She uses auto-ethnography and personal narrative to explore a range of research interests, including African Diaspora Studies and Communication and Cultural Studies. Currently, she is pursuing research that explores the subjective experience of motherhood and African American women.

Elissa Foster (Ph.D., University of South Florida) is Associate Professor and Director of the MA in Health Communication at DePaul University. She also serves as a contracted Medical Educator in the Department of Family Medicine at Lehigh Valley Health Network. Her research focus is on health communication and interpersonal relationships, and she has published in *Qualitative Inquiry, Journal of Ageing and Identity, Women's Studies in Communication*, and the *Southern Communication Journal*, and elsewhere. Her book, *Communicating at the End of Life: Finding Magic in the Mundane* (Erlbaum, 2007), received the Outstanding Scholarly Book award from the Applied Communication Division of NCA for 2009.

Eduardo Gargurevich (Ph.D., University of Maryland) is Professor in the Department of Spanish and Hispanic Studies at Concordia College in Moorhead, Minnesota. He teaches Latin American literature, poetry, and cultural studies. He frequently integrates service-learning and experiential learning when planning and leading study abroad travels. His scholarly contributions include creative works of Latin American fiction and poetry.

Patricia Geist-Martin (Ph.D., Purdue University) is a Professor in the School of Communication at San Diego State University where she teaches organizational communication, health communication, ethnographic research methods, and gendering organizational communication. Her research interests focus on narrative and negotiating identity, voice, ideology, and control in organizations, particularly in health and illness. She has co-authored three books, *Communicating Health: Personal, Political, and Cultural Complexities* (2004); *Courage of Conviction: Women's Words, Women's Wisdom* (1997); and *Negotiating the Crisis: DRGs and the Transformation of Hospitals* (1992). Patricia has published more than sixty articles and book chapters covering a wide range of topics related to gender, health, and negotiating identities.

Jennifer Morey Hawkins (Doctoral Candidate, University of Wisconsin, Milwaukee) studies health communication within interpersonal and intercultural contexts and holds particular interest in sensitive health topics. Representative topics of her research include: HIV/AIDS, mental health, personal health practices, online health information seeking, and pregnancy loss. Jennifer has published in *Health Communication* and has received Top Paper Award at the Western Communication Association conference and Top Student Paper Award the National Communication Association conference. She teaches classes in health communication, interpersonal communication, and public speaking, and trains community members on health campaign message design. Jennifer currently serves as a student representative on the Executive Board for the Organization of the Study of Communication, Language, & Gender.

Kristann Heinz (M.D., RD, University of Pennsylvania) is both a medical doctor and registered dietician. She completed her post-graduate training at the Department of Family Medicine at Lehigh Valley Health Network in Allentown, Pennsylvania. Kristann is board certified through the American

Board of Family Medicine and American Board of Integrated and Holistic Medicine. She is also certified in Medical Acupuncture and has served as a community preceptor in acupuncture for Lehigh Valley Health Network. Kristann practices integrative family medicine and runs a health consulting practice called Physician in the Kitchen where she provides integrative health education with a focus on nutrition.

Sherokee Ilse (B.A., Hamlin University) is a bereaved mother, author, international speaker/trainer, and parent advocate/activist. Her first book, *Empty Arms: Coping With Miscarriage, Stillbirth, and Early Infant Death*, has more than 350,000 copies in print and is given out by clinics and hospitals worldwide to offer support to families making decisions after the news of their loss. Her web site, www.BabiesRemembered.org, offers compassion, support, and empowerment through the resources available to families. Sherokee has worked for more than thirty years to improve the care families receive when a baby dies. Her newest venture, www.LossDoulasInternational.com, certifies well-healed parents and birth professionals to support newly bereaved parents at the time of news-giving and during the early days of loss. She and her husband, David, have two living sons and have had three losses.

Kara L.C. Jones (B.A., Carnegie Mellon University; CAIC, The Leading Clinic; Master-Teacher, Vashon Reiki-Seichim) is mother to three dead sons, a living son, a daughter, and three amazing grandchildren. She is author of the book *Mrs. Duck and Woman* and co-founder of KotaPress and the Creative Grief Studio. Through the Studio, in partnership with Cath Duncan of Remembering For Good, she offers creative grief education through their four-month certification program. In her private practice, she is the coach and heARTist behind the works at GriefAndCreativity.com and MotherHenna.com.

Rebecca Kennerly (Ph.D., Louisiana State University) is Assistant Professor at Georgia Southern University. She is a critical cultural scholar interested in communication and social justice, and the performance of everyday life, the cultural performance of social ritual, and staged aesthetics. Her research interests focus on emergent mourning practices in the U.S. and narrative histories of marginalized groups in South Georgia. She has published in *Text & Performance Quarterly, Forum for Qualitative Social Science: Special Issue on Performative Research*, and the *Iowa Journal of Communication*. Her most recent work, "Service Learning, Intercultural Communication and Advanced Video Praxis: Developing a Sustainable Program of Community Activism with/in a Mexican Migrant Community," appeared in *Teaching Communication Activism*. Rebecca is currently the director of the Vidalia Onion Oral History Project.

Jodi McGivern (RDMS, RVT, University of Iowa) is a graduate of the Franciscan Hospital Radiologic Technology Program and the University of Iowa Medical School Diagnostic Medical Sonography Program. She is an experienced clinician with an active practice in both obstetrical and urological sonography, who serves as a preceptor for sonography trainees and as an instructor for physicians in practice. Since 1999 Jodi has served as the Program Coordinator and Instructor for the Diagnostic Medical Sonography Program at Carl Sandburg College.

Caryn E. Medved (Ph.D., University of Kansas) is Associate Professor at Baruch College. Her research focuses on issues of work–life communication. She has published numerous studies on stay-at-home fathering families and dual-career couples' work–family negotiations, working mothers' identity struggles, single-employee workplace backlash, and young adult work and family socialization. Her research has appeared in outlets such as *Women's Studies Quarterly*, *Women & Language*, *Management Communication Quarterly*, *Communication Yearbook*, and *Sloan Work and Family Encyclopedia* as well as *Journal of Family Communication*. She is the past editor of the *Journal of Family Communication* (Taylor & Francis). Professor Medved is currently conducting a study of stay-at-home fathers and breadwinning mothers funded by the Alfred P. Sloan Foundation and PCS-CUNY.

Michaela D. E. Meyer (Ph.D., Ohio University) is Associate Professor of Communication at Christopher Newport University in Virginia. She is an identity scholar primarily interested in the intersections between communication, culture, media, and interpersonal relationships. She is the author of more than forty academic publications appearing in outlets such as *Sexuality & Culture*, *The Journal of Bisexuality*, *Women's Studies: An Interdisciplinary Journal*, *Feminist Media Studies*, *Review of Communication*, *Communication Quarterly*, *Communication Studies*, *The Ohio Communication Journal*, *The International and Intercultural Communication Annual*, and *The Carolina Communications Annual*.

Julie Novak (Ph.D., North Dakota State University) is Associate Professor in the Department of Communication at Wayne State University. As an applied researcher, she studies lived experiences and practical issues at the nexus of health, risk, and organizational communication. Her research has been published in *Educational Gerontology*, *Journal of Applied Communication Research*, *Handbook of Applied Communication*, and other journals. She has received top papers in the Disabilities Caucus and the Health Division at the National Communication Association Conferences. Her professional experiences in primary health care, nutrition, and breastfeeding services and her personal health experiences of infertility and trauma play a significant role in the perspective she brings to her scholarly work.

Deleasa Randall-Griffiths (Ph.D., Southern Illinois University) is Associate Professor in the Department of Communication Studies at Ashland University and winner of the 2012 Ohio Communication Association's Innovative Teacher Award. She teaches the introductory human communication course, along with courses in interpersonal communication, family communication, performance studies, and international storytelling. Her research interests include health care narratives, language and social interaction, family communication, and multicultural storytelling. Her research appears in *Text & Performance Quarterly* and the *American Journal of Semiotics*.

Elizabeth Root (Ph.D., University of New Mexico) is Assistant Professor at Oregon State University. She began her career as an English as a second/foreign language teacher. Besides teaching refugees, immigrants, and international students in Minnesota, she also taught conversational English classes in both China and South Korea for several years. Elizabeth teaches courses in intercultural communication and qualitative research methods. Her research focuses on issues of university internationalization, cultural identity, and intercultural communication pedagogy.

Desiree Rowe (Ph.D., Arizona State University) is Assistant Professor of Communication Studies at the University of South Carolina, Upstate. Dr. Rowe teaches courses such as Communication and Social Movements, Qualitative Research Methods, and Feminism and Popular Culture. Her research interests include feminist engagements with popular culture, performative writing, and the digital humanities. She has published in *Text & Performance Quarterly*, *Cultural Studies ↔ Critical Methodologies*, and *Qualitative Inquiry*.

Lisa Jo Schilling (M.S., ARNP, PNP-BC, CPN, University of South Florida) is a pediatric nurse practitioner in private practice, adjunct clinical faculty for undergraduate pediatric registered nurse students, and a gynecological teaching assistant. Schilling plans to further her education with a doctor of nursing practice (DNP) degree specializing in pediatric endocrinology with a focus on childhood obesity and future publications. She lives in central Florida with her husband where they are actively trying to grow their family through adoption and infertility treatments.

Benjamin M. Walker (M.F.A., Minnesota State University, Mankato) is Assistant Professor of Communication Studies and the Assistant Director of Forensics at Southwest Minnesota State University, where he teaches a variety of courses and coaches the speech and debate team. Ben's research interests include competitive speech and debate, communication pedagogy, and experiential learning. His work has been published in several peer-reviewed journals.

Julie L. G. Walker (M.A., Minnesota State University, Mankato) is an independent scholar whose research interests include identity negotiations, critical pedagogy, forensics, and the integration of social justice into the basic communication course. To date her research has primarily investigated the relationship between marital surname choice and personal and relational identity negotiations. Julie's research has been presented at meetings of the National Communication Association, the Central States Communication Association, and the Communication and Theater Association of Minnesota, and her work has been published in several scholarly journals.

Lisa Weckerle (Ph.D., University of Texas, Austin) is Associate Professor in the Department of Communication Studies at Kutztown University of Pennsylvania. Dr. Weckerle's research focuses on the adaptation of literature, the role of myth in popular culture, and performance studies. Her previous publications include an article in *The Edith Wharton Review*, as well as book chapters in *Myth in the Modern World: Essays on Intersections With Ideology and Culture* and *The Twilight Saga: Exploring the Global Phenomenon*.

Glossary of Terms

Assisted Reproductive Techniques (ART). Procedures in which pregnancy is attempted through gamete manipulation outside the body, such as in vitro fertilization or assisted hatching.

Dilation and Curettage (D&C). A procedure in which the cervix is gradually widened and the lining of the uterus is gently removed by scraping or suction.

Donor Egg. An egg donated by a woman, either known or anonymous. Generally, the donor relinquishes any rights to any resultant offspring.

Donor Embryo. An embryo donated by a couple, either known or anonymous. Generally, the donor relinquishes any rights to any resultant offspring.

Donor Sperm. Sperm donated by man, either known or anonymous. Generally, the donor relinquishes any rights to any resultant offspring.

Ectopic Pregnancy (Tubal Pregnancy). A pregnancy in which the fertilized ovum has implanted in a location other than the uterus, usually the fallopian tube.

Egg Retrieval. Procedure using ultrasound to guide a needle through the vagina into the ovary to eggs. Usually performed under sedation.

Embryo. The fertilized ovum after it has begun the process of cell division.

Embryo Transfer. A placement of embryos into a women's uterus through the cervix after IVF.

Endometriosis. A condition in which tissue resembling the lining of the uterus is found elsewhere in the body, usually the pelvis.

Estrogen (Estradiol). A hormone that is produced in the ovaries and that plays a role in regulating ovulation and endometrial development.

Fertilization. The penetration of the egg by the sperm and the resulting fusion of genetic material that develops into an embryo.

Fetus. In medical terms, an embryo becomes a fetus at about the end of the seventh week of pregnancy, after major structures (head, torso, limbs) have formed.

Gamete Intrafallopian Transfer (GIFT). A variation of ART in which unfertilized eggs and sperm are placed together in the fallopian tubes, with fertilization taking place in the tube instead of the laboratory dish.

Gestational Mother. In a surrogacy arrangement, the women who carries the pregnancy to term and delivers the baby, which may or may not be genetically related to her.

Impotence. A condition in which a man cannot achieve or sustain an erection long enough to ejaculate inside the vagina.

In Vitro Fertilization (IVF). A form of assisted reproduction in which an egg and sperm are combined in a laboratory dish and the resulting embryo (sometimes called a pre-embryo) is transferred into the fallopian tube.

Infertility. The absence of conception after one year of attempting to become pregnant. Approximately 30% of infertility is due to a female factor and 30% due to a male factor. Another 30% is thought to stem from the combination of parents and the remaining 10% is unknown.

Intrauterine Insemination (IUI). A technique in which sperm are introduced directly into the cervix or the uterus to produce pregnancy, with or without ovarian stimulation to produce multiple ova.

Luteal Phase. The second half of the menstrual cycle, beginning at ovulation (day fourteen in an average twenty-eight-day cycle) and ending with menstruation.

Miscarriage. Also known as spontaneous abortion, the loss of a pregnancy before twenty weeks of gestation. Problems with the development of the fetus occur as a result of chromosomal abnormalities (where there is extra or missing genetic information), defective implantation (inability to adhere to the uterine wall), faulty fertilization (which occurs when the embryo does not develop normally), and placental problems (problematic development or function of placenta or umbilical cord). Parental problems usually occur as a result of anatomical malformations or disease-related issues. Such issues include defective egg or sperm (malformed or too old for proper development to occur), hormonal imbalance (defect in luteal phase of menstrual cycle), infection (including herpes, syphilis, urinary tract infections, heart disease, polio, and chickenpox), immunological factors (incompatibility of parental blood types), uterine disorders (malformation of the uterus), incompetent cervix (as a result of genetics or surgery), and sperm count (high/low, poor quality, diabetes). External causes for miscarriage are usually the result of injury or the environment (such as smoking, poor nutrition, drug abuse). Any number of these factors can play a role in pregnancy loss and, for the most part, each loss is unique.

Molar Pregnancy (Gestational Trophoblastic Disease, GTD). Also known as hydatidiform mole. An abnormal growth that occurs in the uterus and is often mistaken for a pregnancy.

Ova. The female sex cells, or eggs, which are produced by the ovaries.

Placenta. The thick pad of tissue in a pregnant woman's uterus that provides nourishment to and disposes of waste from the growing fetus.

Pregnancy, Chemical. Pregnancy documented by a blood or urine test that shows a rise in the level of human gonadotropin (HCG) hormone.

Pregnancy Loss. The loss of a desired pregnancy.

Reproductive Endocrinologist. An obstetrician/gynecologist (OB/GYN) who specializes in diagnosing and treating infertility.

RESOLVE. A national, nonprofit consumer organization offering education, advocacy, and support to people experiencing infertility.

Secondary Infertility. Infertility after one or more pregnancies.

Spontaneous Abortion (Miscarriage). A pregnancy ending in the spontaneous loss of the embryo or fetus before twenty weeks of gestation.

Stillborn. When a fetus dies in the uterus after the twenty-week mark.

Appendix: Pregnancy Loss in the Media

Pregnancy Loss on Television

All in the Family (Season 1, Episode 6)
American Horror Story (Season 1)
Beverly Hills, 90210 (Season 7, Episode 30)
Big Love (Season 3)
Boardwalk Empire (Season 1)
Bomb Girls (Season 2, Episode 2)
Brothers & Sisters (Season 2, Episode 6; Season 4, Episode 17)
Derek (Season 2, Episode 2)
Desperate Housewives (Season 2, Episode 8)
Downton Abbey (Season 1, Episode 7)
Dynasty (Season 2, Episode 7)
Enlightened (Season 1, Episode 4)
ER (Season 9)
Grey's Anatomy (Season 2, Episode 4; Season 6, Episode 24)
House, M.D. (Season 7, Episode 18)
The L Word (Season 1, Episode 9)
Mad Men (Season 6, Episode 3)
NYPD Blue (Season 9)
Party of Five (Season 2, Episode 18)
Private Practice (Seasons 5 & 6)
The Real Housewives of Miami (Seasons 2 & 3)
Rescue Me (Season 2)
Sex and the City (Seasons 4–6)
Six Feet Under (Season 5, Episode 1)
Teen Mom 2 (Season 4, Episode 1)
The Tudors (Season 2, Episode 5)
Upstairs Downstairs (Season 3, Episode 12)

Pregnancy Loss in Literature

The Cider House Rules (Irving, 1985)
For Colored Girls (Shange, 1997)
The Handmaid's Tale (Atwood, 1998)
The Help (Stockett, 2009)
Gone Girl (Flynn, 2012)
Gone With the Wind (Mitchell, 1964)
Last Night in Twisted River (Irving, 2012)
Luscious Lemon (Swain, 2005)
Marley & Me (Grogan, 2005)
Out of Africa (Dinesen, 1963)
The Red Tent (Diamant, 2007)
Where'd You Go, Bernadette (Semple, 2012)

Pregnancy Loss in Film

Away We Go (Mendes, 2003)
Baby Mama (McCullers, 2008)
Butter (Smith, 2011)
Children of Men (Cuaron, 2006)
Country Strong (Feste, 2011)
The Curious Case of Benjamin Button (Fincher, 2008)
Diary of a Mad Black Woman (Grant, 2005)
Frances Ha (Baumbach, 2013)
Julie & Julia (Ephron, 2009)
Junebug (Morrison, 2005)
Juno (Reitman, 2005)
Mother and Child (Garcia, 2010)
The Odd Life of Timothy Green (Hedges, 2012)
Orphan (Collett-Serra, 2009)
The Other Woman (Roos, 2009)
Prometheus (Scott, 2012)
Rabbit Hole (Mitchell, 2010)
Raising Arizona (Coen & Coen, 1987)
Return to Zero (Hanish, 2014)
Secrets and Lies (Leigh, 2006)
The Time Traveler's Wife (Schwentke, 2009)
21 Grams (Inarritu, 2003)
Up (Giacchino, 2009)
What to Expect When You're Expecting (Jones, 2012)
Young Adult (Reitman, 2011)

Celebrity Accounts of Pregnancy Loss

Beyonce & Jay Z
Michelle Duggar
Bethenny Frankel
Khloe Kardashian
Lisa Ling
Gwyneth Paltrow
Guiliana Rancic
Brooke Shields
Kirstie Alley
Mariah Carey
Nicole Kidman
Jane Seymour
Sharon Stone
Emma Thompson

References

Abboud, L., & Liamputtong, P. (2005). When pregnancy fails: Coping strategies, support networks and experiences with health care of ethnic women and their partners. *Journal of Reproductive and Infant Psychology, 23*, 3–18.

Abelson, R. P. (1981). Psychological status of script concept. *American Psychologist, 36*(7), 715–729.

Adams, T. E. (2008). A review of narrative ethics. *Qualitative Inquiry, 14,* 175–194.

Adams, T. E. (2009). Mothers, faggots, and witnessing (un)contestable experience. *Cultural Studies ↔ Critical Methodologies, 9*, 619–626.

Adolfsson, A., Bertero, C., Larsson, P. G., & Wijma, B. (2004). Guilt and emptiness: Women's experiences of miscarriage. *Health Care for Women International, 25*(6), 543–560. doi:10.1080/07399330490444821

Agar, M. (1985). Institutional discourse. *Text, 5*, 147–168.

Albrecht, T. L., & Adelman, M. B. (1987). Communicating social support: A theoretical perspective. In T. L. Albrecht, M. B. Adelman, & Associates (Eds.), *Communicating social support* (pp. 18–39). Newbury Park, CA: Sage.

Alexander, M. J. (2005). *Pedagogies of crossing: Meditations on feminism, sexual politics, memory, and the sacred.* Durham, NC: Duke University Press.

Allen, M., & Marks, S. (Eds.). (1993). *Miscarriage: Women sharing from the heart.* Hoboken, NJ: Wiley & Sons.

Amankwaa, L. (2003). Postpartum depression among African American women. *Issues in Mental Health Nursing, 24*, 297–316.

American Pregnancy Association. (2013). Stillbirth: Surviving emotionally. Retrieved from http://americanpregnancy.org/preganancyloo/sbsurvivingemotionally.html

Andersen, H. C. (1999). Thumbelina. In M. Ponsot (Trans.) & A. Segur (Ill.), *Golden Book of fairy tales* (pp. 30–36). New York, NY: Golden Books.

Anzaldúa, G. (1981). Speaking in tongues: A letter to third world writers. In C. Moraga & G. Anzaldúa (Eds.), *This bridge called my back: Writings by radical women of color* (pp. 165–174). Watertown, MA: Persephone Press.

Armstrong, D. (2001). Exploring fathers' experiences of pregnancy after a prior perinatal loss. *The American Journal of Maternal/Child Nursing (MCN), 26,* 147–153.

Arrington, M. I. (2000). Sexuality, society, and senior citizens: An analysis of sex talk among prostate cancer support group members. *Sexuality & Culture, 4,* 45–74.

Austin, J. L. (1975). *How to do things with words.* Cambridge: Harvard University Press.

Bachmann, G. A. (1990). Hysterectomy: A critical review, *Journal of Reproductive Medicine, 35,* 839–863.

Baddeley, J., & Singer, J. (2009). A social interaction model of bereavement narrative disclosure. *Review of General Psychology, 13*(3), 202–218. doi:10.1037/a0015655

Baesler, E. J. (1995). Construction and test of an empirical measure for narrative coherence and fidelity. *Communication Reports, 8*(2), 97–101.

Bahktin, M. (1981). *The dialogic imagination.* Austin, TX: University of Texas Press.

Barad, K. (2007). *Meeting the universe halfway: Quantum physics and the entanglement of matter and meaning.* Durham, NC: Duke University Press.

Bateson, M. C. (2001). *Composing a life.* New York, NY: Grove Press.

Beach, M. C., Inui, T., & the Relationship-Centered Care Research Network. (2006). Relationship-centered care: A constructive reframing. *Journal of General Internal Medicine, 21,* S3–S8.

Beall, J. (2008). Infertility. In D. Haase (Ed.), *Greenwood encyclopedia of folk tales and fairy tales* (p. 485). Westport, CT: Greenwood Press.

Beauboeuf-Lafontant, T. (2007). You have to show strength: An exploration of gender, race, and depression. *Gender and Society, 21*(1), 28–51.

Belenky, M. F., Clinchy, B. M., Goldberger, N. R., & Tarule, J. M. (1986). *Women's way of knowing: The development of self, voice, and mind.* New York, NY: Basic Books.

Berlant, L. (2007). Starved. *South Atlantic Quarterly, 106,* 433–444.

Berlant, L. (2011). *Cruel optimism.* Durham, NC: Duke University Press.

Berry, K., & Warren, J. T. (2009). Cultural studies and the politics of representation: Experience ↔ subjectivity ↔ research. *Cultural Studies ↔ Critical Methodologies, 9,* 597–607.

Black, R. B. (1991). Women's voices after pregnancy loss: Couples' patterns of communication and support. *Social Work in Health Care, 16*(2), 19–36. doi:10.1300/J010v16n02_03

Bochner, A. (2001). Narrative's virtues. *Qualitative Inquiry, 7,* 131–157.

Bochner, A. (2014). *Coming to narrative: A personal history of paradigm change in the human sciences.* Walnut Creek, CA: Left Coast Press.

Borg, S., & J. Lasker (1982/1989). *When pregnancy fails: Coping with miscarriage, stillbirth and infant death.* New York, NY: Routledge.

Borisoff, D., & Merrill, L. (1998). *The power to communicate: Gender differences as barriers* (3rd ed.). Prospect Heights, IL: Waveland.

Boston Women's Health Book Collective. (1992). *The new our bodies, ourselves.* New York, NY: Simon & Schuster.

Bowman, J. (2013). Black Vietnam vets finally getting PTSD treatment. KDVR. Retrieved from http://kdvr.com/2013/02/15/black-vietnam-vets-finally-getting-ptsd-treatment

Bowman, M., & Bowman, R. L. (2002). Performing the mystory: A textshop in auto-performance. In N. Stucky & C. Wimmer (Eds.), *Teaching performance studies* (pp. 161–174). Carbondale: Southern Illinois University Press.

Brann, M. (2011). No time to grieve: Losing my life's love and regaining my own strength. In M. Brann (Ed.), *Contemporary case studies in health communication: Theoretical & applied approaches* (pp. 21–31). Dubuque, IA: Kendall/Hunt.

Brann, M. (2013). Helping patients get what they need: Persuading health care providers of perceived threat and positive outcome expectations. In C. J. Liberman (Ed.), *Casing persuasive communication* (pp. 237–248). Dubuque, IA: Kendall/Hunt.

Brashers, D. E. (2001). Communication and uncertainty management. *Journal of Communication, 51*(3), 477–497. doi:10.1093/joc/51.3.477

Brashers, D. E. (2007). A theory of communication and uncertainty management. In B. B. Whaley & W. Samter (Eds.), *Explaining communication: Contemporary theories and exemplars* (pp. 201–218). Mahwah, NJ: Erlbaum.

Brashers, D. E., Neidig, J. L., & Goldsmith, D. J. (2000). Social support and the management of uncertainty for people living with HIV or AIDS. *Health Communication, 16*(3), 305–331. doi:10.1207/S15327027HC1603_3

Brier, N. (2004). Anxiety after miscarriage: A review of the empirical literature and implications for clinical practice. *Birth: Issues in Perinatal Care, 31*, 138–142.

Brier, N. (2008). Grief following miscarriage: A comprehensive review of the literature. *Journal of Women's Health, 17*(3), 451–464. doi:10.1089/jwh.2007.0505

Brody, H. (2002). *Stories of sickness* (2nd ed.). Oxford, England: Oxford University Press.

Brooks, J. (2001). The lasting trauma of stillbirth. *WebMD*. Retrieved from http://web-md.com/baby/news/200101724/lasting-trauma-of-stillbirth

Bruner, J. (1986). *Actual minds, possible worlds.* Cambridge, MA: Harvard University Press.

Bruner, J. (1990). *Acts of meaning.* Cambridge, MA: Harvard University Press.

Bruner, J. (2002). *Making stories: Law, literature, life.* Cambridge, MA: Harvard University Press.

Bruner, J. (2004). Life as narrative. *Social Research, 71*(3), 691–710.

Burke, K. (April, 1938). Literature as equipment for living. *Direction, 1,* 10–13.

Burke, K. (1973). *The philosophy of literary form* (3rd ed.). Berkeley: University of California Press.

Burke, K. (1989). *On symbols and society.* Chicago, IL: University of Chicago Press.

Burnell, K. J., Hunt, N., & Coleman, P. G. (2009). Developing a model of narrative analysis to investigate the role of social support in coping with traumatic war memories. *Narrative Inquiry, 19,* 91–105.

Bury, M. (2001). Illness narratives: Fact or fiction. *Sociology of Health & Illness, 23,* 263–285.

Bushnell, C. (Writer), Star, D. (Writer), & King, M. P. (Director). (1998–2004). *Sex and the City* [Television series]. In D. Star (Producer). New York, NY: HBO.

Bute, J. J. (2011). When public and private intermingle ... Reflections on (re)production. *Health Communication, 26,* 104–106.

Butler, J. (1995). Melancholy gender/Refused identification. In M. Berger, B. Wallis, & S. Watson (Eds.). *Constructing masculinity* (pp. 21–36). London: Routledge

Butler, J, (2004). *Precarious life: The powers of mourning and violence.* London: Verso.

Buzzanell, P., & Ellingson, L. (2005). Contesting narratives of workplace maternity. In L. Harter, P. Japp, & C. Beck (Eds.), *Narratives, health, and healing: Communication theory, research, & practice* (pp. 277–294). Mahwah, NJ: Erlbaum.

Callister, L. C. (2006). Perinatal loss: A family perspective. *The Journal of Perinatal & Neonatal Nursing, 20*(3), 227–234.

Campbell, J. (2008). *The hero with a thousand faces* (3rd ed.). Bollingen series. Novato, CA: New World Library.

Campbell, J., Moyers, B., & Flowers, S. (Eds.). (1988). *The power of myth.* New York, NY: Doubleday.

Carey, J. (1989). *Communication as culture: Essays on media and society.* New York, NY: Routledge.

Casper, W. J., Weltman, D., & Kwesiga, E. (Eds.). (2007). Beyond family-friendly: The construct and measurement of singles-friendly work culture. *Journal of Vocational Behavior, 70,* 478–501.

Charon, R. (2001). Narrative medicine: A model for empathy, reflection, profession, and trust. *JAMA, 286,* 1897–1902.

Charon, R. (2006). *Narrative medicine: Honoring the stories of illness.* New York, NY: Oxford University Press.

Charon, R. (2009). Narrative medicine as witness for the self-telling body. *Journal of Applied Communication Research, 37,* 118–131.

Chira, S. (1994, June 26). When hope died. *The New York Times.* Retrieved from http://www.nytimes.com

Chozick, A. (2014, February 28). Outrage over sexist remarks turns into a political fund-raising tool. *The New York Times.* Retrieved from http://www.nytimes.com

Christ, C. P. (1995). *Odyssey with the goddess: A spiritual quest in Crete.* New York, NY: Continuum.

Clift-Matthews, V. (2007). How much change in 50 years? *British Medical Journal, 15,* 64.

Coles, R. (1989). *The call of stories: Teaching and the moral imagination.* Boston, MA: Houghton Mifflin.

Collins, P. H. (1991). *Black feminist thought.* New York, NY: Routledge.

Conway, K., & Russell, G. (2000). Couples' grief and experience of support in the aftermath of miscarriage. *British Journal of Medical Psychology, 73*(4), 531–545. doi:10.1348/000711200160714

Corbet-Owen, C. (2003). Women's perceptions of partner support in the context of pregnancy loss(es). *South African Journal of Psychology, 33*(1), 19–27. doi:10.1177/008124630303300103

Corbet-Owen, C., & Kruger, L. (2001). The health system and emotional care: Validating the many meanings of spontaneous pregnancy loss. *Families, Systems & Health, 19*, 411–427.

Cosgrove, L. (2004). The aftermath of pregnancy loss: A feminist critique of the literature and implications for treatment. In J. Chrisler (Ed.), *From menarche to menopause: The female body in feminist therapy* (pp. 107–122). Binghamton, NY: Haworth Press.

Cote-Arsenault, D., Bidlack, D., & Humm, A. (2001). Women's emotions and concerns during pregnancy following perinatal loss. *The American Journal of Maternal/Child Nursing (MCN), 26, 3*, 129–134.

Crossman, K. (2013). State of North Carolina to pay $10 million to women who were victims of forced sterilization. *Healthy Black Woman: Healthy Mind Body & Soul.*, from http://www.healthyblackwoman.com/north-carolina-eugenics-victims-to-receive-10-million-settlement/

Cutrona, C. E., & Russell, D. W. (1990). Type of social support and specific stress: Toward a theory of optimal matching. In B. R. Sarason, I. G., Sarason, & G. R. Pierce (Eds.), *Social support: An interactional view* (pp. 319–366). New York, NY: Wiley.

Danquah, M. N. (1998). *Willow weep for me: A black woman's journey though depression.* New York, NY: One World.

Davies, R. (2004). New understandings of parental grief: Literature review. *Journal of Advanced Nursing, 46*, 506–513.

Day, M. V., Kay, A. C., Holms, J. G., & Napier, J. L. (2011). System justification and the defense of committed relationship ideology. *Journal of Personality and Social Psychology, 101*(2), 291–306.

DelVecchio Good, M. J. (1998). *American medicine: The quest for competence.* Berkeley: University of California Press.

Denzin, N. K. (1997). *Interpretive ethnography: Ethnographic practices for the 21st century.* Thousand Oaks, CA: Sage.

DePaulo, B. M., & Morris, W. L. (2005). Singles in society and in science. *Psychological Inquiry, 16*, 57–83. doi:10.1207/s15327965pli162&3_01

Dinshaw, C., Edelman, L., Ferguson, R. A., Freccero, C., Freeman, E., Halberstam, J., et al. (2007). Theorizing queer temporalities: A roundtable discussion. *GLQ: A Journal of Lesbian and Gay Studies, 13*, 177–195.

Doka, K. J. (1989). Disenfranchised grief. In K. J. Doka (Ed.), *Disenfranchised grief: Recognizing hidden sorrow* (pp. 3–11). Lexington, MA: Lexington Books.

DuBose, T. (2006). Sonography: What is it? Words are golden. *ADVANCE for Imaging and Radiation and Therapy Professionals, 19*(14), 12., Retrieved September 9, 2013, from http://www.uams.edu/chrp/sonography/Sonography_what_is_it_06May22-Advance_fini.pdf

Dubriwny, T. (2013). *The vulnerable, empowered woman: Feminism, postfeminism, and women's health.* New Brunswick, NJ: Rutgers University Press.

du Pré, A. (2013). *Communicating about health: Current issues and perspectives* (4th ed.). New York, NY: Oxford University Press.

Ellingson, L. (2009). *Engaging crystallization in qualitative research: An introduction.* Los Angeles, CA: Sage.

Ellingson, L. L., & Buzzanell, P. M. (1999). Listening to women's narratives of breast cancer treatment: A feminist approach to patient satisfaction with physician–patient communication. *Health Communication, 11,* 153–183.

Ellis, C. (1999). Bringing emotion and personal narrative into medical social science. *Health, 3,* 229–237.

Ellis, C., Adams, T. E., & Bochner, A. P. (2011). Autoethnography: An overview. *Historical Social Research, 36,* 273–290.

Ellis, C., & Bochner, A. P. (1992). Telling and performing personal stories: The constraints of choice in abortion. In C. Ellis & M. G. Flaherty (Eds.), *Investigating subjectivity: Research on lived experience.* Newbury Park, CA: Sage.

Elson, J. (2003). Hormonal hierarchy: Hysterectomy and stratified stigma. *Gender and Society, 17*(5), 750–770.

Engelhard, I. M., van den Hout, M. A., & Arntz, A. (2001). Posttraumatic stress disorder after pregnancy loss. *General Hospital Psychiatry, 23,* 62–66.

Evans, L., Lloyd, D., Considine, R., & Hancock, L. (2002). Contrasting views of staff and patients regarding psychosocial care for Australian women who miscarry: A hospital-based study. *Australian and New Zealand Journal of Obstetrics and Gynaecology, 42,* 155–160.

Everett, H. (2002). *Roadside crosses in contemporary memorial culture.* Denton: University of North Texas Press.

Fairchild, J. L. (2009). *What might have been: The communication of social support and women's post-miscarriage narrative reconstruction* (Unpublished doctoral dissertation). University of Kentucky, Lexington.

Fairchild, J., & Arrington, M. I. (2012). Depictions of husbands in miscarriage accounts. *Illness, Crisis, and Loss, 20,* 363–373.

Fairchild, J., Nickell, D. F., & Arrington, M. I. (2008, April). *No Hallmark card: Post-miscarriage social support among female friends.* Paper presented to the Gender Studies Division, Southern States Communication Association, Savannah, GA.

Fasset, D. L., & Warren, J. P. (2006). *Critical communication pedagogy.* Thousand Oaks, CA: Sage.

Fernandez, R., Harris, D., & Leschied, A. (2011). Understanding grief following pregnancy loss: A retrospective analysis regarding women's coping responses. *Illness, Crisis & Loss, 19,* 143–163.

Finn, H. (2011). *The baby chase: An adventure in fertility.* New York, NY: Byliner.

Fisher, W. R. (1987). *Human communication as narration: Toward a philosophy of reason, value, and action.* Columbia: University of South Carolina Press.

Fiske, J. (2011). *Television culture.* New York, NY: Routledge.

Fliehr, R. (1956). Management of the elderly primigravida. *Obstetrics & Gynecology, 8,* 494–499.

Florence + the Machine. (2011). No light, no light. *Ceremonials* [CD]. Santa Monica, CA: Island Records.

Flory, N., Bissonnette, F., & Binik, Y. M. (2005). Psychosocial effects of hysterectomy: Literature review. *Journal of Psychosomatic Research, 59*, 117–129.

Footprints Ministry. (2006). Who we are. Retrieved from http://angelfire.com/ny5/fotprintsministry/

Foster, E. (2005). Desiring dialectical discourse: A feminist ponders the transition to motherhood. *Women's Studies in Communication, 28*, 57–83.

Foster, E. (2010). My eyes cry without me: Illusions of choice and control in the transition to motherhood. In S. Hayden & L. O'Brien Hallstein (Eds.), *Contemplating maternity: Discourses of choice and control* (pp. 139–158). Lanham, MD: Lexington Press.

Foucault, M. (1977). *Discipline and punish: The birth of the prison.* New York, NY: Random House.

Fox, R. (2010). Tales of a fighting bobcat: An auto-archaeology of gay identity formation and maintenance. *Text & Performance Quarterly, 30*, 122–142.

Frank, A. (1994). Reclaiming an orphan genre: The first-person narrative of illness. *Literature and Medicine, 13*, 1–21.

Frank, A. (2013). *The wounded storyteller* (2nd ed.). Chicago, IL: University of Chicago Press. (Originally published 1995)

Frankel, R. M., & Quill, T. (2005). Integrating biopsychosocial and relationship-centered care into mainstream medical practice: A challenge that continues to produce positive results. *Families, Systems, & Health, 23*, 413–421.

Freedman, M. (2009). *Mama Mia: A memoir of mistakes, magazines, and motherhood.* Sydney, Australia: HarperCollins.

Frontgia, T. (1991). Archetypes, stereotypes, and the female hero: Transformations in contemporary perspectives. *Mythlore, 67*, 15–18.

Frost, J., Bradley, H., Levitas, R., Smith, L., & Garcia, J. (2007). The loss of possibility: Scientisation of death and the special case of early miscarriage. *Sociology of Health and Illness, 29*, 1003–1022.

Frye, J. (1986). *Living stories, telling lives: Women and the novel in contemporary experience.* Ann Arbor: University of Michigan Press.

Galinsky, E. (2013, May 26). A work–life ways to go. *The Daily Beast. Retrieved May 14, 2014* from http://www.thedailybeast.com/articles/2013/05/26/a-work-life-ways-to-go.html

Galvin, K., & Patrick, D. (2009). *Gay male partners achieving fatherhood: Stories of communicative complexities and challenges.* Paper presented at the National Communication Association, Chicago, IL.

Gannon, S. (2006). The (im)possibilities of writing the self-writing: French poststructuralist theory and autoethnography. *Cultural Studies ↔ Critical Methodologies, 6*, 474–495.

Garel, M., Blondel, B., Lelong, N., Bonenfant, S., & Kaminski, M. (1994). Long-term consequences of miscarriage: The depressive disorders and the following pregnancy. *Journal of Reproductive and Infant Psychology, 12*, 233–240.

Garro, L., & Mattingly, C. (2000). Narrative as construct and construction. In C. Mattingly & L. Garro (Eds.)., *Narrative and the cultural construction of illness and healing* pp. 1–49. Los Angeles, CA: University of California Press

Geller, P. A., Psaros, C., & Kornfield, S. L. (2010). Satisfaction with pregnancy loss aftercare: Are women getting what they want? *Archives of Women's Mental Health, 13*, 111–124.

Gergen, K. (1991) *The saturated self.* New York, NY: Basic Books

Gilbert, K., & Smart, L. (1992). *Coping with infant or fetal loss: The couple's healing process.* New York, NY: Bruner/Mazel.

Gillespie, R. (2003). Childfree and feminine: Understanding the gender identity of voluntarily childless women. *Gender and Society, 17*(1), 122–136.

Goffman, E. (1986). *Stigma: Notes on the management of a spoiled identity.* New York, NY: Touchstone Books.

Gold, K. J. (2007). Navigating care after a baby dies: A systematic review of parent experiences with health care providers. *Journal of Perinatology, 27*, 230–237.

Goodall, H. L. (2004). Narrative ethnography as applied communication research. *Journal of Applied Communication Research, 32*(3), 185–194.

Grimm, J., & W. (2009a). Briar Rose. *The complete Grimm's fairy tales* (pp. 121–123). New York, NY: digireads.com.

Grimm, J., & W. (2009b). Rapunzel. *The complete Grimm's fairy tales* (pp. 36–38). New York, NY: digireads.com.

Greenspan, M. (2004). *Healing through the dark emotions.* Boston, MA: Shambhala.

Groer, A. (October 24th, 2012). Indiana GOP Senate hopeful Richard Mourdock says God intended rape pregnancies, *Washington Post.*

Grosz, E. (2005). *Time travels: Feminism, nature, power.* Durham, NC: Duke University Press.

Halberstam, J. (2005). *In a queer time & place: Transgender bodies, subcultural lives.* New York, NY: NYU Press.

Hale, B. (2007). Culpability and blame after pregnancy loss. *Journal of Medial Ethics, 33*, 24–27.

Hall, J., & Stevens, P. (1991). Rigor in feminist research. *Advances in Nursing Science, 13 (3)*, 16–29.

Haney, C. A., Leimer, C., & Lowrey, J. (1997). Spontaneous memorialization: Violent death and emerging mourning ritual. *Omega: The Journal of Death and Dying, 35*(2), 159–171.

Hanisch, (1970). The personal is political. In Firestone & Koedt (Eds.), *Notes from the second year: Women's liberation* p. X. New York, NY: By the Editors.

Harries, E. W. (2004). The mirror broken: Women's autobiography and fairy tales. In D. Hasse (Ed.), *Fairy tales and feminism: New approaches* (pp. 99–112). Detroit, MI: Wayne State University Press.

Harris, P. (Producer), & Mendes, S. (Director), (2009). *Away We Go.* [Motion Picture] USA: Focus Features

Harter, L. M. (2009). Narratives as dialogic, contested, and aesthetic performances. *Journal of Applied Communication Research, 37*, 140–150.

Harter, L. M., & Bochner, A. P. (2009). Healing through stories: A special issue on narrative medicine. *Journal of Applied Communication Research, 37*, 113–117.

Harter, L. M., Japp, P., & Beck, C. (2005). Vital problematics in narrative theorizing. In L. Harter, P. Japp, & C. Beck (Eds.), *Narratives, health, and healing: Communication theory, research, and practice* (pp. 1–29). Mahwah, NJ: Erlbaum.

Harter, L. M., Patterson, S., & Gerbensky-Kerber, A. (2010). Narrating "new normals" in health care contexts. *Management Communication Quarterly, 24*(3), 465–473. doi:10.1177/0893318910370271

Harvey, J., Moyle, W., & Creedy, D. (2001). Women's experience of early miscarriage: A phenomenological study. *Australian Journal of Advanced Nursing, 19*, 8–14.

Hawkins, A. H. (1999a). *Reconstructing illness: Studies in pathography.* West Lafayette, IN: Purdue University Press.

Hawkins, A. H. (1999b). Pathography: Patient narratives of illness. *Western Journal of Medicine, 171*, 127–129.

Herkes, B. (2002). A bereavement counseling service for parents: Part 1. *British Journal of Midwifery, 10*, 79–82.

Hesse-Biber, S. (2007). *Handbook of feminist research: Theory and praxis.* Thousand Oaks, CA: Sage.

Hewlett, S. A. (1986). *A lesser life: The myth of women's liberation in America.* New York, NY: William Morrow.

Hinson Langford, C. P., Bowsher, J., Maloney, J. P., & Lillis, P. P. (1997). Social support: A conceptual analysis. *Journal of Advanced Nursing, 25*, 95–100.

Hobson, D. (1982). *Crossroads: The drama of a soap opera.* London, England: Methuen.

Hogeland, L. (1998). *Feminism and its fictions: The consciousness-raising novel and the women's liberation movement.* Philadelphia: University of Pennsylvania Press.

Hollander, E. M. (2004). Am I all right? *Journal of Loss and Trauma, 9*, 201–204.

hooks, b. (1994). *Teaching to transgress: Education as the practice of freedom.* New York, NY: Routledge.

Hughes, C. B., & Page-Lieberman J. (1989). Father experiences a perinatal loss. *Death Studies, 13*, 537–556.

Hullet, C. R. (2005). Grieving families: Social support after the death of a loved one. In E. B. Ray (Ed.), *Health communication in practice. A case study approach* (pp. 211–221). Mahwah, NJ: Erlbaum.

Hutchon, D. J. R. (1998). Understanding miscarriage or insensitive abortion: Time for more defined terminology? *American Journal of Obstetrics and Gynecology, 179*, 397–398.

Hydén, L. (1997). Illness and narrative. *Sociology of Health & Illness, 19*, 48–69.

Ilse, S. (2013). *Empty arms: Coping with miscarriage, stillbirth, and early infant death.* Maple Plain, MN: Wintergreen Press. (Original work published 1982)

Ilse, S., & Burns, L. H. (1985). *Miscarriage: A shattered dream*. Maple Plain, MN: Wintergreen Press.

Jack's Mannequin (2011). Release me. *People and Things* [CD]. Santa Monica, CA: Sire Records.

Jay-Z. (2012). Glory. (Recorded by Jay-Z). New York, NY: Roc Nation.

Jeane, D. G. (1989). Folk art in rural Southern cemeteries. *Southern Folklore, 46,* 159–174.

Jenner, K., & Seacrest, R. (Producers), (2011–2012). *Khloe & Lamar* [Television series]. Los Angeles, CA: Bunim/Murray Productions.

Jeong, H.-G., Lim, J.-S., Lee, M.-S., Kim, S.-H., Jung, I.-K., & Joe, S.-H. (2013). The association of psychological factors and obstetric history with depression in pregnant women: Focus on the role of emotional support. *General Hospital Psychiatry, 35,* 354–358.

Jewson, N. D. (1976). The disappearance of the sick man from medical terminology. *Sociology, 10,* 225–244.

Jones, C., & Shorter-Gooden, K. (2003). *Shifting: The double lives of black women in America*. New York, NY: HarperCollins.

Jones, R. F. (1993). Preface. In M. Allen & S. Marks (Eds.), *Miscarriage: Women sharing from the heart* (p. xi). Hoboken, NJ: Wiley & Sons.

Jurkovic, D., Overton, C., & Bender-Atik, R. (2013). Diagnosis and management of first-trimester miscarriage. *British Medical Journal, 346,* 3676.

Kapoor, K. (2013). Abu. Retrieved from http://www.kamalkapoor.com/nams-meaings-African-baby-boy-names.asp

Kavanaugh, K., & Hershberger P. (2005). Perinatal loss in low-income African American parents. *Journal of Obstetric, Gynecologic, & Neonatal Nursing, 34,* (5), 595–605.

Kennerly, R. (1999, 2000). *Getting messy: In the field and at the crossroads with roadside shrines* [Performance]. Black Box Theatre, Louisiana State University, Baton Rouge.

Kennerly, R. (2002). Getting messy: In the field and at the crossroads with roadside shrines. *Text and Performance Quarterly, 22*(4), 229–260.

Kennerly, R. (2003). *Getting messy: In the field and at the crossroads with roadside shrines* [Performance]. Black Box Theatre, Georgia Southern University, Statesboro.

Kennerly, R. (2008). Locating the gap between grace and terror: Performative research and spectral images of (and on) the road [85 paragraphs]. *Forum for Qualitative Social Science, 9*(2), Art. 52. Retrieved from http://www.qualitative-research.net/fqs-texte/2-08/08-2-52-e.htm

Kennerly, R. (2009). Locating community, memory and meaning-making in the performative gap: An experiment in aesthetics, autoethnography, and the ethic of the unfinished. *Iowa Journal of Communication, 41*(1), 1–30.

Kennerly, R., & Fenske, M. (2001). Theatron: The interpenatrable boundaries between literature, cultural studies, and ethnography. [Installation]. National Communication Association Annual Convention, Marriott Marquis Hotel, Atlanta, GA.

Kiesinger, C. (2002). My father's shoes: The therapeutic value of narrative reframing. In A. P. Bochner & C. Ellis (Eds.)., *Ethnographically speaking: Autoethnography, literature and aesthetics* (pp. 95–114). Walnut Creek, CA: AltaMira.

Kinser, A. (2004). Negotiating spaces for/through third wave feminism. *NWSA, 16*, 124–151.

Kleinman, A. (1988). *The illness narratives: Suffering, healing, and the human condition.* New York, NY: Basic Books.

Kluger-Bell, K. (1998). *Unspeakable losses: Understanding the experience of pregnancy loss, miscarriage and abortion.* New York, NY: William Morrow Paperbacks.

Koedt, A., Levine, E., & Rapone, A. (1973). *Radical feminism.* New York, NY: Quadrangle.

Kohn, I., & Moffitt, P. L. (2000). *A silent sorrow: Pregnancy loss: Guidance and support for you and your family.* New York, NY: Routledge.

Kong, G. W. S., Lok, I. H., Lam, P. M., Yip, A. S. K., & Chung, T. K. H. (2010). Conflicting perceptions between health care professionals and patients on psychological morbidity following miscarriage. *Australian and New Zealand Journal of Obstetrics and Gynaecology, 50*, 562–567.

Kristeva, J. (1981). Women's time. *Signs, 7*, 13–35.

Kristeva, J., & Guberman, R. (1998). *Time and sense.* New York, NY: Columbia University Press.

Kundera, M. (1991). *Immortality* (P. Kussi, Trans.). New York, NY: Grove Press. (Original work published 1988)

Laing, R. D. (1969). *The politics of the family and other essays.* New York, NY: Vintage Books.

Langellier, K. M. (1999, April). Personal narrative, performance, performativity: Two or three things I know for sure. *Text and Performance Quarterly, 19*, 125–144.

Langellier, K. M., & Peterson, E. E. (2004). *Storytelling in daily life: Performing narrative.* Philadelphia: Temple University Press.

Lapp, L. K., Agbokou, C., Peretti, C. C., & Ferreri, F. (2010). Management of post traumatic stress disorder after childbirth: A review. *Journal of Psychosomatic Obstetrics and Gynecology, 3*, 113–122. doi:10.3i09/0167482X.2010.503330

Lasker, J., & Lin, S. Q. (1996). Patterns of grief reaction after pregnancy loss. *American Journal of Orthopsychiatry, 66*(2), 262–271.

Lasker, J., & Toedter, L. (2003). The impact of ectopic pregnancy: A 16-year follow-up study. *Health Care for Women International, 24*(3), 209–220. doi:10.1080/07399330303997

Lauritzen, P. (1990). What price parenthood? *The Hastings Report, 20*(2), 38–46.

Layne, L. (1990). Motherhood lost: Cultural dimensions of miscarriage. *Women & Health, 16*, 69–98.

Layne, L. (1997). Breaking the silence: An agenda for a feminist discourse of pregnancy loss. *Feminist Studies, 23*(2), 289–315.

Layne, L. (2003a). *Motherhood lost.* New York, NY: Routledge.

Layne, L. (2003b). Unhappy endings: A feminist reappraisal of the women's health movement from the vantage of pregnancy loss. *Social Science & Medicine, 56*, 1881–1891.

Lefkowitz, M. (1990). The myth of Joseph Campbell. *The American Scholar, 59*(3), 429–434.

Leon, I. (1990). *When a baby dies: Psychotherapy for pregnancy and newborn loss.* New Haven: Yale University Press.

Letherby, G. (2002). Childless and bereft? Stereotypes and realities in relation to "voluntary" and "involuntary" childlessness and womanhood. *Sociological Inquiry, 72*(1), 7–20.

Letherby, G., & Williams, C. (1999). Non-motherhood: Ambivalent autobiographies. *Feminist Studies, 25*(3), 719–728.

Lieberman, M. R. (1972). "Some day my prince will come": Female acculturation through the fairy tale. *College English, 34*(3), 383–395.

Lim, C. E. D., & Cheng, N. C. L. (2011). Clinician's role of psychological support in helping parents and families with pregnancy loss. *Journal of the Australian Traditional-Medicine Society, 17,* 215–217.

Limbo, R., & Kobler, K. (2010). The tie that binds: Relationships in perinatal bereavement. *The American Journal of Maternal Child Nursing (MCN), 35,* 316–321.

Lindemann-Nelson, H. (1997). How to do things with stories. *Stories and their limits: Narrative approaches to bioethics.* London: Routledge.

Lindemann-Nelson, H. (2001). *Damaged identities and narrative repair.* Ithaca, NY: Cornell University Press.

Lindlof, T. R., & Taylor, B. C. (2002). *Qualitative communication research methods* (2nd ed.). Thousand Oaks, CA: Sage.

Lipman, D. (1999). *Improving your storytelling.* Littlerock, AR: August House.

Long, B. W., & Strine, M. (1989). Reading intertextually: Multiple mediations and critical practice. *Quarterly Journal of Speech, 75*(4), 467–475.

Lorde, A. (2007). The transformation of silence into language and action. In *Sister Outsider: Essays and Speeches.* Berkeley, CA: Crossing Press.

Lundqvist, A., Nilstun, T., & Dykes, A.-K. (2002). Both empowered and powerless: Mothers' experiences of professional care when their newborn dies. *Birth, 29,* 192–199.

Lupton, D. (2003). *Medicine as culture* (2nd ed.). London, England: Sage.

Maguire, M., Maines, N., Robinson, E., & Wilson, D. (2006). So Hard (Recorded by the Dixie Chicks). On *Taking the Long Way* (CD). Nashville, TN: Columbia Records.

Maker, C., & Ogden, J. (2003). The miscarriage experience: More than just a trigger to psychological morbidity? *Psychology and Health, 18,* 403–415.

Markovic, M., Manderson, L., & Warren, N. (2008). Pragmatic narratives of hysterectomy among Australian women. *Sex Roles, 58,* 467–476.

Mansell, A. (2006). Early pregnancy loss. *Emergency Nurse, 14,* 26–28.

Matthew Populis' mother arrested. (1995). *Sunday Advocate* [Baton Rouge, LA], p. 3B.

Mattingly, C., & Garro, L. (Eds.), (2000). *Narrative and cultural construction of illness and healing.* Berkeley: University of California Press.

McCabe, E. (2011, June). Depressive realism: An interview with Lauren Berlant. *Hypocrite Reader, 5.* Retrieved from http://hypocritereader.com/5/depressive-realism

McCreight, B. S. (2001). Parinatal grief and emotional labour: A study of nurses' experiences in the gynae wards. *International Journal of Nursing Studies, 42,* 439–448.

McCreight, B. S. (2008). Perinatal loss: A qualitative study in Northern Ireland. *OMEGA, 57,* 1–19.

McGuinness, D. (2012). Beyond grief: Understanding post traumatic stress disorder (PTSD). Retrieved from http://unspokengrief.com/grief-and-ptsd/

Medved, C. (2004). The everyday accomplishment of work and family: Exploring practical actions in daily routines. *Communication Studies* 55(1) pp. 128–145.

Medved, C. E. (2006). The everyday accomplishment of work and family: Exploring practical actions in daily routines. *Communication Studies, 55,* 128–145.

Medved, C. E., Brogan, S., McClanahan, A. M., Morris, J. F., & Shepherd, G. J. (2006). Work and family socializing communication: Messages, gender, and power. *Journal of Family Communication, 6,* 161–180.

Medved, C. E., & Kirby, E. L. (2005). Family CEOs: A feminist analysis of corporate mothering discourses. *Management Communication Quarterly, 18,* 435–478.

Meyer, M. D. E. (2007). On remembering the queer self: The impact of memory, trauma and sexuality on interpersonal relationships. *Sexuality & Culture, 11,* 18–30.

Milbauer, J. A. (1989). Southern folk traits in cemeteries of northern Oklahoma. *Southern Folklore, 46,* 75–85.

Miller, M., Geist-Martin, P., & Cannon Beatty, K. (2005). Wholeness in a breaking world: Narratives as sustenance for peace. In L. Harter, P. Japp, & C. Beck (Eds.), *Narratives, health, and healing: Communication theory, research, & practice* (pp. 295–316). Mahwah, NJ: Erlbaum.

Miller, S. (1997). Multiple paradigms for nursing: Postmodern feminisms. In S. E. Thorne & V. E. Hayes (Eds.), *Nursing praxis: Knowledge and action* (pp. 140–156). Thousand Oaks, CA: Sage.

Mishler, E. (1984). *The discourse of medicine: Dialectics of medical interviews.* New York, NY: Greenwood Publishing Group.

Modiba, L. M. (2008). Experiences and perceptions of midwives and doctors when caring for mothers with pregnancy loss in a Gauteng hospital. *Health SA Gesondheid, 13*(4), 29–40.

Moore, L. (2012, August 20). Rep. Todd Akin: The statement and the reaction. *The New York Times.*

Mosley, W. (2012). *The gift of fire/On the head of a pin.* New York, NY: Tor Books.

Moulder, C. (1999). Miscarriage: Preparing SHOs for their role in hospital care. *Journal of Obstetrics & Gynaecology, 19,* 54–55.

Murdock, M. (1990). *The heroine's journey.* Boston, MA: Shambhala.

Murphy, F. A. (1998). The experience of early miscarriage from a male perspective. *Journal of Clinical Nursing, 7,* 325–332.

Myers, D. T. (2001). The rush to motherhood: Pronatalist discourse and women's autonomy. *Signs, 26,* 735–773.

Nathanson, D. L. (1996, Spring–Summer). What's a script? *Bulletin of the Tompkins Institute, 3,* 1–4. Retrieved from http://tomkins.org/uploads/whatsascript.pdf

National Institutes of Health. (2011). *Miscarriage*. Retrieved from http://www.nlm.nih. gov/medlineplus/ency/article/001488.htm

Neidig, J. R., & Dalgas-Pelish, P. (1991). Parental grieving and perceptions regarding health care professionals' interventions. *Pediatric Nursing, 14*, 179–191.

Neria, Y., & Litz, B. T. (2004). Bereavement by traumatic means: The complex synergy of trauma and grief. *Journal of Loss and Trauma, 9*, 73–87.

Neumann, E. (1991). *The great mother: An analysis of the archetype*. Princeton, NJ: Princeton University Press.

Nicholson, S. (2011). The problem of woman as hero in the work of Joseph Campbell. *Feminist Theology, 19*(2), 182–193.

Nicolopoulou, A. (2008). The elementary forms of narrative coherence in young children's storytelling. *Narrative Inquiry, 18*(2), 299–325.

Nikcevic, A. V., Tunkel, S. A., & Nicolaides, K. H. (1998). Psychological outcomes following missed abortions and provision of follow-up care. *Ultrasound in Obstetrics and Gynecology, 11*, 123–128.

Olde, E., van der Hart, O., Kleber, R., & van Son, M. (2006). Posttraumatic stress following childbirth: A review. *Clinical Psychology Review, 26*(1), 1–16. Retrieved from http://dx.doi.org/10.1016/j.cpr.2005.07.002

O'Leary, J. (2004). Grief and its impact on prenatal attachment in the subsequent pregnancy. *Archive of Women's Mental Health, 7*, 7–18.

Paulsell, S. (2007). Annunciation. *Literary Review, 50*(2), 46–52.

Pecchioni, L. L. (2012). Interruptions to cultural life scripts: Cancer diagnoses, contextual age, and life narratives. *Research on Aging, 34*(6), 758–780. doi:10.1177/0164027512449748

Peck, E., & Senderowitz, J. (Eds.). (1974). *Pronatalism: The myth of mom & apple pie*. New York, NY: Thomas Y. Crowell.

Pelias, R. J. (1999). *Writing performance: Poeticizing the researcher's body*. Carbondale: Southern Illinois University Press.

Pelias, R. J. (2002). For father and son: An ethnodrama with no catharsis. In A. Bochner & C. Ellis (Eds.), *Ethnographically speaking: Autoethnography, literature, and aesthetics* (pp. 35–43). Walnut Creek, CA: AltaMira Press.

Pelias, R. (2005). Performative writing as scholarship: An apology, an argument, and an-ecdote. *Cultural Studies, Critical Methodologies, 5*(4), 415–424.

Pennebaker, J. W., & Seagal, J. D. (1999). Forming a story: The health benefits of narrative. *Journal of Clinical Psychology, 55*(10), 1243–1254.

Peppers, L., & Knapp, R. (1980). *Motherhood and mourning: Perinatal death*. New York, NY: Praeger.

The Personal Narratives Group. (Ed.). (1989). Introduction. *Interpreting women's lives: Feminist theory and personal narratives*. Bloomington: Indiana University Press.

Peters, K., Jackson, D., & Rudge, T. (2011). Fostering resilience in couples. *Contemporary Nurse, 40*(1), 130–140.

Polkinghorne, D. (1988). *Narrative knowing and the human sciences.* Albany, NY: State University of New York Press.

Pollock, D. (1998). Performing writing. In P. Phelan & J. Lane (Eds.), *The ends of performance* (pp. 73–103). New York, NY: NYU Press.

Pollock, D. (1999). *Telling bodies performing birth: Every narrative of childbirth.* New York, NY: Columbia University Press.

Pollock, D. (2006). Marking new directions in performance ethnography. *Text and Performance Quarterly, 26*(4), 325–329.

Polly Klaas Foundation. (n.d.). Polly's story. Retrieved from http://www.pollyklaas.org/about/polly-story.html?gclid=CIjD6a3dg

Price, S. (2008). Stepping back to gain perspective: Pregnancy loss history, depression, and parenting capacity in the early childhood longitudinal study, birth cohort (ECLS-B). *Death Studies, 32,* 97–122.

Puddifoot, J., & Johnson, M. (1997). The legitimacy of grieving: The partner's experience at miscarriage. *Social Science and Medicine, 45,* 837–845.

Radway, J. (1984). *Reading the romance: Feminism and the representation of women in popular culture.* Chapel Hill: University of North Carolina Press.

Ramazani, J. (1994). *Poetry of mourning: The modern elegy from Hardy to Heaney.* Chicago, IL: University of Chicago Press.

Reagan, L. (2003). From hazard to blessing to tragedy: Representations of miscarriage in twentieth-century America. *Feminist Studies, 29*(2), 357–377.

Reagan, R. (1988). Proclamation 5890—Pregnancy and Infant Loss Awareness Month, 1988. Retrieved from http://www.regan.utexas.edu/archives/speeches/1988/102588b.htm

Rebillot, P. (1993). *The call to adventure.* New York, NY: HarperCollins.

Register, C. (1975). American feminist literary criticism: A bibliographical introduction. In J. Donovan (Ed.), *Feminist literary criticism: Explorations in theory* (pp. 1–28). Lexington: University of Kentucky Press.

Renner, C. H., Verdekal, S., Brier, S., & Fallucca, G. (2000). The meaning of miscarriage to others: Is it unrecognized loss? *Journal of Personal and Interpersonal Loss, 5,* 65–76.

RESOLVE: The National Infertility Association. (2011). Myths about African Americans and infertility. Retrieved August 12, 2011 from http://www.resolve.org/national-infertility-awareness-week/myths-about-african-americans-and-infertility.html

Reuters, (2012, May 17). More minority babies than whites in U.S.: Census Bureau. *Chicago Tribune.* p. X.

Rhimes, S. (Creator). (2005–2014). *Grey's Anatomy* [Television series]. In S. Rhimes (Producer). Los Angeles, CA: ABC Television.

Richardson, L. (1990). Narrative and sociology. *Journal of Contemporary Ethnography, 19,* 116–135.

Ricouer, P. (1984). *Time and narrative.* Chicago, IL: University of Chicago Press

Ricoeur, P. (1980). Narrative time. *Critical Inquiry, 7,* 169–190.

Ried, K., & Alfred, A. (2013). Quality of life, coping strategies and support needs of women seeking traditional Chinese medicine for infertility and viable pregnancy in Australia: A mixed methods approach. *BMC Women's Health, 13*, 17–27.

Riessman, C. K. (1993). *Narrative analysis.* Newbury Park, CA: Sage.

Riessman, C. K. (2002). Analysis of personal narratives. In J. F. Gubrium & J. A. Holstein (Eds.), *Handbook of interview research: Context and method* (pp. 695–710). Thousand Oaks, CA: Sage. doi:10.4135/9781412973588

Riessman, C. K. (2003). Performing identities in illness narrative: Masculinity and multiple sclerosis. *Qualitative Research, 3*(1), 5–33.

Riessman, C. K. (2008). *Narrative methods for the human sciences.* Thousand Oaks, CA: Sage.

Robinson, M., Baker, L., & Nackerud L. (1999). The relationship of attachment theory and perinatal loss. *Death Studies, 23*, (3), 257–270.

Rockwood, C. (Ed.). (1997). *Fodor's Greece.* New York, NY: Fodor's.

Rodman Aronson, K. M., & Schaler Buchholz, E. (2001). The post-feminist era: Still striving for equality in relationships. *The American Journal of Family Therapy, 29*, 109–124.

Ronai, C. R. (1997). Discursive constraint in the narrated identities of childhood sex abuse survivors. In C. R. Ronai & B. A. Zsembik (Eds.), *Everyday sexism in the third millennium,* (pp. 123–136). New York, NY: Routledge.

Roos, D. (Writer & Director). (2009). *The Other Woman* [Motion Picture]. In M. A. Brooke (Producer). New York, NY: Incentive Filmed Entertainment.

Rowlands, I. J., & Lee, C. (2010). "The silence was deafening": Social and health service support after miscarriage. *Journal of Reproductive and Infant Psychology, 28*, 274–286.

The Russian. (1999). Kip the enchanted cat. In M. Ponsot (Trans.) & A. Segur (Ill.), *Golden Book of fairy tales* (pp. 55–58). New York, NY: Golden Books.

Safran, D., Miller, W., & Beckman, H. (2006). Organizational dimensions of relationship-centered care. *Journal of General Internal Medicine, S1*, S9–S15.

Sakalys, J. (2000). The political role of illness narratives. *Journal of Advanced Nursing, 31*, 1469–1475.

SCBS Baby Club. (2010). Baby names meaning "gift." Retrieved from http://scbsfm. blogspot.com/2010/09/baby-names-meaning-gift.html

Schleifer, R. (1993). Walter Benjamin and the crisis of representation: Multiplicity, meaning, and athematic death. In S. W. Goodwin & E. Bronfen (Eds.), *Death and representation* (pp. 312–333). London: Johns Hopkins UP.

Schneider, R. (1997). *The explicit body in performance.* New York, NY: Routledge.

Seacrest, R., & Murray, J. (Producers). (2007–2014). *Keeping up With the Kardashians* [Television series]. Los Angeles, CA: Bunim/Murray Productions.

Seacrest, R., & Murray, J. (Producers). (2011–2012). *Kourtney and Kim Take New York* [Television series]. New York, NY: Bunim/Murray Productions.

Séjourné, N., Callahan, S., & Chabrol, H. (2010). Support following miscarriage: What women want. *Journal of Reproductive and Infant Psychology, 28*, 403–411.

Selzer, R., (1989). *The doctor stories.* New York, NY: Macmillan.

Seybert, B. (2009). Amber Hagerman. *Amber Alert.* Retrieved from http://www.amber-alertcreator.com/

Sharf, B. (2005). How I fired my surgeon and embraced an alternate narrative. In L. Harter, P. Japp, & C. Beck (Eds.), *Narratives, health, and healing: Communication theory, research, & practice* (pp. 325–342). Mahwah, NJ: Erlbaum.

Sharf, B. (2009). Observations from the outside in: Narratives of illness, healing, and mortality in everyday life. *Journal of Applied Communication Research, 37,* 132–139.

Sharf, B. F., Harter, L. M., Yamasaki, J., & Haidet, P. (2011). Narrative turns epic: Continuing developments in health narrative scholarship. In T. L. Thompson, R. Parrott, & J. F. Nussbaum (Eds.), *The Routledge handbook of health communication* (pp. 36–52). New York, NY: Routledge.

Shreffler, K. M., Hill, P. W., & Cacciatore, J. (2012). Exploring the odds of divorce following miscarriage or stillbirth. *Journal of Divorce & Remarriage, 53,* 91–107.

Siegel, D. L. (1997). The legacy of the personal: Generating theory in feminism's third wave. *Hypatia, 12,* 46–75.

Silverman, P. R., & Klass, D. (1996). Examining the dominant model—introduction: What's the problem? In D. Klass, P. R. Silverman, & S. L. Nickman (Eds.), *Continuing bonds: New understandings of grief* (pp. 3–23). Philadelphia: Taylor & Francis.

Simmons, R. K., Singh, G., Maconochie, N., Doyle, P., & Green, J. (2006). Experience of miscarriage in the UK: Qualitative findings from the National Women's Health Survey. *Social Science & Medicine, 63,* 1934–1946.

Society of Diagnostic Medical Sonographers. (2006). Code of ethics for the profession of diagnostic medical sonography. Retrieved September 2, 2013, from http://www.sdms.org/about/codeofethics.asp

Sontag, S. (2003). *Regarding the pain of others.* New York, NY: Farrar, Straus & Giroux.

Sowards, S., & Renegar, V. (2004). The rhetorical functions of consciousness raising in third-wave feminism. *Communication Studies, 55,* 535–552.

Spry, T. (2001). Performing autoethnography: An embodied methodological practice. *Qualitative Inquiry, 7,* 706–732.

Star, D. (Writer), & Attias, D. (Director). (1990–2000). *Beverly Hills, 90210* [Television series]. In A. Spelling, E. D. Vincent, & D. Star (Producers). Los Angeles, CA: Fox.

Stone, L. (1997). *Close to the bone: Memoirs of hurt, rage, and desire.* New York: Grove Press.

Stone, L. (1998). *Close to the bone: Memoirs of hurt, rage, and desire.* New York, NY: Grove Press.

Stratton, K., & Lloyd, L. (2008). Hospital-based interventions at and following miscarriage: Literature to inform a research–practice initiative. *Australian and New Zealand Journal of Obstetrics and Gynaecology, 48,* 5–11.

Streep, P. (1994). *Sanctuaries of the goddess: The sacred landscapes and objects.* Boston, MA: Bulfinch Press.

Street, R. L. (2003). Communication in medical encounters: An ecological perspective. In T. L. Thompson, A. M. Dorsey, K. I. Miller, & R. Parrot (Eds.), *Handbook of health communication* (pp. 63–89). Mahwah, NJ: Erlbaum.

Sunwolf & Frey, L. R. (2001). Storytelling: The power of narrative communication and interpretation. In W. P. Robinson & H. Giles (Eds.), *The new handbook of language and social psychology* (pp. 119–135). Hoboken, NJ: Wiley.

Swain, H. (2004). *Luscious Lemon*. New York, NY: Gallery Books.

Swan, T. B., & Benack, S. (2012). Renegotiating identity in unscripted territory: The predicament of queer men in heterosexual marriages. Journal of GLBT Family Studies, 8(1), 46–66. doi:http://dx.doi.org/10.1080/1550428X.2012.641371

Sweet Honey in the Rock. (1995). Sing oh barren one. *Sacred Ground* [CD]. Redway, CA: EarthBeat.

Taylor, E. N. (2003). Throwing the baby out with the bathwater. *Women & Politics, 24*(4), 49–75. doi:10.1300/J014v24n04_03

Taylor, T. (Writer & Director). (2011). *The Help* [Motion Picture]. In M. M. Al-Mazrouel (Producer). Clarksdale, MS: Dreamworks.

Thompson, T. L. (2009). The applicability of narrative ethics. *Journal of Applied Communication Research, 37*, 188–195.

Thorstensen, K. A. (2000). Midwifery management of first trimester bleeding and early pregnancy loss. *Journal of Midwifery & Women's Health, 45*, 481–497.

Toller, P. (2011). Bereaved parents' experiences of supportive and unsupportive communication. *Southern Communication Journal, 76*, 17–34.

Tompkins, S. S. (1979). Script theory: Differential magnification of affects. In H. E. Howe Jr. & R. A. Dienstbier (Eds.), *Nebraska Symposium on Motivation* (Vol. 26). Lincoln: University of Nebraska Press.

Trinh, T. M-ha. (1991). *When the moon waxes red: Representation, gender, and cultural politics.* New York, NY: Routledge.

Ulmer, G. (1989). *Teletheory: Grammatology in the age of video*. New York, NY: Routledge.

Ulmer, G. (1994). *Heuretics: The Logic of Invention*. Baltimore: Johns Hopkins UP.

U.S. Equal Employment Opportunity Commission. (1978). The Pregnancy Discrimination Act of 1978. Retrieved from http://www1.eeoc.gov//laws/statutes/preganancy.cfm?renderfor print=1

Van, P. (2001). Breaking the silence of African American women: Healing after pregnancy loss. *Health Care for Women International, 22*, 229–243.

Van, P. (2012/2013). Conversations, coping, & connectedness: A qualitative study of women who have experienced involuntary pregnancy loss. *OMEGA, 65*(1), 71–85.

Vedder, E. (2007). Rise. *Into the Wild* [CD]. Seattle, WA: J Records.

Villarosa, L. (2004, April). Baby hung. *Essence*, 172–176.

Volkan, V. D. (1975). Re-grief therapy. In B. Schoenberg, I. Gerber, A. Wiener, A. H. Kutscher, D. Peretz, & A. C. Carr (Eds.), *Bereavement: Its psycho-social aspects* (pp. 334–350). New York, NY: Columbia University Press.

Weed, L. L. (1964). Medical records, patient care, and medical education. *Irish Journal of Medical Science, 39*, 271–282. doi:10.1007/BF02945791

Welch, M., & Herrmann, D. (1980). Why miscarriage is so misunderstood: New medical and emotional findings. *Ms. Magazine, 8*(8), 14–22.

Wilson, C., & Leese, B. (2013). Do nurses and midwives have a role in promoting the well-being of patients during their fertility journey? A review of the literature. *Human Fertility, 16*, 2–7.

Winter, M. J. (2012). Remembering Polly. *Cloverdale.* Retrieved from http://cloverdale. towns.pressdemocrat.com/2012/02/photos/remembering.polly

Wong, M. K. Y., Crawford, T. J., Gask, L., & Grinyer, A. (2003). A qualitative investigation into women's experiences after a miscarriage: Implications for the primary healthcare team. *British Journal of General Practice, 53*, 697–702.

World Health Organization. (1946). Preamble to the constitution of the World Health Organization. (Official Records of the World Health Organization, no. 2.) Retrieved from http://www.ncbi.nlm.nih.gov/pmc/articles/PMC2567708/

Yu, S. (2011). Reclaiming the personal: Personal narratives of third-wave feminists. *Women's Studies, 40*, 873–889.

Zal, H. M. (2001). *The sandwich generation: Caught between growing children and aging parents.* New York, NY: Perseus.

Zimmerman, B. (1984). The politics of transliteration: Lesbian personal narratives. *Signs: Journal of Women in Culture and Society, 9*, 663–682.

Index

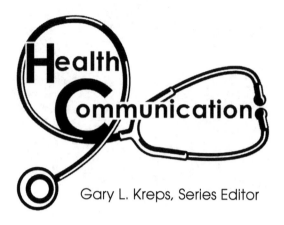

Gary L. Kreps, Series Editor

This series examines the powerful influences of human and mediated communication in delivering care and promoting health.

Books analyze the ways that strategic communication humanizes and increases access to quality care as well as examining the use of communication to
encourage proactive health promotion. The books describe strategies for addressing major health issues, such as reducing health disparities, minimizing health risks,
responding to health crises, encouraging early detection and care, facilitating informed health decisionmaking, promoting coordination within and across health
teams, overcoming health literacy challenges, designing responsive health information technologies, and delivering sensitive end-of-life care.

All books in the series are grounded in broad evidence-based scholarship and
are vivid, compelling, and accessible to broad audiences of scholars, students,
professionals, and laypersons.

For additional information about this series or for the submission of manuscripts,
please contact:

Gary L. Kreps
University Distinguished Professor and Chair, Department of Communication
Director, Center for Health and Risk Communication
George Mason University Science & Technology 2, Suite 230, MS 3D6
Fairfax, VA 22030-4444
gkreps@gmu.edu

To order other books in this series, please contact our Customer Service Department:

(800) 770-LANG (within the U.S.)
(212) 647-7706 (outside the U.S.)
(212) 647-7707 FAX

Or browse online by series:
www.peterlang.com